Aberdeenshire Lib
www.aberdeenshire.gov.
Renewals Hotline 01224 661511
Downloads available from
www.aberdeenshirelibraries.lib.overdrive.com

KT-464-455

DMT: The Spirit Molecule

"Strassman's important research contributes to a growing awareness that we inhabit a multidimensional universe that is far more complex and interesting than the one our scientific theories have shown us. It is of the utmost importance that we face the implications of this discovery, for it has so much to tell us about who we are and why we are here."

John Mack, author of
Abduction and *Passport to the Cosmos*

"The most extensive scientific study of the mental and perceptual effects of a psychedelic drug since the 1960s. Strassman provides fascinating insight into the world of psychiatric research as he seeks to understand these most mysterious substances and their profound effects on human consciousness."

Ralph Metzner, Ph.D., author of
Ayahuasca: Consciousness and the Spirits of Nature

"This book is essential reading for anyone with an interest in the mind, philosophy, the nature of reality, and spirituality. The world's foremost expert on DMT has created a masterpiece of the genre, as he brilliantly leads the reader through a series of startling revelations about the nature of the universe, revealed behind the doorway once DMT turns the key."

Karl Jansen, M.D., Ph.D., author of
K. Ketamine: Dreams and Realities

"*DMT: The Spirit Molecule* points the way beyond the present impasse of the reigning "drug abuse" paradigm. We owe a debt of gratitude to Strassman for persevering in the face of bureaucratic obstacles to conduct important research into the human pharmacology of DMT and elucidate it for the general public, in both scientific and humanistic terms."

Jonathan Ott, author of
The Age of Entheogens and
Hallucinogenic Plants of North America

ABERDEENSHIRE LIBRARIES

2080636

DMT:
The Spirit
Molecule

DMT: The Spirit Molecule

A Doctor's Revolutionary Research into the Biology of Near-Death and Mystical Experiences

Rick Strassman, M.D.

Park Street Press
Rochester, Vermont

Park Street Press
One Park Street
Rochester, Vermont 05767
www.InnerTraditions.com

Park Street Press is a division of Inner Traditions International

Copyright © 2001 by Rick J. Strassman, M.D.

All rights reserved. No part of this book may be reproduced or utilized in any form or
by any means, electronic or mechanical, including photocopying, recording, or by any
information storage and retrieval system, without permission in writing from the publisher.

Library of Congress Cataloging-in-Publication Data
Strassman, Rick.
    DMT : the spirit molecule : a doctor's revolutionary research into the biology
 of near-death and mystical experiences / Rick Strassman.
        p. cm.
    Includes bibliographical references.
    ISBN 978-0-89281-927-0 (alk. paper)
    ISBN 0-89281-927-8 (alk. paper)
    1. Dimethyltryptamine. 2. Pineal gland—Secretions. I. Title.

    RM666.D564 S77 2000
    615'.7883—dc21

                                                                00-050498

Printed and bound in the United States

20 19

Text design and layout by Rachel Goldenberg

This book was typeset in Bodoni with Bodoni Open as the display typeface

**615.
788**

To the volunteers, and all their relations

*We do not possess imagination enough
to sense what we are missing.*

Jean Toomer[1]

Contents

Acknowledgments   xi

Introduction   xv

Prologue: First Sessions   1

Part I: The Building Blocks

1 ■ Psychedelic Drugs: Science and Society   21

2 ■ What DMT Is   42

3 ■ The Pineal: Meet the Spirit Gland   56

4 ■ The Psychedelic Pineal   67

Part II: Conception and Birth

5 ■ 89-001   89

6 ■ Labyrinth   99

Part III: Set, Setting, and DMT

7 ■ Being a Volunteer   121

8 ■ Getting DMT   136

9 ■ Under the Influence   143

Part IV: The Sessions

10 ■ Introduction to the Case Reports   153

11 ■ Feeling and Thinking   156

12 ■ Unseen Worlds   176

13 ■ Contact Through the Veil: 1   185

14 ■ Contact Through the Veil: 2   202

15 ■ Death and Dying   220

16 ■ Mystical States   233

17 ■ Pain and Fear   247

Part V: Taking Pause

18 ■ If So, So What?   266

19 ■ Winding Down   278

20 ■ Stepping on Holy Toes   294

Part VI: What Could and Might Be

21 ■ DMT: The Spirit Molecule   310

22 ■ The Futures of Psychedelic Research   329

Epilogue   343

Notes   346

Acknowledgments

Countless colleagues, committees, and agencies helped with all stages of this research. Several deserve special mention. The late Daniel X. Freedman, M.D., from UCLA's Department of Psychiatry, advocated for these projects at all levels and was instrumental in my obtaining crucial early funding. Staff at the U.S. Food and Drug Administration and the U.S. Drug Enforcement Administration were extraordinarily flexible and responsive to the unusual circumstances of this research. Clifford Qualls, Ph.D., the University of New Mexico biostatistician, spent endless hours, days, and weeks crunching numbers at the Research Center, at his home, and at mine. David Nichols, Ph.D., from Purdue University, made the DMT, without which the research never would have occurred.

At every turn, the University of New Mexico School of Medicine provided academic, physical, and administrative support for my work. Walter Winslow, M.D., chairman of the Department of Psychiatry, gave me great latitude as one of his only clinical research scientists at the time. Samuel Keith, M.D., continued with outstanding administrative and academic assistance and counsel after Dr. Winslow retired. Alan Frank, M.D., chair of the university's Human Research Ethics Committee, handled my requests with consistency and evenhandedness.

To the UNM General Clinical Research Center I express my appreciation for their decade of assistance in all my studies: melatonin, DMT, and psilocybin. Jonathan Lisansky, M.D., a UNM Psychiatry and Research Center colleague, originally introduced me to the late Glenn Peake, M.D., Scientific Director of the GCRC. Together they enticed me to Albuquerque in 1984. Philip Eaton, M.D., effortlessly took over the reins of the GCRC after Dr. Peake's sudden death, and barely blinked an eye when I told him I had decided to study psychedelic drugs. David Schade, M.D., Joy McLeod, and Alberta Bland helped with me with skillful laboratory support throughout the years. Lori Sloane of the Computing Center kept all the machines running at top efficiency with what seemed to be amazing ease, and taught me to use programs that otherwise would have taken me years to understand.

Many thanks to the inpatient and outpatient nursing staff, kitchen personnel, and administrative staff, especially Kathy Legoza and Irene Williams. Laura Berg, M.S.N, and Cindy Geist, R.N., provided heroic, cheerful, and disciplined nursing support for all the studies. Katy Brazis, R.N., also contributed her skills to the early psychiatric interviews.

A generous research grant from the Scottish Rite Foundation for Schizophrenia Research helped establish the earliest phases of the DMT project's scientific merit. Later, more substantial funding for the DMT and psilocybin research came from the National Institute on Drug Abuse, a division of the U.S. National Institutes of Health.[1]

For the writing of this book, John Barlow and the Rexx Foundation, as well as Andrew Stone, provided crucial financial kindling, while support from the Barnhart Foundation later set the project blazing forth. Rick Doblin at the Multidisciplinary Association for Psychedelic Studies graciously and generously administered the Stone and Barnhart support. Ned Naumes of the Barnhart Foundation and Sylvia Thiessen and Carla Higdon at MAPS seamlessly coordinated the movement in and out of grant monies.

Friends, colleagues, students, teachers, and mentors over the years have contributed ideas and support to this project: Ralph Abraham, Debra Asis, Alan Badiner, Kay Blacker, Jill and Lewis Carlino, Ram Dass, David Deutsch, Norman Don, Betty Eisner, Dorothy and James Fadiman, Robert Forte, Shefa Gold, Alex Grey, Charles Grob, Stan Grof, John Halpern, Diane Haug, Mark Galanter, Mark Geyer, Chris Gillin, George Greer, Abram Hoffer,

Carol and Rodney Houghton, Daniel Hoyer, Oscar Janiger, David Janowsky, Karl Jansen, Sheperd Jenks, Robert Jesse, Robert Kellner, Herbert Kleber, Tad Lepman, Nancy Lethcoe, Paul Lord, David Lorimer, Luis Eduardo Luna, John Mack, Dennis and Terence McKenna, Herbert Meltzer, David Metcalf, Ralph Metzner, Nancy Morrison, Ethan Nadelmann, Ken Nathanson, Steven Nickeson, Oz, Bernd Michael Pohlman, Karl Pribram, Jill Purce, Rupert Sheldrake, Alexander and Ann Shulgin, Daniel Siebert, Wayne Silby, Zachary Solomon, Myron Stolaroff, Juraj and Sonja Styk, Steven Szára, Charles Tart, Requa Tolbert, Tarthang Tulku, Joe Tupin, Eberhard Uhlenhuth, Andrew Weil, Samuel Widmer, and Leo Zeff. My former wife, Marion Cragg, was there for me and the research through all its twists and turns, providing valuable advice and counsel.

Several people additionally read all or part of the manuscript and commented liberally and helpfully on the work-in-progress: Robert Barnhart, Rick Doblin, Rosetta Maranos, Tony Milosz, Norm Smookler, Andrew Stone, Robert Weisz, and Bernard Xolotl.

Many thanks to Daniel Perrine for rendering the best possible images of the book's molecular structures. And to Alex Grey, deep appreciation for the cover art, and for leading me to Inner Traditions, where Jon Graham liked what he saw in my proposal. Rowan Jacobsen has been everything an editor can be, and then some. Nancy Ringer's peerless copyediting made many improvements to the text.

I am grateful to my former Zen Buddhist community's late abbot, and to the monastic and extended lay communities for their teaching, guidance, and a powerful model of mystical pragmatism.

My deepest thanks go to my family, for without my parents, Alvin and Charlotte Strassman; my brother, Marc Strassman; and my sister, Hanna Dettman, none of this would have been possible.

Finally, I salute, bow, and stand in awe of the volunteers. Their courage to hitch themselves to the spirit molecule's wings, their faith in the research team watching over their bodies and minds while they ventured forth, and their grace under the most austere and unforgiving environment imaginable for taking psychedelic drugs will serve as an inspiration for generations of fellow seekers.

Introduction

In 1990 I began the first new research in the United States in over twenty years on the effects of psychedelic, or hallucinogenic, drugs on humans. These studies investigated the effects of N,N-dimethyltryptamine, or DMT, an extremely short-acting and powerful psychedelic. During the project's five years, I administered approximately four hundred doses of DMT to sixty human volunteers. This research took place at the University of New Mexico's School of Medicine in Albuquerque, where I was tenured Associate Professor of Psychiatry.

I was drawn to DMT because of its presence in all of our bodies. I believed the source of this DMT was the mysterious pineal gland, a tiny organ situated in the center of our brains. Modern medicine knows little about this little gland's role, but it has a rich "metaphysical" history. Descartes, for example, believed the pineal was the "seat of the soul," and both Western and Eastern mystical traditions place our highest spiritual center within its confines. I therefore wondered if excessive pineal DMT production was involved in naturally occurring "psychedelic" states. These might include birth, death and near-death, psychosis, and mystical experiences. Only later, when the study was well underway, did I also begin considering DMT's role in the "alien abduction" experience.

The DMT project was founded on cutting-edge brain science, especially that which dealt with the psychopharmacology of serotonin. However, my own background, which included a decades-long relationship with a Zen Buddhist training monastery, powerfully affected how we prepared people for, and supervised, their drug sessions.

DMT: The Spirit Molecule reviews what we know about psychedelic drugs in general, and DMT in particular. It then traces the DMT research project from its earliest intimations through a maze of committees and review boards to its actual performance.

Although all of us believed in the potentially beneficial properties of psychedelic drugs, the studies were not intended to be therapeutic, and so our research subjects were healthy volunteers. The project generated a wealth of biological and psychological data, much of which I have already published in the scientific literature. On the other hand, I have written nearly nothing about volunteers' stories. I hope the many excerpts I have included here, taken from over one thousand pages of my notes, will provide a sense of the remarkable emotional, psychological, and spiritual effects of this chemical.

Problems inside and outside of the research environment led to the end of these studies in 1995. Despite the difficulties we encountered, I am optimistic about the possible benefits of the controlled use of psychedelic drugs. Based upon what we learned in the New Mexico research, I offer a wide-ranging vision for DMT's role in our lives and conclude by proposing a research agenda and optimal setting for future work with DMT and related drugs.

The late Willis Harman possessed one of the most discerning minds to apply itself to the field of psychedelic research. Earlier in his career, he and his colleagues administered LSD to scientists in an attempt to bolster their problem-solving skills. They found that LSD demonstrated a powerfully beneficial effect on creativity. This landmark research remains the first and only scientific project to use psychedelics to enhance the creative process. When I met Willis thirty years later, in 1994, he was president of the Institute of Noetic Sciences, an organization founded by the sixth man to walk on the moon, Edgar Mitchell. Mitchell's mystical experience, stimulated by viewing Earth on his return home, inspired him to study phenomena outside the range of traditional science that nevertheless might yield to a broader application of the scientific method.

During a long walk together along the central California coastal range one day, Willis said firmly, "At the very least, we must enlarge the discussion about psychedelics." It is in response to his request that I include in this book highly speculative ideas and my own personal motivations for performing this research.

This approach will satisfy no one in every respect. There is intense friction between what we know intellectually, or even intuitively, and what we experience with the aid of DMT. As one of our volunteers exclaimed after his first high-dose session, "Wow! I never expected *that!*" Or as Dogen, a thirteenth-century Japanese Buddhist teacher, said, "We must always be disturbed by the truth."

Enthusiasts of the psychedelic drug culture may dislike my conclusion: that DMT has no beneficial effects in and of itself; that rather, the context in which people take it is at least as important. Proponents of drug control may condemn what they read as encouragement to take psychedelic drugs and a glorification of the DMT experience. Practitioners and spokespersons of traditional religions may reject the suggestion that spiritual states can be accessed, and mystical information gained, through drugs. Those who have undergone "alien abduction," and their advocates, may interpret my suggestion that DMT is intimately involved in these events as a challenge to the "reality" of their experiences. Opponents and supporters of abortion rights may find fault with my proposal that a pineal DMT release at forty-nine days after conception marks the entrance of the spirit into the fetus. Brain researchers may object to the suggestion that DMT affects the brain's ability to *receive* information, rather than only generating those perceptions. They also may dismiss the proposal that DMT can allow our brains to perceive dark matter or parallel universes, realms of existence inhabited by conscious entities.

However, if I did not describe all the ideas behind the DMT studies, and the entire range of our volunteers' experiences, I would not be telling the entire tale. And without the radical proposals I offer in an attempt to understand volunteers' sessions, *DMT: The Spirit Molecule* might have, at best, little effect on the scope of discussion about psychedelics; at worst, the book would reduce the field. Nor would I be honest if I did not share my own speculations and theories, which are based on decades of study and listening to hundreds of DMT sessions. This is why I did it. This is what happened. This is what I think about it.

It is so important for us to understand consciousness. It is just as important to place psychedelic drugs in general, and DMT in particular, into a personal and cultural matrix in which we do the most good, and the least harm. In such a wide-open area of inquiry, it is best that we reject no ideas until we actually disprove them. It is in the interest of enlarging the discussion about psychedelic drugs that I've written *DMT: The Spirit Molecule.*

DMT:
The Spirit
Molecule

Prologue:
First Sessions

One morning in December 1990, I gave both Philip and Nils an injection of a large dose of intravenous DMT. These two men were the first people in the study to receive DMT, and they were helping me determine the best dose and manner of injecting it. They were our "human guinea pigs."

Two weeks earlier, I had given the very first dose of DMT to Philip. As I will describe, the intramuscular injection, into his shoulder, didn't give completely satisfactory results. We then switched to the intravenous route, and Nils received the drug that way for the first time a week later. Nils's reaction indicated that the dose we gave him was too low. So today Philip and Nils were going to receive substantially higher doses of intravenous DMT.

It was hard to believe we really were giving DMT to human volunteers. A two-year process of obtaining permission and funding, which I felt would never end, was finally over. Attaining the goal never seemed as likely as the continual struggle to do so.

1

Philip and Nils both had previous experience with DMT, and I was glad they did. About a year before starting our study, they had attended a ceremony in which a Peruvian folk healer gave all participants *ayahuasca*, the legendary DMT-containing tea. The two men were enthusiastic about this orally active form of DMT and were eager to smoke pure DMT the next day, when a member of the workshop made it available. They wanted to feel its effects in a much more immediate and intense manner than the tea form allowed.

Philip's and Nils's experiences smoking DMT were typical: a startlingly rapid onset of effects, a kaleidoscopic display of visual hallucinations, and a separation of consciousness from the physical body. And, most curiously, there was a feeling of "the other" somewhere within the hallucinatory world to which this remarkable psychedelic allowed them entrance.

Their prior experience with DMT was a very important aspect of bringing them in as the first volunteers. Philip and Nils were familiar with the effects of DMT. Even more crucial, they were familiar with the effects of smoking the drug, which would help them gauge the adequacy of the two different administration methods I was considering, intramuscular (IM) or intravenous (IV), in reproducing the full effects of the smoking route. Since recreational users of DMT usually smoke it, I wanted to approximate as closely as possible the effects as they occur when taken in this manner.

On the day Philip received the first dose of DMT by the intramuscular route, I already was thinking ahead. Perhaps the IM method might be too slow and mild compared to smoking the drug. What I had read about IM DMT suggested it took up to a minute to start working, substantially longer than when it was smoked. However, since all but one of the previously published human research papers on DMT reported giving it intramuscularly, I was obliged to begin this way. This older literature suggested that the dose I was to give Philip, 1 milligram per kilogram (mg/kg), about 75 mg, probably would be a moderately high dose.

Philip was forty-five years old when he began participating in our research. Bespectacled, bearded, and of medium height and build, he was an internationally known clinical psychologist, psychotherapist, and workshop leader. He was soft-spoken but direct, and he elicited great affection from his friends and clients.

At the time, Philip was beginning a divorce that would become especially long and difficult. His life had been marked by many deep changes, losses, and gains, and he seemed to take the good and the bad with the same equanimity. He liked to say that the title of his self-help best-seller would be *Surviving Your Life.*

At least five years had passed since I last gave an IM injection of anything to anyone, and I was nervous about administering the first dose of DMT this way. What if I missed? The last time I gave such an injection, I probably had been giving the antipsychotic drug haloperidol to an agitated patient with psychosis. These patients often had their arms and legs tied down by psychiatric orderlies or the police beforehand, to make sure their disorganized and frightened behavior didn't end in violence. This also kept the patients' arms in a relatively stable position for my injection.

I tried remembering the confidence with which I previously gave IM shots, since I had performed hundreds in the past. The secret was to think of the syringe as a dart. We were taught in medical school to pretend you were throwing this dart into the rounded deltoid muscle of the shoulder, or the gluteus maximus muscle of the buttocks. A single, fluid motion, lightening the pressure just as the needle pierced the muscle through the skin, usually produced excellent results. We practiced on grapefruits.

Philip, however, was neither a grapefruit nor an acutely psychotic patient delivered up to me for involuntary tranquilization. He was a professional colleague, friend, and research volunteer on equal footing with me and my staff. Philip was to be the scout. Cindy, our research nurse, and I were to remain at "base camp," to hear about where he went after his return.

Practicing my technique in the air, I walked down the hall and entered Philip's room.

Philip lay in bed; his new girlfriend, Robin, sat nearby. The cuff of a blood pressure machine was loosely wrapped around his arm. We would check his heart rate and blood pressure frequently throughout the session.

I explained what was going to happen: "I'll wipe your shoulder with some alcohol. Take as much time as you need to collect yourself. Then I'll inject the needle into your arm, draw back to make sure I'm not in a blood vessel, and then push in the plunger on the syringe. It might sting, or it might not. I don't really know. You ought to feel something in a minute or less. But I'm not sure what that something will be. You're the first."

Philip closed his eyes for a moment as he prepared to venture into unknown territory, worlds only he would perceive, leaving us behind to look after his life functions. He opened his eyes widely to briefly gaze at us one more time, then closed them again, took a deep breath, and on his exhalation said, "I'm ready."

The injection went without a hitch.

After a little more than a minute, Philip opened his eyes and began breathing deeply. He looked as if he were in an altered state of consciousness. His pupils were large, he began groaning, and the lines of his face smoothed. He closed his eyes while Robin held his hand. He laid extremely still and remained silent, eyes closed. What was happening? Was he all right? His blood pressure and heart rate seemed fine, but what about his mind? Did we overdose him? Was he having any effect at all?

About 25 minutes after the injection, Philip opened his eyes and looked up at Robin. Smiling, he said,

I could have done more.

We all breathed a sigh of relief.

Fifteen minutes later, or 40 minutes after the injection, Philip started speaking slowly and haltingly.

I never lost touch with my body. Compared to smoking DMT, the visuals were less intense, the colors were not as deep, and the geometric patterns did not move as fast.

He sought my hand for comfort. My hands were damp from nervousness, and he laughed good-naturedly at my anxiety, which was clearly greater than his!

Upon arising to go the bathroom, Philip was shaky. He drank some grape juice, ate a little container of yogurt, and filled out the rating scale. He felt "spaced-out," fuzzy in his mind, awkward, while we walked to and from another building where I had some business. It was important to be with him, to observe how he functioned for the next couple of hours. Philip seemed well enough three hours after his DMT shot for Robin to drive him home. We said good-bye in the hospital parking lot, and I told him to expect a call that night.

When we spoke, Philip told me that Robin and he went to eat lunch after leaving the hospital. He immediately became more alert and focused. On the ride home, he felt euphoric, and colors seemed brighter everywhere he looked. He sounded quite happy.

Philip sent me a written report a few days later. Most important was his last comment:

I expected to jump to a higher level, to leave the body and ego consciousness, the jump into cosmic space. But this did not happen.

This threshold to which Philip referred is what we now call the "psychedelic threshold" for DMT. You cross it when there is a separation of consciousness from the body and psychedelic effects completely replace the mind's normal contents. There is a sense of wonder or awe, and a feeling of undeniable certainty in the reality of the experience. This clearly had not occurred with 1 mg/kg intramuscular DMT.

It was great to have Philip in this explorer's role. He was psychologically mature and stable and was familiar with the effects of psychedelics in general, and DMT in particular. He could make clear, understandable comparisons between different drugs and different ways of receiving them. His case was powerful validation of our decision to enroll only experienced psychedelic users.

Philip's report left no doubt that IM DMT effects lagged behind those of smoked DMT. I considered giving a higher dose. However, even if full peak effects developed, I doubted that this route would ever give the "rush" that is another hallmark of smoked DMT. During this "rush," which usually happens in the first 15 to 30 seconds after smoking DMT, the shift from normal consciousness to an overwhelming psychedelic reality takes place with breathtaking speed. It is this "nuclear cannon" effect that users find so frighteningly attractive. We definitely needed a more rapid way of getting DMT into the system.

Most recreational DMT users smoke it in a pipe, sprinkled on marijuana or a non-psychoactive herb. This is not the ideal method of getting DMT into your body. The drug often catches fire, which is disconcerting when you are trying to inhale as much of the vapor as possible. The smell of burning DMT is intensely nauseating, like that of burning plastic. As the drug takes effect and the room seems to begin breaking up into crystalline shards, your body following suit, it becomes nearly impossible to know if you are inhaling or exhaling. In that state of intoxication, imagine trying to breathe into your lungs as much of this flaming, foul-odored blob of chemical as possible!

The fastest and most efficient way to administer DMT is by injection. Intramuscular injections depend on the relatively limited blood flow through muscles to drain away the drug, and it is the slowest type of injection. Drugs also may be given into the skin, or subcutaneously, where the slightly richer blood flow makes for a faster, though usually painful, method. Injection into a vein is the best method. From the intravenous, or IV, injection site, drug-rich blood returns to the heart. The heart pumps this blood through the lungs; from there it reenters the heart and then makes its way out to the rest of the body, including the brain. The time for this entire process, what physiologists call "arm-to-tongue time," is usually about 16 seconds.[1]

I consulted with my colleague who had made the DMT, David Nichols, Ph.D., at Purdue University in Indiana. He agreed that I needed to switch to the intravenous route. Reflecting upon our mutual anxiety about this change in plans, he added dryly, "I'm glad it's you and not me."

It was time to consult with Dr. W., the physician at the U.S. Food and Drug Administration (FDA) who, after helping guide the project through the two-year regulatory process, was now overseeing its performance. When I asked his opinion, he laughed and said, "You are the only research scientist in the world giving DMT. You're the expert. You decide."

He was right, but I was nervous about entering such uncharted territory so quickly, after giving just one dose of DMT. There was only one previously published report that described giving DMT intravenously, but this was to psychiatric patients, not normal volunteers.[2] That 1950s project studied severely impaired patients with schizophrenia, most of whom were unable to report much about their experiences. In fact, one unfortunate woman's pulse was not detectable for a short while after she received IV DMT. It was in deference to this report that I was so cautious about heart function in all prospective volunteers.[3]

Dr. W. recommended trying about one-fifth the IM dose when switching to the IV route. "That will probably give you lower blood and brain levels of DMT than you produced by giving it intramuscularly, and you should have some room to maneuver," he said. "You probably won't overdose anyone this way." In our case, that meant converting the IM dose of 1 mg/kg to 0.2 mg/kg intravenous DMT.

Philip and Nils both had eagerly volunteered for this new and uncharted phase of the research: finding a satisfactory dose of IV DMT in normal volunteers. Since both had smoked DMT previously, we would be able to compare directly the effects of IV to smoked drug. And, in Philip's case, we could compare IV to IM routes.

Nils was thirty-six years old when he began in our research. As a younger man, Nils had enlisted in the Army, desiring to specialize in explosives. However, he quickly saw that he was unfit for the armed services, and he applied for an early discharge for psychological reasons. Philip happened to be the psychologist who performed this evaluation on Nils, and they had remained friends afterward.

Nils was keenly interested in mind-altering drugs and always was looking for a neglected plant or animal product that might produce such effects. He had written several popular pamphlets, including one announcing his discovery of the psychedelic properties of the venom of the Sonoran Desert toad. This venom contains high levels of 5-methoxy-DMT, a compound closely related to DMT. When smoked, this toad product is quite impressive.

Nils was a long and lanky fellow, charming and fun to be around. He had taken LSD many times, having "lost track after the 150th dose." The first time he had smoked DMT, at Philip's house the year before, he was powerfully moved. He said,

It made strong telepathic impressions, causing mental bonds with the people around me. This was confusing and overwhelming. I became very excited as an inner voice spoke to me. This was my intuition directly relating to me. It was the most intense experience of my life. I want to go back. I saw a different space with bright bands of color. I couldn't raise my hands, I tripped so hard. It is a mental Mecca, an excellent reference point for all other psychedelics. Those around me looked like alien space insects. I realized they were all part of it, too.

Nils received 0.2 mg/kg intravenous DMT about a week after Philip's first IM dose. My feelings were similar to those I had for Philip's injection; that is, while the actual day was a landmark, it also seemed like a dry run, a rehearsal for the real thing. It was very likely we would go beyond this dose.

On the day of Nils's 0.2 mg/kg session, I found him lying on the hospital bed in his research center room, underneath his familiar Army sleeping bag. He took this bag with him whenever he traveled, both literally and figuratively: when he would journey on the road, or when he would take a psychedelic drug trip.

Cindy and I sat on either side of Nils. I gave him a brief preview of what to expect. He nodded for me to begin.

Halfway through the injection, Nils said,

Yes, I taste it.

Nils turned out to be one of the few volunteers who could taste intravenous DMT as the drug-rich blood rushed through his mouth and tongue on the way to his brain. It was a metallic, slightly bitter taste.

I thought, "This seems fast enough."

My notes are sketchy as to the effects of this dose of IV DMT on Nils. This may have been due to his taciturn nature, or because neither of us were especially impressed with the intensity of the experience. He did remark, however, that 0.2 mg/kg was "maybe one-third to one-fourth" a full dose, relative to his experience smoking DMT. Perhaps feeling a little overconfident from how easy these first two sessions—Philip's IM, and Nils's IV—had been, I decided to proceed immediately to triple Nils's IV dose: from 0.2 to 0.6 mg/kg.

My confidence was premature. In retrospect, a more cautious move to doubling it, to 0.4 mg/kg, would have been more reasonable. Thankfully, I didn't jump to 0.8 mg/kg, which would have happened had I followed Nils's suggestion that 0.2 mg/kg was a fourth of a full dose.

This morning, both Philip and Nils were going to get 0.6 mg/kg IV DMT.

It was sunny, cold, and windy in Albuquerque that day, and I was glad to be working inside. I entered Nils's room in the Research Center. He was lying under his sleeping bag, awaiting the first 0.6 mg/kg dose. Cindy already had placed a small needle into a forearm vein, the portal through which I would inject the DMT solution directly into his blood. She sat on his right side, and I on his left, where the tubing from the IV line dangled off his arm. Philip also was here; he was scheduled to receive the same dose later in the morning if all went well with Nils. He sat at the foot of the bed, curious about what Nils was to experience, and ready to provide moral support for all of us. Little did we suspect we'd need him for physical backup, too.

I infused the solution of DMT somewhat more quickly than I did for Nils's previous 0.2 mg/kg dose, over 30 seconds rather than a minute. I thought a faster injection might allow for less dilution of the DMT in the bloodstream. This then would generate higher peak levels of DMT in the blood and, therefore, the brain. After the infusion of drug was complete, Nils said excitedly,

I can taste it. . . . Here it is!

Immediately after blurting this out, he began tossing and turning under his sleeping bag. He then sat up with a start, exclaiming,

I'm going to vomit!

He gazed at us, stunned and uncertain. Cindy and I looked at each other at the same time, realizing we had nothing into which he could throw up. We hadn't foreseen that our test subjects might need to vomit. He mumbled,

But I didn't have any breakfast . . . so there's nothing to throw up.

Nils became agitated and pulled the pillow and sleeping bag over his face. He curled into the fetal position, away from us and the blood pressure machine, kinking the tubing that connected the cuff to the unit. We could not get a reading at either 2 or 5 minutes, when we knew his blood pressure and heart rate would be at their highest, and potentially most dangerous, levels. He tried climbing out of the bed with a mostly purposeless flailing of his arms and legs—but this was a substantial mass of limbs in someone 6'4". His hands were cold and clammy as Cindy, Philip, and I joined forces and maneuvered him back into the now-too-small-seeming bed. At 6 minutes, he retched into a basin we found in the closet. Because he had to sit up to do so, we were able to reposition him in the bed, and we obtained a blood pressure and heart rate recording. At this point, 10 minutes after the injection, his readings were surprisingly normal.

He reached out to Cindy, touching her arm and sweater. It looked as if he were about to stroke her hair, but quickly seemed to forgot what he was going to do. Nils then stared at me, saying,

I need to look at you now, not Philip or Cindy.

I did my best to look calm, answering his gaze with my own, praying quietly that he would be all right. At 19 minutes, he sat up on his elbows and laughed. He looked very "stoned": large pupils, lopsided grin, mumbling incoherently.

He finally said,

I think the best high dose is between 0.2 and 0.6.

We all laughed, and the tension in the room dropped a few notches. Nils still had his wits about him, at least at that moment.

He continued,

There was the movement of the self. I am disappointed that it's ending. It was a cafeteria of colors. A familiar feeling. Yes, I've returned. "They" were there and we recognized each other.

I asked, "Who?"

No one or thing identifiable as such.

He still seemed quite under the influence. I did not want to press him. He shook his head and added,

Coming down from the high was very colorful, but it was boring compared to the peak. At the peak, I knew I was back where I had been when

I smoked it last year. It was a lonely feeling leaving there.

I thought I had gotten really sick. I felt you hovering over me, like I was dying, and you all were trying to resuscitate me. I hoped everything was all right. I was just trying to catch what was happening inside.

He paused, then concluded,

I'm tired. I'd like to nap, but I'm not really sleepy.

Nils had little to say beyond this, other than that he was ravenously hungry, wisely having skipped breakfast. He ate heartily while filling out our rating scale. So even Nils thought 0.6 mg/kg was "too much"!

I spent a few minutes in the nurses' lounge, reflecting upon what we had just seen. From a cardiac point of view, Nils's blood pressure and heart rate had risen only moderately, although we missed the readings at their presumed peak. Thus, there seemed likely to be no physical harm from administering 0.6 mg/kg IV DMT. However, I was not sure if the thinness of Nils's report was because he could not remember what had happened, or because of his style of keeping to himself most of what had taken place.

We clearly had broken through the "psychedelic threshold." The suddenness and intensity of onset, the irrefutable nature of the experience, the inhabited sense Nils described, all added up to a "full" DMT trip. But was it too far beyond the psychedelic barrier? Nils was a self-acknowledged "hard head," requiring higher doses than many to attain comparable levels of altered perceptions from the same drug. How would Philip fare?

Philip and I walked down the Research Center's brightly lit hall. We passed Nils at the nurses' station, looking for more food. He felt great. It was reassuring to see how well he looked so quickly after his harrowing jump off the psychic cliff.

I asked Philip, "Are you sure you want the same dose?"

"Yes." There was absolutely no hesitation.

I was not so sure.

If Philip declined undergoing an experience similar to Nils's, my anxiety would have become more tolerable. Perhaps he would settle for 0.5 or 0.4 mg/kg. This would be easy enough to do—I could simply stop short of emptying the entire syringe full of DMT solution. While I believed 0.6 mg/kg most likely was physically safe, the potentially shattering mental effects loomed in front of all of us even more dramatically than they had before Nils's session. However, Philip was not to be outdone by his friend and fellow "psychonaut." He was ready for *his* 0.6 mg/kg dose.

This tendency in our volunteers, to persevere even under the possibility of an annihilating psychedelic experience, was marked. It was most apparent during our tolerance study, which took place the next year, in 1991, in which volunteers received four large doses of DMT, each separated by only 30 minutes. Not one volunteer, no matter how worn out, refused that fourth and final high dose of DMT.

Philip's desire to take the same dose as Nils confronted me with a scientific, personal, and ethical dilemma. My training had taught me that one should not shy away from prescribing a little too much of a medication if the circumstances called for doing so. For example, very high doses might be necessary for a full therapeutic response in otherwise treatment-resistant patients. In addition, it was important to learn about toxic effects, to be able to recognize them quickly in various circumstances. This latter point is even more important when studying a new experimental drug.

It was within my authority and responsibility as the principal investigator of the project to tell Philip I did not want him to repeat a Nils-like 0.6 mg/kg DMT experience. However, Nils seemed fine now. Most importantly, he was the first and only person to get this dose. I had planned on two 0.6 mg/kg sessions that morning so that I could determine if this dose caused similar responses in two different people.

I liked Philip, and he did want his 0.6 mg/kg dose. But how much of a role did our friendship play? I didn't want to do as he requested just so that I wouldn't jeopardize our relationship, but I wanted his participation in this early stage of the study to be worth his while. He was, in some ways, "doing us a favor." Philip lived far from Albuquerque, and asking him to return once more to get 0.6 mg/kg, if 0.4 or 0.5 were not a full-enough dose, would have inconvenienced him. There were many competing priorities. I hoped I made the right decision by agreeing to give Philip 0.6 mg/kg.

Entering his room, Philip and I said hello to Cindy and Robin, Philip's girlfriend, who were already there, waiting for us. He made himself comfortable on the bed. Another 0.6 mg/kg IV DMT session was about to begin.

Philip's bare and sterile room featured brightly waxed linoleum floors, salmon pink walls, and tubes for oxygen, suctioning of secretions, and water exiting from behind the bed. He had taped a poster of *Avalokitesvara*, the one-thousand-armed Buddhist saint of compassion, on the outside of the closed wooden bathroom door that faced his bed. A television attached by a maze of cables hung from the ceiling, looking down at his mechanized, narrow bed, which was covered with thin hospital sheets. The air conditioning hummed loudly. He lay down on the bed and made himself as comfortable as possible.

Cindy smoothly and skillfully placed an intravenous line into one forearm vein. The blood pressure cuff was also wrapped around this arm. Philip's other arm had inserted into it a larger IV line from which we could draw blood, so we could measure concentrations of DMT in his blood after administering it. This line was attached to a clear plastic bag that dripped sterile saltwater into the vein so that there would be no clotting in the blood-drawing tube. Cindy and I sat on either side of Philip, not sure what to expect in light of Nils's earlier reaction. Robin sat off to the side, near the foot of the bed.

Philip, fresh from Nils's unnerving session only an hour ago, needed little preparation. He knew what to expect from us while he was lying in his bed under the influence. He had seen that we would help him immediately if he seemed in need of assistance. We wished him luck. He closed his eyes, lay back, took some deep breaths, and said, "I'm ready."

I watched the second hand of the clock on the wall, waiting for it to hit the "6" so that I could time the 30-second injection to finish when the second hand hit the "12," which would be "time zero." It was nearly 10 A.M.

Just as I finished inserting the needle of the syringe into Philip's line, but before depressing the plunger and emptying the DMT solution into Philip's vein, there was a loud, insistent knocking on the door. I looked up, paused, removed the needle from the line, capped it, and placed it on the nightstand next to Philip's bed.

The director of the Research Center laboratory was waiting outside the door. I stepped into the hall, out of earshot from the room. He said that the previous blood samples for DMT analyses were collected incorrectly, and that we needed to change how we did this. I told him we would modify our technique accordingly.

I let myself back into Philip's room and took the chair by the side of his bed once more. He seemed unaware of the interruption, having begun the inward turning and letting go that we found allows for the smoothest possible entry into the DMT realms. For him, the trip had already begun.

I apologized for the interruption and, trying to lighten the mood, said, "Where were we now?" Philip replied with only a grunt; he opened his eyes, nodded for me to proceed, and closed them again. I uncapped the syringe and reinserted the needle into his IV tubing. Cindy nodded that she was ready, too.

I said, "Okay, here's the DMT."

I slowly and carefully began infusing 0.6 mg/kg DMT into Philip's vein.

Halfway through the injection, Philip's breath caught in his throat, sounding like a cough that never quite got out. We quickly learned that whenever this catching in the throat followed a high-dose injection, we were in for a wild ride.

Quietly, I let Philip know, "It's all in."

Twenty-five seconds after the infusion was complete, he began groaning,

I love, I love . . .

His blood pressure rose moderately, but his heart rate jumped to 140 beats per minute, up from his resting level of 65. This increase in pulse is equivalent to that which might occur after racing up three or four flights of stairs. But in this case, Philip hadn't moved an inch.

At 1 minute, Philip sat up, looking at Cindy and me with saucer-sized eyes. His pupils were hugely dilated. His movements were automatic, jerky, puppetlike. There seemed to be "no one home" behind Philip's actions.

He leaned toward Robin and stroked her hair:

I love, I love . . .

Twice that morning, then: a volunteer in a dazed DMT state, attracted to a woman's hair. Nils to Cindy's, Philip to Robin's. Perhaps it was the most powerful image of living, organic, familiar reality available when one looked around a dreary hospital room in such a highly psychedelic state.

To our relief, he laid back down without prompting or assistance. His skin was cold and clammy, as had been Nils's. His body was in a classic "fight-or-flight" reaction: high blood pressure and heart rate, blood moving from the skin deeper into the vital internal organs, but all while he was performing almost no actual physical activity. It was difficult to draw Philip's blood—the high levels of stress hormones caused the tiny muscles lining the veins to clamp down, reducing unnecessary blood flow to the skin.

At 10 minutes, Philip began to sigh,

How beautiful, how beautiful!

Tears began streaming down his cheeks.

Now that was what you would call a transcendent experience. I died and went to heaven.

By 30 minutes after the injection, his pulse and blood pressure were normal.

It was flying within a vastness. There was no relative space or size.

I asked, "What did you feel when your breath caught in your throat?"

I felt a cold, contracting feeling in my throat. It frightened me. I thought maybe I would stop breathing. The thought, "Let go, surrender, let go," was there for a split second, then the rush of the drug swept even that away.

"Do you recall sitting up and stroking Robin's hair?"

I did what?

Forty-five minutes after the injection, drinking tea and no longer feeling any effects of the drug, Philip could not remember sitting up, looking at us, or touching Robin. Soon thereafter, he seemed comfortable and we were confident Robin could look after him.

Philip and I spoke the following evening. He felt a little run down, but had slept very well. His dreams were "more interesting than usual," although not particularly bizarre. Nevertheless, he could not remember any of them. He worked a full ten hours the next day, although "not at full steam." However, he said, "Nobody but I would have noticed I was tired."

Amazingly, these are all the notes I have from that session and the next day's report. This contrasts strikingly with Philip's usually quite eloquent descriptions of his drug sessions. Perhaps his getting through the morning safely was the most important information we needed to learn.

Driving home that evening into the mountains outside of Albuquerque, I used the time to think about the day's events. I was glad that both Nils and Philip had emerged intact from their 0.6 mg/kg IV DMT encounters. However, I had not learned much about what their experiences were really like. Their reports were remarkably brief and lacked detail.

Why were Nils's and Philip's reports so sparse?

One possibility was "state-specific memory." This refers to the phenomenon in which events experienced in an altered state of consciousness can be recalled clearly only upon reentering that state, and not in the normal one. This happens under the influence of substances such as alcohol, marijuana, or prescription drugs like the sedatives Valium, Xanax, or barbiturates. It also results from non-drug-induced altered states, such as hypnosis or dreams. In Philip's and Nils's cases, this explanation would be likely if they later recalled more of their 0.6 mg/kg sessions while working with lower, more manageable doses of DMT. However, this did not occur to any extent in either man during their subsequent participation in the project.

Another possibility is that Nils and Philip suffered a brief delirium, an "acute organic brain syndrome," or "acute confusional state." *Delirium* derives from the Latin *de*, meaning "from" or "out of," and *lira*, "a furrow"; literally, "going out of the furrow," or "out of it." Delirium can result from physical factors such as fever, head injury, lack of oxygen, or low blood sugar. In addition, a profoundly traumatic psychological experience may produce a delirious state, such as what happens in survivors of severe trauma or disasters.

I was uncertain to what degree "psychological trauma" contributed to Nils's and Philip's confusion in, and inability to remember much of, their

DMT sessions. How much was a psychological reaction to the drug's effects, rather than a direct effect of the drug itself? That is, climbing a ladder to view a scene of unimaginable shock value might throw one into a delirious or confused state, but it is not the ladder but rather the view the ladder provides that is responsible. Was what Nils and Philip saw so bizarre, so incomprehensible, so utterly aberrant that their minds simply turned off to spare them from seeing clearly what was there? Maybe it was better to forget.

In either case, whether too much drug or too much experience, whatever 0.6 mg/kg IV DMT did to these two seasoned psychedelic veterans, it came down to just this: "too much." As Philip said later,

It was a cosmic blowtorch, a tempest of color, bewildering, like I was thrown overboard into a storm and was spinning out of control, being tossed like a cork.

I called Dave Nichols again to discuss the DMT dose. What should be a lower "high" dose? A reduction to 0.5 mg/kg would be lowering the dose by only one-sixth, while 0.4 mg/kg was fully one-third less. We went back and forth. While I wanted to make certain the high dose elicited a full effect, I did not want to psychologically traumatize our volunteers. I was feeling a little tentative after the day's events with Philip and Nils. "First, do no harm" is the overriding dictum for medicine in general, and even more so for human research. Creating a group of psychically damaged volunteers was not an option. Keeping the effects of Philip's and Nils's 0.6 mg/kg sessions in the forefront of our discussion, we decided to make 0.4 mg/kg the top DMT dose for the study.

A few days later, I called the early DMT pioneer Dr. Stephen Szára to discuss these dosage issues. Dr. Szára had discovered the psychedelic effects of DMT by injecting it into himself in his laboratory in Budapest, Hungary, in the mid-1950s. (During the first phases of human psychedelic research, it was common for the researchers themselves to "go first.") He now was completing a long and distinguished career at the U.S. National Institute on Drug Abuse in Washington, D.C.

I asked him, "Did you ever give too much DMT to your volunteers?"

Dr. Szára thought for a moment, then answered in his refined Eastern European accent, "Yes. They could not remember anything. They could not bring back memories of the experience. The only thing that remained with them was the feeling that something frightening had happened. We did not believe it worthwhile administering those kinds of doses."

It is fascinating how many of the themes that would emerge over the next five years appeared that December morning when I administered 0.6 mg/kg IV DMT doses to Philip and Nils. We hear about near-death and spiritual experiences, and contact with "them" in the DMT realms. I felt conflicting priorities around friendship and research goals. The drawbacks of the hospital setting and medical model quickly were apparent. The need to give full psychedelic doses was already tempered by an awareness of their potential for negative reactions. There was a far-flung network of colleagues and regulators who variously assisted the project. All were there in some form or another in Philip's and Nil's 0.6 mg/kg IV DMT sessions.

Let's now turn to the background for this research, the vast amount we know about psychedelic drugs, and the way our science and society have used that information. Then we can begin to understand the unique role DMT plays in our bodies, and the astonishing functions it may serve in our lives.

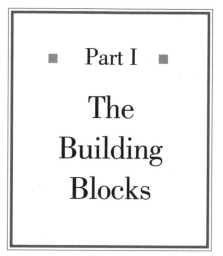

■ Part I ■

The
Building
Blocks

Psychedelic Drugs:
Science and Society

The history of human use of plants, mushrooms, and animals for their psychedelic effects is far older than written history, and probably predates the appearance of the modern human species. Ronald Siegel and Terence McKenna, for example, suggest that our apelike ancestors imitated other animals by eating things that caused unusual behavior. In this way, they discovered the earliest mind-altering substances.

There is growing physical evidence that many ancient cultures used psychedelics for their effects on consciousness. Archaeologists have uncovered ancient African images of mushrooms sprouting from a human body, and recent discoveries of prehistoric northern European rock art strongly suggest the influence of psychedelically altered consciousness.

Some authors have proposed that language developed out of psychedelically enhanced appreciation of, and associations with, early hominid mouth sounds. Others suggest that psychedelic states formed the basis of humans' earliest awareness of religious experience.

The visions, ecstatic states, and flights of imagination made possible by psychedelic drugs gave these substances an important role in many ancient cultures. Hundreds of years of anthropological research have demonstrated that these societies used psychedelics to maintain social solidarity, aid the healing arts, and inspire artistic and spiritual creativity.

New World aboriginal people used, and continue to use, a wide range of mind-altering plants and mushrooms. Most of what we know about psychedelics comes from investigating chemicals first found in Western Hemisphere materials: DMT, psilocybin, mescaline, and several LSD-like compounds.

The depth and breadth of psychedelic plant use by New World residents surprised and alarmed European settlers. Their reaction may have been due to the relative lack of psychedelic plants and mushrooms in Europe. Just as important was the association of mind-altering substances with witchcraft. The Church effectively suppressed information about the use of those materials in both the Old and New Worlds and persecuted bearers and practitioners of that knowledge. It is only in the last fifty years that we have realized that Mexican Indian use of magic mushrooms did not entirely die out in the sixteenth century.

In Europe, there was little interest in, or access to, psychedelic plants or drugs until the end of the late 1800s. Some authors described their own "psychedelic" reactions to opium or hashish, but the amount required for psychedelic effects was difficult to consume, excessive, or dangerous. This situation began to change with the discovery of mescaline in *peyote*, a New World cactus.

German chemists isolated mescaline from peyote in the 1890s. The more literary among those exploring its effects hailed its ability to open the gates of an "artificial paradise." However, medical and psychiatric interest in mescaline was surprisingly restrained, and researchers published only a limited number of papers by the end of the 1930s. The unpleasant nausea and vomiting that often occur with mescaline may have had something to do with the lack of interest in it.

Another reason for the minimal enthusiasm about mescaline may have been that there was no scientific or medical context in which to understand its effects. Freudian psychoanalysis was that era's predominant force in psychiatry. While Freud himself was strongly attracted to mind-altering drugs such as cocaine and tobacco, his students were less so. In addition, Freud distrusted religion and believed spiritual or religious experience was a defense against childish fears and wishes. This attitude probably did little to encourage investigation of mescaline, with its trappings of Native American spirituality. Then LSD made its revolutionary appearance.

In 1938 the Swiss chemist Albert Hofmann was working with ergot, a rye fungus, in the natural products division of Sandoz Laboratories, even then a major pharmaceutical company. He hoped to find a drug that might help stop uterine bleeding after childbirth. One of these ergot-based compounds was LSD-25, or lysergic acid diethylamide. It had little effect on the uterus of laboratory animals, and Hofmann shelved it. Five years later, "a curious presentiment" called Hofmann back to examine LSD, and he accidentally discovered its powerful psychedelic properties.

The remarkable thing about LSD was that it brought on psychedelic effects at doses of *millionths* of a gram, which meant that it had more than one thousand times the strength of mescaline. In fact, Hofmann nearly overdosed himself with what he thought was too small a quantity to possibly be mind-altering: a quarter milligram. Hoffman and his Swiss colleagues were quick to publish their findings in the early 1940s. Because of the highly altered state of mind LSD produced, and the traditional psychiatric context in which researchers explored it, scientists decided to emphasize its "psychosis-mimicking" properties.[1]

The years after World War II were exciting ones for psychiatry. In addition to LSD, scientists also discovered the "antipsychotic" properties of chlorpromazine, or Thorazine. Thorazine made it possible for severely mentally ill patients to improve enough that they could leave asylums in unprecedented numbers. This and other antipsychotic medications finally allowed doctors to make progress in treating some of our most disabling illnesses.

The contemporary field of "biological psychiatry" was born in those years. This discipline, which studies the relationship between the human mind and its brain chemistry, was the child of these two strange bedfellows: LSD and Thorazine. And serotonin was the matchmaker.

In 1948 researchers discovered that serotonin carried in the bloodstream was responsible for contracting the muscles lining veins and arteries. This was vitally important in understanding how to control the bleeding process. The name for serotonin came from the Latin *sero*, "blood," and *tonin*, "tightening."

A few years later, in the mid-1950s, investigators discovered serotonin in the brain of laboratory animals. Subsequent experiments demonstrated its precise localization and its effects on electrical and chemical functions of individual nerve cells. Drugs or surgery that modified serotonin-containing areas of an animal's brain profoundly altered sexual and aggressive behavior as well as sleep, wakefulness, and a diverse array of basic biological functions. The presence and function of serotonin in the brain and in animal behavior clinched its role as the first known neurotransmitter.[2]

At the same time, scientists showed that LSD and serotonin molecules looked very much like each other. They then demonstrated that LSD and serotonin competed for many of the same brain sites. In some experimental situations, LSD blocked the effects of serotonin; in others, the psychedelic drug mimicked serotonin's effects.

These findings established LSD as the most powerful tool available for learning about brain-mind relationships. If LSD's extraordinary sensory and emotional properties resulted from changing the function of brain serotonin in specific and understandable ways, it might be possible to "chemically dissect" particular mental functions into their basic physiological components. Other mind-altering drugs with comparably well-characterized effects on different neurotransmitters could lead to a decoding of the varieties of conscious experience into their underlying chemical mechanisms.

Dozens of investigators around the world administered a dizzying array of psychedelic drugs to thousands of healthy volunteers and psychiatric patients. For more than two decades, generous government and private funding supported this effort. Researchers published hundreds of papers and dozens of books. Many international conferences, meetings, and symposia discussed the latest findings in human psychedelic drug research.[3]

Sandoz Laboratories distributed LSD to researchers so they might induce a brief psychotic state in normal volunteers. Scientists hoped such experiments might shed light on naturally occurring psychotic disorders like schizophrenia.

Sandoz also recommended giving LSD to psychiatric interns to help them establish a sense of empathy for their psychotic patients. These young doctors were amazed by this temporary encounter with insanity. The raw encounter with their own previously unconscious memories and feelings led these psychiatrists to believe that these mind-loosening properties might enhance psychotherapy.

Numerous research publications suggested that the normal mechanisms of talk therapy were much more effective with the addition of a psychedelic drug. Dozens of scientific articles described remarkable success in helping previously untreatable patients suffering from obsessions and compulsions, post-traumatic stress, eating disorders, anxiety, depression, alcoholism, and heroin dependence.

The rapid breakthroughs described by researchers using "psychedelic psychotherapy" spurred other investigators to study these drugs' beneficial effects in despairing and pain-ridden terminally ill patients. While there was little effect on the underlying medical conditions, psychedelic psychotherapy in these patients had striking psychological effects. Depression lifted, requirements for pain medication fell dramatically, and patients' acceptance of their disease and its prognosis improved markedly. In addition, patients and their families seemed able to address deep-seated and emotionally charged issues in ways never before possible. The rapid accleration of psychological growth resulting from this new treatment appeared quite promising in these cases where time was of the essence. Some therapists believed that a transformative, mystical, or spiritual experience was responsible for many of these "miraculous" responses to psychedelic psychotherapy.[4]

In addition, it soon became apparent that the experiences described by volunteers under deep psychedelic influences were strikingly similar to those of practitioners of traditional Eastern meditation. The overlap between consciousness alteration induced by psychedelic drugs and that induced by meditation attracted the attention of writers outside of academics, including the English novelist and religious philosopher Aldous Huxley. Huxley underwent his own remarkably positive mescaline and LSD experiences under the watchful eye of the Canadian psychiatrist Humphrey Osmond, who visited him in Los Angeles in the 1950s. Huxley soon wrote about his drug sessions and the musings they inspired in him. His writings on the nature and value of the psychedelic experience were compelling and eloquent, inspiring many individuals' attempts to attain, and researchers to elicit, spiritual enlightenment through psychedelic drugs. Despite that fact that his ideas stimulated a massive movement toward popular experimentation with the psychedelics, Huxley was a staunch advocate of the theory that only an elite group of intellectuals and artists should have access to them. He did not believe that the common man or woman was capable of using psychedelics in the safest and most productive ways possible.[5]

However, terminal illness studies and discussions of similarities between psychedelic drug effects and mystical experiences brought religion and science together in an uneasy mix. The research was moving further away from Sandoz's original agenda.

Complicating things further was LSD's escape from the laboratory in the 1960s. Reports of emergency room visits, suicides, murders, birth defects, and broken chromosomes filled the media. The highly publicized abandonment of scientific research principles by Timothy Leary, Ph.D., and his research team at Harvard University ultimately resulted in their dismissals. These events reinforced the growing suspicion that even the scientists had lost control of these powerful psychoactive drugs.[6]

The media exaggerated and emphasized psychedelic drugs' negative physical and psychological effects. Some of these reports resulted from poor research; others were simply fabricated. Subsequent publications cleared psychedelics from serious toxicity, including chromosome damage. However, these follow-up studies generated much less fanfare than did the original damaging reports.

Papers in the psychiatric literature describing "bad trips," or adverse psychological reactions to psychedelics, also multiplied, but are similarly limited. In order to address these concerns in my own study, I read every paper describing such negative effects and published the results. It was clear that rates of psychiatric complications were extraordinarily low in controlled research settings, for both normal volunteers and psychiatric patients. However, when psychiatrically ill or unstable individuals took impure or unknown psychedelics, combined with alcohol and other drugs, in an uncontrolled setting with inadequate supervision, problems occurred.[7]

In response to the public's anxiety about uncontrolled LSD use, and over the objections of nearly every investigator in the field, the United States Congress passed a law in 1970 making LSD and other psychedelics illegal. The government told scientists to return their drugs, paperwork requirements for obtaining and maintaining new supplies of psychedelics for research became a time-consuming and confusing burden, and there was little hope for new projects. Money for studies dried up and researchers abandoned their experiments. With the new drug laws in place, interest in human psychedelic research died off almost as rapidly as it had begun. It was as if the psychedelic drugs became "un-discovered."

Considering the intense pace of human research with psychedelics just thirty years ago, it is amazing how little today's medical and psychiatric training programs teach about them. Psychedelics were *the* growth area in psychiatry for over twenty years. Now young physicians and psychiatrists know nearly nothing about them.

By the time I was a medical student in the mid-1970s, less than ten years after the drug laws changed, psychedelics were the topic of just two lectures in my four years of study. Even this may have been more information than students received at most other medical schools, because there was a research group performing animal studies at the Albert Einstein College of Medicine in New York City, where I trained. In the mid-1990s,

I taught a psychedelic drug research seminar to senior psychiatric residents at the University of New Mexico—probably the only one of its kind in the country in decades.

The lack of academic attention to psychedelics may have been partly due to the absence of any ongoing human research. However, it is common for physicians-in-training to learn about previously popular theories and techniques, even if they no longer are in favor. The psychedelic drugs, however, seemed to have dropped out of all psychiatric dialogue.

Most new theories, techniques, and drugs in the clinical psychiatric field follow a predictable course of evolution as they are introduced, tested, and refined for further application. Therefore, it was not at all surprising that conflicting results began to emerge as more data accumulated during the first wave of human psychedelic research. Enthusiasm predictably slowed for claims that psychedelics could produce a "model psychosis" or "cures" in intractable psychotherapy cases. The natural process within psychiatric research is for scientists to refine research questions, methods, and applications. This never happened with the psychedelic drugs. Instead, their study went through a highly unnatural evolution. They began as "wonder drugs," turned into "horror drugs," then became nothing.

I believe that medical students and psychiatric trainees learn so little about psychedelic drugs not because research *did* end, but because of *how* it ended. This process deeply demoralized academic psychiatry, which then turned its back on psychedelic drugs.

Psychedelic research was a bruising and humiliating chapter in the lives of many of its most prominent scientists. These were the best and the brightest psychiatrists of their generation. Many of today's most respected North American and European psychiatric researchers, in both academics and industry, now chairmen of major university departments and presidents of national psychiatric organizations, began their professional lives investigating psychedelic drugs. The most powerful members of their profession discovered that science, data, and reason were incapable of defending their research against the enactment of repressive laws fueled by opinion, emotion, and the media.

Once these laws passed, government regulators and funding agencies quickly withdrew permits, drugs, and money. The same psychedelic drugs that researchers thought wcrc uniquc kcys to mental illncss, and that had launched dozens of careers, became feared and hated.

Another problem was that psychedelics were becoming an embarrassing source of contention even within psychiatry itself. Biology-based psychiatrists had little patience with colleagues who "found religion" and touted the spiritual effects of these drugs. These latter researchers viewed their brain-only associates as narrow-minded and repressed. Psychiatry has never been especially comfortable with spiritual issues, and in fact, an entirely new division appeared in the field to contend with results from psychedelic research: the "transpersonal" area of theory and practice. Thus, at least some psychedelic researchers may have been quietly relieved that they no longer had to face many of the complex, contradictory, and confusing effects these drugs produced in their patients, themselves, and their colleagues.

Why would anyone want to lecture on this embarrassing chapter in academic psychiatry to an auditorium packed with two hundred sharp-witted medical students? This early group of psychedelic researchers was for the most part professional scientists, not zealots. They knew enough not to publicly criticize the behavior of their colleagues and benefactors. Better to live and learn.[8]

Now that we have reviewed some important background of the psychedelics, let's look at what they do.

Psychedelics exert their effects by a complex blending of three factors: *set, setting,* and *drug.*

Set is our own makeup, both long term and immediate. It is our past, our present, and our potential future; our preferences, ideas, habits, and feelings. Set also includes our body and brain.

The psychedelic experience also hinges on *setting:* who or what is or isn't in our immediate surroundings; the environment we're in, whether natural or urban, indoor or outdoor; the quality of the air and ambient sound around us; and so on. Setting also partakes of the *set* of who is with us while we take the drug, whether they be a friend or a stranger, relaxed or tense, a supportive guide or a probing scientist.

Then, there is the *drug.*

First, what do we call it? Even among researchers there is little agreement over this crucial point. Some don't even use the word *drug*, preferring instead *molecule, compound, agent, substance, medicine,* or *sacrament.*

Even if we agree to call it a drug, look at how many different names it has: *hallucinogen* (producing hallucinations), *entheogen* (generating the divine), *mysticomimetic* (mimicking mystical states), *oneirogen* (producing dreams), *phanerothyme* (producing visible feelings), *phantasticant* (stimulating fantasy), *psychodysleptic* (mind-disturbing), *psychotomimetic* and *psychotogen* (mimicking or producing psychosis, respectively), and *psychotoxin* and *schizotoxin* (a poison causing psychosis or schizophrenia, respectively).

This focus on name is not trivial. If everyone agreed about what a psychedelic is or does, there certainly would not be so many words for the same drug. The multitude of labels reflects the deep-seated and ongoing debate about psychedelic drugs and their effects.

Scientists rarely acknowledge the importance of the name they give to psychedelics, even though they know how powerfully expectations modify drug effects. All undergraduate psychology students learn this in their introductory psychology courses when they review landmark studies published in the 1960s. These experiments injected volunteers with adrenaline, the "fight-or-flight" hormone, under different sets of expectations. Adrenaline caused a calm and relaxed state in volunteers told they were receiving a sedative. If told that the experimental drug was stimulating, volunteers felt the more typical anxiety and energy.[9]

Thus, what we call a drug we take, or give, influences our expectations of what that drug will do. It also modifies the effects themselves, and how we interpret and deal with them. No other drug's name feeds back so powerfully upon the responses they elicit as do the psychedelics, because they greatly magnify our suggestibility.

In addition to what we call psychedelics, the terms we apply to the people involved in their use also impact set and setting, and therefore drug response. As one who takes the drug, are we *research subjects* or *volunteers*? *Clients* or *celebrants*? As the one giving them, are we *guides, sitters,* or *research investigators*? *Shamans* or *scientists*?

Try this mental exercise: Consider how you might look forward to your day as a "research subject" under the influence of a "psychotomimetic agent." Then reconsider: How would you feel about your role as a "celebrant" in a "ceremony" involving an "entheogenic sacrament"? How would these different contexts affect your interpretation of the hallucinations and intense mood swings brought on by the drug? Would you be "going crazy" or having an "enlightenment experience"?

If you were administering psychedelics, what types of behavior would you anticipate in your research subject, and what sorts would you ignore? Much would depend upon whether you were giving a "schizotoxin" or a "phantasticant." You might encourage an "out-of-body experience" in a "shamanic" context, but abort the same effects by giving an antipsychotic antidote in a "psychotomimetic" one.[10]

Hallucinogen is the most common medical term for psychedelic drugs, and it emphasizes the perceptual, mostly visual effects of these drugs. However, while perceptual effects of psychedelics are usual, they are not the only effects, nor are they necessarily the most valued. The visions actually may be distractions from the more sought-after properties of the experience, such as intense euphoria, profound intellectual or spiritual insights, and the dissolving of the body's physical boundaries.

I prefer the term *psychedelic*, or mind-manifesting, over *hallucinogen*. Psychedelics show you what's in and on your mind, those subconscious thoughts and feelings that are are hidden, covered up, forgotten, out of sight, maybe even completely unexpected, but nevertheless imminently present. Depending upon set and setting, the same drug, at the same dose, can cause vastly different responses in the same person. One day, very little happens; another day, you soar, full of ecstatic and insightful discoveries; the next, you struggle through a terrifying nightmare. The generic nature of *psychedelic*, a term wide open to interpretation, suits these effects.

Psychedelic has taken on its own cultural and linguistic life. It now can refer to a particular style of art, clothing, or even an especially intense set of circumstances. When it comes to rational discourse about drugs, *psychedelic* also stirs up powerful 1960s-based emotions and conflicts over unrelated political and sociological issues. Many of us now think "counterculture," "rebellious," "liberal," or "left-wing" when we see the term "psychedelic." I will take my chances, however, and use it throughout this book. I think it is the best term we have. I hope not to offend anyone who finds the word objectionable.

No matter what we call them, most of us agree that the psychedelic drugs are physical, chemical things. It is at this most basic level that we can begin to understand what they are and what they do.

The diagrams accompanying the following descriptions show the chemical structure of various psychedelic compounds. The balls represent atoms, the most common of which is carbon, which is not labeled. "N" signifies nitrogen; "P," phosphorous; and "O," oxygen. Numerous hydrogen atoms are attached to other atoms in the molecules; however, there are so many that they would unnecessarily clutter up the diagram, so I have not included them here.

There are two main chemical families of psychedelic drugs: the phenethylamines and the tryptamines.[11]

The phenethylamines build upon the "parent compound" phenethylamine.

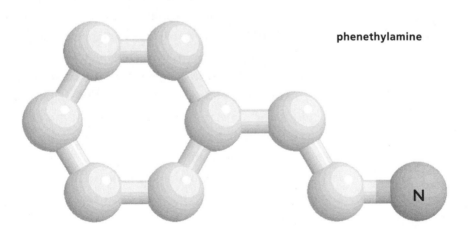

phenethylamine

The best-known phenethylamine is mescaline, which is derived from the peyote cactus of the American Southwest.

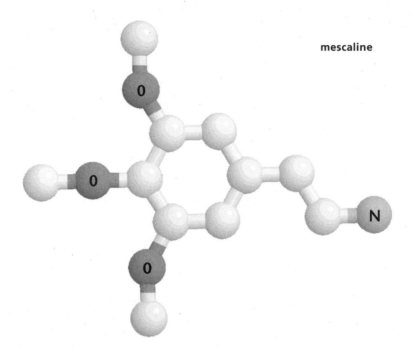

mescaline

Another famous phenethylamine is MDMA, or "Ecstasy."

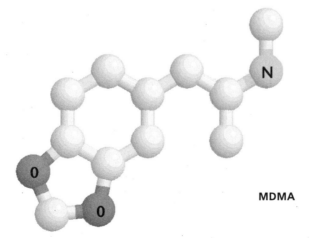

MDMA

The other main chemical family of psychedelic drugs is the tryptamines. These all possess a nucleus, or basic building block, of tryptamine. Tryptamine is a derivative of tryptophan, an amino acid present in our diet.

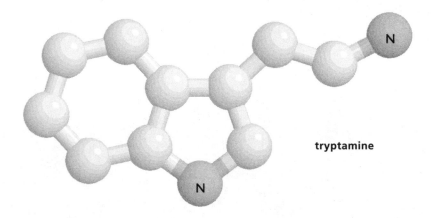

tryptamine

Serotonin is a tryptamine—5-hydroxy-tryptamine, to be exact—but it is not psychedelic. It contains one more oxygen atom than does tryptamine.

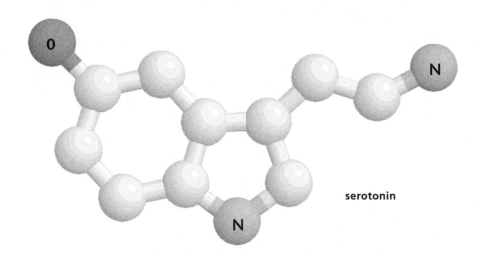

serotonin

DMT is also a tryptamine and is the simplest psychedelic. Simply add two methyl groups to the tryptamine molecule and the result is "di-methyl-tryptamine": DMT.[12]

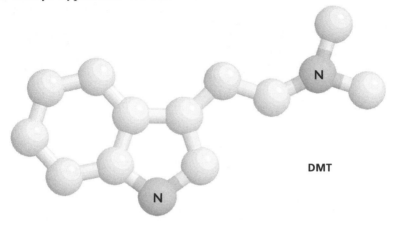

DMT

The "grandfather" of all modern psychedelics, LSD, contains a tryptamine core, as does ibogaine, the African psychedelic with highly publicized anti-addictive properties.

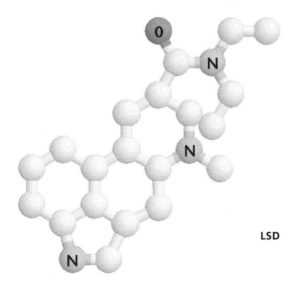

LSD

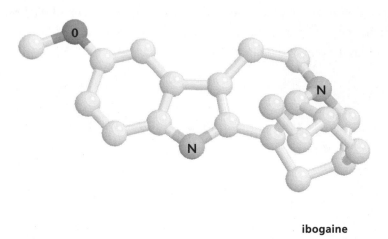

ibogaine

One of the best-known tryptamine psychedelics is psilocybin, the active ingredient of "magic mushrooms."

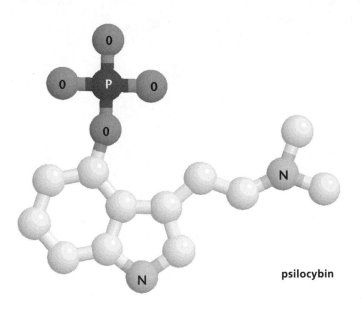

psilocybin

When these mushrooms are ingested, the body removes a phosphorous atom from the psilocybin, converting it to psilocin.

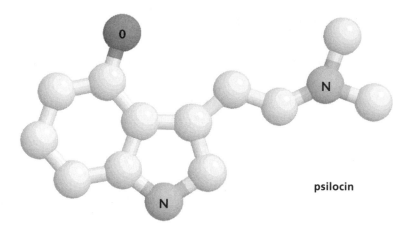

psilocin

Psilocin differs from DMT by only one oxygen. I like to think of psilocybin/psilocin as "orally active DMT."

Another important tryptamine is 5-methoxy-DMT, or 5-MeO-DMT. It differs from DMT by the addition of only one methyl group and one oxygen.

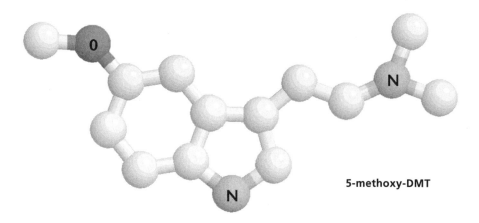

5-methoxy-DMT

Many of the plants, fungi, and animals containing DMT also possess 5-MeO-DMT. As with DMT, those who use 5-MeO-DMT usually smoke it.[13]

In addition to their chemical *structure*, psychedelics also possess *activity*. This is where chemistry becomes *pharmacology*, the study of drug action.

One way to describe psychedelics' activity is by how quickly they work and how long they last.

DMT and 5-MeO-DMT effects are remarkably rapid in onset and brief in duration. We gave DMT through a vein, or intravenously, in which case volunteers felt it within several heartbeats. They were "highest" at 1 to 2 minutes and were "back to normal" within 20 to 30 minutes.

LSD, mescaline, and ibogaine are longer-acting. Effects begin 30 to 60 minutes after swallowing them. The effects of LSD and mescaline may last 12 hours, ibogaine up to 24 hours. Psilocybin effects are slightly shorter; they begin within 30 minutes and last 4 to 6 hours.

Another more basic aspect of pharmacology is "mechanism of action," or how drugs affect brain activity. This is a crucial issue, because it is by altering brain function that psychedelics change consciousness.

The earliest psychopharmacological experiments in humans and animals suggested that LSD, mescaline, DMT, and other psychedelic drugs exerted their primary effects on the brain's serotonin system. Animal research, in contrast to human studies, has continued over the last thirty years and has established conclusively this neurotransmitter's crucial role.

Serotonin has reigned as the royal neurotransmitter for decades, and there's little sign of change. The new, safer, and more effective antipsychotic medications all have unique effects on serotonin. The new generation of antidepressants, of which Prozac is the most famous, also specifically modify the function of this neurotransmitter.

We now believe that psychedelics mimic the effects of serotonin in some cases and block them in others. Researchers are now concerned with determining which of the twenty or so different types of serotonin receptors psychedelics attach to. These multiple docking sites for serotonin exist in high concentrations on nerve cells in brain areas regulating a host of important psychological and physical processes: cardiovascular, hormone, and temperature regulation, as well as sleep, feeding, mood, perception, and motor control.

Now that we've looked at what psychedelics "are" and "do" in the worlds of objective and measurable data, let's turn our attention how they *feel* to us, for it is only in the mind that we notice their effects.

It is important to remember that while we understand a great deal about the pharmacology of psychedelics, we know nearly nothing about how changes in brain chemistry *directly* relate to subjective, or inner, experience. This is as true for psychedelics as it is for Prozac. That is, we are far from comprehending how activating particular serotonin receptors translates into a new thought or emotion. We don't "feel" a serotonin receptor blockade; rather, we feel ecstasy. We don't "see" frontal lobe activation; instead, we observe angels or demons.

It is impossible to predict accurately what will happen after taking a psychedelic drug on any particular day. Nevertheless, we will generalize about their subjective effects because we must gain a sense of a "typical" response. We can do this by averaging all of our own and others' experiences, all of the "trips" that have gone before us. (By "trip" I mean the full effects of a typical psychedelic drug like LSD, mescaline, psilocybin, or DMT. A trip is difficult to define, but we certainly know when we are having one!)

The following descriptions do not apply to "mild" psychedelics such as MDMA or usual-strength marijuana, nor do they describe responses to low doses of psychedelics, for which effects are similar to those of other non-psychedelic drugs, like amphetamine.

Psychedelics affect all of our mental functions: perception, emotion, thinking, body awareness, and our sense of self.

Perceptual or sensory effects often, but not always, are primary. Objects in our field of vision appear brighter or duller, larger or smaller, and seem to be shifting shape and melting. Eyes closed or open, we see things that have little to do with the outside world: swirling, colorful, geometric cloud patterns, or well-formed images of both animate and inanimate objects, in various conditions of motion or activity.

Sounds are softer or louder, harsher or gentler. We hear new rhythms in the wind. Singing or mechanical sounds appear in a previously silent environment.

The skin is more or less sensitive to touch. Our ability to taste and smell becomes more or less acute.

Our emotions overflow or dry up. Anxiety or fear, pleasure or relaxation, all feelings wax and wane, overpoweringly intense or frustratingly absent. At the extremes lie terror or ecstasy. Two opposite feelings may exist together at the same time. Emotional conflicts become more painful, or a new emotional acceptance takes place. We have a new appreciation of how others feel, or no longer care about them at all.

Our thinking processes speed up or slow down. Thoughts themselves become confused or clearer. We notice the absence of thoughts, or it is impossible to contain the flood of new ideas. Fresh insights about problems come, or we become hopelessly stuck in a mental rut. The significance of things takes on more importance than the things themselves. Time collapses: in the blink of an eye, two hours pass. Or time expands: a minute contains a never-ending march of sensations and ideas.

Our bodies are hot or cold, heavy or light; our limbs grow or shrink; we move upward or downward through space. We feel the body no longer exists, or that the mind and body have separated.

We feel more or less in control of our "selves." We experience others influencing our minds or bodies—in ways that are beneficial or frightening. The future is ours for the taking, or fate has determined everything and there is no point in trying.

Psychedelics affect every aspect of our consciousness. It is this unique consciousness that separates our species from all others below, and that gives us access to what we consider the divine above. Maybe that's another reason why the psychedelics are so frightening and so inspiring: They bend and stretch the basic pillars, the structure and defining characteristics, of our human identity.

These are the psychedelic drugs. There exists a complex and rich context for viewing them, a perspective that few appreciate. They are not new substances, and we know an enormous amount about them. They ushered in the modern era of biological psychiatry, and their highly publicized abuse prematurely ended an extraordinarily rich human research endeavor.

It was into this seething matrix of conflict, ambivalence, and controversy that I looked for a point of traction and a clear line of sight in order to formulate my own research agenda. Where could I get a toehold? In which direction should I look? I needed a key with which to open the lock keeping psychedelic research buried.

Out of this virtual swamp emerged one small obscure molecule: DMT. Its call was one I could not ignore, even though I had little idea of how I might get to it. Nor could I possibly expect where it would lead me once I found it.

2

What DMT Is

N, N-dimethyltryptamine, or DMT, is the remarkable main character of this book. While chemically simple, this "spirit" molecule provides our consciousness access to the most amazing and unexpected visions, thoughts, and feelings. It throws open the door to worlds beyond our imagination.

DMT exists in all of our bodies and occurs throughout the plant and animal kingdoms. It is a part of the normal makeup of humans and other mammals; marine animals; grasses and peas; toads and frogs; mushrooms and molds; and barks, flowers, and roots.

Psychedelic alchemist Alexander Shulgin devotes an entire chapter to DMT in *TIHKAL: Tryptamines I Have Known and Loved.* He aptly entitles this chapter "DMT Is Everywhere" and declares: "DMT is . . . in this flower here, in that tree over there, and in yonder animal. [It] is, most simply, almost everywhere you choose to look." Indeed, it is getting to the point where one should report where DMT is *not* found, rather than where it *is*.[1]

DMT is most abundant in plants of Latin America. There, humans have known of its amazing properties for some tens of thousands of years. However, it is only in the last 150 years that we have gained some inkling of the antiquity of DMT's relationship with our species.

Beginning in the mid-1800s, explorers of the Amazon, particularly Richard Spruce from England and Alexander von Humboldt from Germany, described the effects of exotic mind-altering snuffs and brews prepared from plants by indigenous tribes. In the twentieth century, the American botanist Richard Schultes continued this dangerous yet exciting line of fieldwork. Especially striking were the effects of, and the manner of administering, the psychoactive snuffs.

Latin American indigenous tribes continue to use these snuffs and have given them many names, including *yopo, epena,* and *jurema.* They take huge doses, sometimes an ounce or more. One dramatic technique is for one's snuffing partner to blow the powdery mixtures with considerable force through a tube or pipe into the other's nose. The energy of the blast may be sufficient to drop the recipient to the ground.

Spruce and von Humboldt reported that natives were immediately incapacitated by these psychedelic snuffs. Neither, however, went so far as to see for themselves what they were like. It was enough to watch the intoxicated Indians, twitching, vomiting, and babbling incoherently. These early explorers heard tales of fantastic visions, "out-of-body travel," predictions of the future, location of lost objects, and contact with dead ancestors or other disembodied entities.

Another plant mixture, this one consumed as a beverage, seemed to produce similar effects at a slower pace. This brew also went by several names, including *ayahuasca* and *yagé.* This drink inspired much rock art and paintings drawn on the walls of native shelters—what would be called "psychedelic" art today.

Spruce and von Humboldt brought samples of these New World psychedelic plants back home to Europe. There the plants lay undisturbed for decades, as neither the interest nor the technology existed for further analysis of their chemical makeup or effects.

While psychedelic plants languished in natural history museum archives, Canadian chemist R. Manske, in unrelated research, synthesized a new drug called N,N-dimethyltryptamine, or DMT. As he described in a 1931 scientific article, Manske had made several compounds derived by chemically modifying tryptamine. He was interested in these products because they occurred in a toxic North American plant, the strawberry shrub. DMT was one of these.[2]

As far as anyone knows, Manske made DMT, noted its structure, and then placed his supply in some isolated corner of his laboratory, where it quietly collected dust. No one yet knew about DMT's existence in mind-altering plants, its psychedelic properties, or its presence in the human body. There was little interest in psychedelics in scientific circles until decades later, after World War II.

In the early 1950s, the discoveries of LSD and serotonin rocked the staid foundations of Freudian psychiatry and laid the groundwork for the new world of neuroscience. Curiosity about psychedelic drugs was intense among the growing circle of scientists who called themselves "psychopharmacologists." Chemists began probing the barks, leaves, and seeds of plants first described as psychedelic a hundred years earlier, seeking their active ingredients. The tryptamine family was a logical place to focus, as both serotonin and LSD are tryptamines.

Success was not long in coming. In 1946, O. Gonçalves isolated DMT from a South American tree used for psychedelic snuffs and published his findings in Spanish. In 1955, M. S. Fish, N. M. Johnson, and E. C. Horning published the first English-language paper describing DMT's presence in another closely related snuff-producing tree. However, although they knew that DMT was a constituent of plants that produced psychedelic effects, scientists didn't know if DMT itself was psychoactive.[3]

In the 1950s, Hungarian chemist and psychiatrist Stephen Szára read about the profoundly mind-altering effects of LSD and mescaline. He ordered some LSD from Sandoz Laboratories so he could begin his own studies into the chemistry of consciousness. Since Szára was behind the Iron Curtain, the Swiss drug company was unwilling to risk letting their powerful LSD falling into Communist hands, and they turned down his request. Undaunted, he looked up recent papers describing DMT's presence in psychedelic Amazonian snuffs. He then synthesized some DMT in his Budapest laboratory in 1955.

Szára swallowed ever-increasing doses of DMT, but felt nothing. He tried taking up to one full gram, hundreds of thousands of times more than an active dose of LSD. He wondered whether something in his gastrointestinal system was preventing oral DMT from working. Maybe it needed to be injected. His hunch predated the later discovery that there is a mechanism in the gut that breaks down oral DMT as quickly as it is swallowed—a mechanism South American natives found a way to bypass thousands of years ago.

In the spirit of "who goes first," Szára gave himself an intramuscular, or IM, injection of DMT in 1956. In this case, he used about half of what we now know to be a "full" dose:

In three or four minutes I started to experience visual sensations that were very similar to what I had read in descriptions by Hofmann [about LSD] and Huxley [about mescaline]. . . . I got very, very excited. It was obvious this was the secret.[4]

After later doubling the dose, he had this to say:

[Physical] symptoms appeared, such as a tingling sensation, trembling, slight nausea, [widening of the pupils], elevation of the blood pressure and increase of the pulse rate. At the same time, eidetic phenomena [after-images or "trails" of visually perceived objects], optical illusions, pseudo-hallucinations, and later real hallucinations appeared. The hallucinations consisted of moving, brilliantly colored oriental motifs, and later I saw wonderful scenes altering very rapidly. The faces of the people seemed to be masks. My emotional state was elevated sometimes up to euphoria. My consciousness was completely filled by hallucinations, and my attention was firmly bound to them; therefore I could not give an account of the events happening around me. After 45 minutes to 1 hour the symptoms disappeared, and I was able to describe what had happened.[5]

Szára quickly recruited thirty volunteers, mostly young Hungarian physician colleagues. They all received full psychedelic doses.[6]

One male physician reported:

The whole world is brilliant. . . . The whole room is filled with spirits. It makes me dizzy. . . . Now it is too much! . . . I feel exactly as if I were flying. . . . I have the feeling that this is above everything, above the earth.

It is comforting to know I am back on earth again. . . . Everything has a spiritual tinge but is so real. . . . I feel that I have landed. . . .

A female physician stated:

How simple everything is. . . . In front of me are two quiet, sunlit Gods. . . . I think they are welcoming me into this new world. There is a deep silence as in the desert. . . . I am finally at home. . . . Dangerous game; it would be so easy not to return. I am faintly aware that I am a doctor, but this is not important; family ties, studies, plans, and memories are very remote from me. Only this world is important; I am free and utterly alone.

The Western world had discovered DMT, and DMT had entered into its consciousness.

Despite the occasional bad trip among his volunteers, Szára liked the short-acting DMT. It was relatively easy to use, fully psychedelic, and experiments could be done in just a few hours. After escaping Hungary with his DMT supply in the late 1950s, he met a Berlin colleague who enrolled him in an LSD study. Finally Szára could try this fabled psychedelic. While he found the effects interesting, its twelve-hour duration was too long for his liking.

Upon emigrating to the United States, Szára's primary research interest continued to be DMT. It served him well in his new job at the National Institutes of Health in Bethesda, Maryland, where he worked for over three decades. He served as the Director of Preclinical Research at the National Institute on Drug Abuse for many years before retiring in 1991.

Other groups confirmed and expanded Szára's discovery that DMT must be injected to work. However, it is surprising how little detailed information researchers other than Szára gave regarding its psychological properties.

For example, after Szára left Hungary, his former laboratory reported only that DMT in normal volunteers caused "a [psychotic] state . . . dominated by colored hallucinations, loss of time and space reality, euphoria, some delusional experiences and sometimes by anxiety and clouding of consciousness."[7]

One of the busiest American centers for human psychedelic research was the Public Health Service Hospital in Lexington, Kentucky. There, men serving prison sentences for narcotic law violations received dozens of mind-altering drugs, hoping their research participation might lead to more favorable treatment. However, all we read about the effects of DMT in these studies is that "the mental effects consisted of anxiety, hallucinations (usually visual) and perceptual distortions."[8]

Even less revealing were studies at the U.S. National Institute of Mental Health. Here, a group of research subjects with experience using psychedelics needed only to provide a number indicating "how high" they were on a full dose of DMT. The authors do comment, however, that most of these seasoned volunteers were "higher than they had ever been."[9]

The "psychedelic subculture" discovered DMT soon after the research community did, but the earliest reports of its effects earned it the title of a "terror drug." William Burroughs, author of *The Naked Lunch,* was one of the earliest field users of DMT. Burroughs's and his British colleagues' encounters with it were unpleasant. Leary relates Burroughs's tale of a psychiatrist and his friend who injected DMT together in a London apartment. The friend began panicking and, to the psychiatrist, appeared to transform into a "writhing, wiggling reptile." "The doctor's dilemma: where to make an intravenous injection [of an antidote] in a squirming, oriental-martian snake?"[10] This is as good an example of the power of a negative set and setting as there is: two people high on injected DMT in a seedy flat at the same time, one being responsible for the other. "Terror" drug, indeed.

It was difficult for DMT to shake its frightening reputation, even after Leary's later positive descriptions of its effects. DMT did see some popularity among those who appreciated its short duration. Some bold individuals thought it possible to take DMT during lunch, and so it gained the dubious nickname, "businessman's trip."[11]

Despite Szára's and others' steady production of research papers about DMT, it remained mostly a pharmacological curiosity: intense, short-lived, and found in plants. Clearly, LSD had a leg up on DMT when it came to making a significant impression on the psychiatric research community. This all changed, however, when researchers discovered DMT in the brains of mice and rats, and then uncovered the pathways by which these animals' bodies made this powerful psychedelic.

Did DMT exist in the *human* body? It seemed likely, because scientists had discovered DMT-forming enzymes in samples of human lung tissue while searching for those same enzymes in other animals.

The race was on. In 1965 a research team from Germany published a paper in the flagship British science journal *Nature* announcing that they had isolated DMT from human blood. In 1972 Nobel-prize winning scientist Julius Axelrod of the U.S. National Institutes of Health reported finding it in human brain tissue. Additional research showed that DMT could also be found in human urine and the cerebrospinal fluid bathing the brain. It was not long before scientists discovered the pathways, similar to those in lower animals, by which the human body made DMT. DMT thus became the first *endogenous* human psychedelic.[12]

Endogenous means that a compound is made in the body: *endo*, "within," and *genous*, "generated" or "formed." Endogenous DMT, then, is DMT made within the body. There are other endogenous compounds with which we've become familiar over the years. For example, *endo*genous mo*rphine*-like compounds are *endorphins*.

However, the discovery of DMT in the human body stimulated much less fanfare than did that of endorphins. As we will see later in this chapter, anti-psychedelic-drug sentiment sweeping the country at the time actually turned researchers *against* studying endogenous DMT. The discoverers of endorphins, in contrast, won Nobel Prizes.

The crucial question then naturally arose: "What is DMT doing in our bodies?"

Psychiatry's answer was: "Perhaps it causes mental illness."

This reply was reasonable, considering psychiatry's mandate to understand and treat serious psychopathology. However, it fell short of all the other possible scientifically meritorious answers. By limiting themselves to investigating DMT's role in psychosis, scientists lost a unique opportunity to probe deeper into the mysteries of consciousness.

Scientists believed that LSD and other "psychotomimetics" induced a short-term "model psychosis" in normal volunteers. They thought that by finding an "endogenous psychotomimetic," the cause of, and potential cures for, serious mental illnesses might be at hand. DMT, as the first known endogenous psychotomimetic, suggested the search might be over. For example, one could give DMT to normal volunteers to induce psychosis, and eventually develop new medications to block its effects in them. Subsequently, psychiatric patients would receive this "anti-DMT." If excessive naturally produced DMT was causing the patient's psychosis, this anti-DMT would have antipsychotic effects.

These DMT investigations just were getting up to speed when, in 1970, Congress passed the law placing it and other psychedelics into a highly restricted legal category. It became nearly impossible to conduct any new human DMT research. Soon after, in 1976, a paper published by scientists at the U.S. National Institute of Mental Health, or NIMH, tolled the death knell for human DMT studies. The authors were topflight researchers, several of whom had given DMT to humans. They correctly concluded that the evidence relating DMT to schizophrenia was complex and uncertain. However, rather than suggesting more refined and careful research into the areas of disagreement, the authors concluded:

> Like any good scientific theory, the DMT model of schizophrenia will ultimately live or die by the data that it heuristically generates. We hope that, within the foreseeable future, forthcoming data will give this theory either a new lease on life or a decent burial.[13]

This "decent burial" came soon enough. Within a year or two, the last paper on human DMT research appeared. Few scientists shed tears to mark its passing.

Was DMT buried alive by those whose careers and reputations were endangered by a controversial area of research? The DMT-psychosis field was no different from any other biological psychiatry research endeavor investigating complex and uncertain relationships between the mind and brain. Encouraging its abandonment appears to have been as much politically as scientifically motivated.

In general, there were two types of studies investigating the DMT-psychosis theory. One compared blood levels of DMT between ill patients and normal volunteers. The other study design compared the subjective effects of psychedelic drugs to those of naturally occurring psychotic states. The NIMH team that discounted the theory of a DMT-psychosis relationship, leading to the demise of human DMT research, critiqued both approaches. They pointed to the lack of consistent differences between blood levels of DMT in normal volunteers and psychotic patients; they also rejected claims that the effects of DMT and symptoms of schizophrenia demonstrated enough similarities to justify additional research.

First, let's discuss the blood level data. Essentially all DMT studies measured its concentration in blood drawn from forearm veins. However, it seems unreasonable to expect these levels to accurately reflect DMT's function in extraordinarily small, highly specialized, distinct brain areas. Finding a close relationship between blood levels and brain effects would be even less likely if the DMT originated in the brain in the first place.

This difficulty is one that all scientists recognize, even for such well-known brain chemicals as serotonin. Dozens of studies have failed to convincingly relate serotonin levels in blood drawn from the forearm to psychiatric diagnoses with presumed abnormalities in brain serotonin. Therefore, it was unlikely, using DMT blood levels, that any real conclusions could be drawn regarding differences between normal and psychotic individuals. If psychiatric researchers demand such data for all brain chemicals, where is the call to bury serotonin?

In the case of comparing schizophrenia to DMT intoxication, the case becomes even murkier. Schizophrenia is a remarkably complex syndrome. There are several forms, such as "paranoid," "disorganized," and "undifferentiated." There are many stages, including "early," "acute," "late," and "chronic." There are even "prodromal" symptoms that exist before the illness becomes severe enough to diagnose. In addition, symptoms of schizophrenia develop over months and years, and individuals modify their behavior to deal with their unusual experiences. These adaptations in turn create new symptoms and behaviors.

To expect a single drug given one time to a normal person to mimic schizophrenia is not reasonable. No one today contends that this is possible. Rather, the consensus even then was that the syndromes of psychedelic drug intoxication and schizophrenia possessed significant overlap. Hallucinations and other sensory distortions, altered thought processes, extreme and rapid shifts in mood, disturbances in the sense of bodily and personal identity—all these may occur in *some* cases of schizophrenia and psychedelic states.

In psychiatry, there are always both similarities and differences between the diseases we seek to understand and the models we use to study them. We are always in search of better models, but we use the ones we have, keeping in mind their shortcomings. The NIMH group's rejection of DMT effects as producing a "valid" psychotic state was not consistent with accepted psychiatric research theory, practice, or the data.[14]

If the scientific basis for discontinuing human DMT research was so meager, why, then, was it stopped? What was the meaning behind the "life and death," "lease on life," and "decent burial" rhetoric? The data begged for further clarification. Instead, these federal scientists distanced themselves from an extraordinarily promising field and encouraged others to do the same.

DMT was in the wrong place at the wrong time. Rational research into its function was swept aside by the anti-psychedelic furor that accompanied these drugs' uncontrolled use and abuse. This move to limit access to psychedelic drugs in order to respond to widespread public health fears affected DMT research in the same way it did research into LSD and other psychedelics. Political concerns overwhelmed scientific principles.[15]

Stuck in the quicksand of trying to prove its role in schizophrenia, and trampled underfoot in the stampede of anti-psychedelic sentiments, no one studying DMT dared continue asking the most obvious and pressing question, which the first round of human research had failed to address. It was a riddle I could not ignore:

"What is DMT doing in our bodies?"

DMT is the simplest of the tryptamine psychedelics. Compared to other molecules, DMT is rather small. Its weight is 188 "molecular units," meaning that it is not significantly larger than glucose, the simplest sugar in our bodies, which weighs 180, and only ten times heavier than a water molecule, which weighs 18. By comparison, consider the weight of LSD at 323, or of mescaline at 211.[16]

DMT is closely related to serotonin, the neurotransmitter that psychedelics affect so widely. The pharmacology of DMT is similar to that of other well-known psychedelics. It affects receptor sites for serotonin in much the same way that LSD, psilocybin, and mescaline do. These serotonin receptors are widespread throughout the body and can be found in blood vessels, muscle, glands, and skin.

However, the brain is where DMT exerts its most interesting effects. There, sites rich in these DMT-sensitive serotonin receptors are involved in mood, perception, and thought. Although the brain denies access to most drugs and chemicals, it takes a particular and remarkable fancy to DMT. It is not stretching the truth to suggest that the brain "hungers" for it.

The brain is a highly sensitive organ, especially susceptible to toxins and metabolic imbalances. A nearly impenetrable shield, the blood-brain barrier, prevents unwelcome agents from leaving the blood and crossing the capillary walls into the brain tissue. This defense extends even to keeping out the complex carbohydrates and fats that other tissues use for energy. The brain burns instead only the purest form of fuel: simple sugar, or glucose.

However, a few essential molecules undergo "active transport" across the blood-brain barrier. Little specialized carrier molecules ferry them into the brain, a process that requires a significant amount of precious energy. In most cases, it is obvious why the brain actively transports particular compounds into its hallowed ground; amino acids required for maintaining brain proteins, for example, are allowed in.

Twenty-five years ago, Japanese scientists discovered that the brain actively transports DMT across the blood-brain barrier into its tissues. I know of no other psychedelic drug that the brain treats with such eagerness. This is a startling fact that we should keep in mind when we recall how readily biological psychiatrists dismissed a vital role for DMT in our lives. If DMT were only an insignificant, irrelevant by-product of our metabolism, why does the brain go out of its way to draw it into its confines?[17]

Once the body produces or takes in DMT, certain enzymes break it down within seconds. These enzymes, called monoamine oxidases (MAO), occur in high concentrations in the blood, liver, stomach, brain, and intestines. The widespread presence of MAO is why DMT effects are so short-lived. Whenever and wherever it appears, the body makes sure it is used up quickly.[18]

In a way, DMT is "brain food," treated in a manner similar to how the brain handles glucose, its precious fuel source. It is part of a "high turnover" system: quick in, quick used. The brain actively transports DMT across its defense system and just as rapidly breaks it down. It is as if DMT is necessary for maintaining normal brain function. It is only when levels get too high for "normal" function that we start undergoing unusual experiences.

Now that we have reviewed the history and science behind DMT, let's return to the most pressing question, one that no one has adequately answered: "What is DMT doing in our bodies?" More specifically, let's ask, "Why do we make DMT in our bodies?"

My answer is: *"Because it is the spirit molecule."*

What, then, is a spirit molecule? What must it do, and how might it do it? Why is DMT the prime candidate?

Visionary artist Alex Grey has sketched an inspiring rendition of the DMT molecule. Alex's art helped me begin thinking about these questions much more clearly. Let's look at it carefully and consider how it reflects the necessary properties of such a chemical.

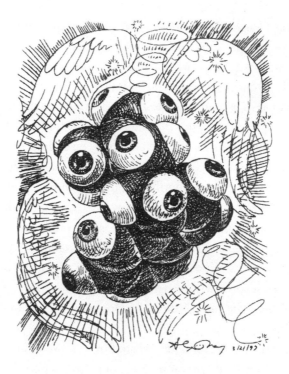

A spirit molecule needs to elicit, with reasonable reliability, certain psychological states we consider "spiritual." These are feelings of extraordinary joy, timelessness, and a certainty that what we are experiencing is "more real than real." Such a substance may lead us to an acceptance of the coexistence of opposites, such as life and death, good and evil; a knowledge that consciousness continues after death; a deep understanding of the basic unity of all phenomena; and a sense of wisdom or love pervading all existence.

A spirit molecule also leads us to spiritual realms. These worlds usually are invisible to us and our instruments and are not accessible using our normal state of consciousness. However, just as likely as the theory that these worlds exist "only in our minds" is that they are, in reality, "outside" of us and freestanding. If we simply change our brain's receiving abilities, we can apprehend and interact with them.

Furthermore, keep in mind that a spirit molecule is not spiritual in and of itself. It is a tool, or a vehicle. Think of it as a tugboat, a chariot, a scout on horseback, something to which we can hitch our consciousness. It pulls us into worlds known only to itself. We need to hold on tight, and we must be prepared, for spiritual realms include both heaven and hell, both fantasy and nightmare. While the spirit molecule's role may seem angelic, there is no guarantee it will not take us to the demonic.

Why is DMT so attractive a candidate for being the spirit molecule?

Its effects are extraordinarily and fully psychedelic. We have read some of the earliest reports of these properties from unprepared and unsuspecting research subjects who participated in the first clinical studies in the 1950s and 1960s. We will read much more about how truly mind-boggling are DMT's effects in our own very experienced and well-prepared volunteers.

Equally important is that DMT occurs in our bodies. We produce it naturally. Our brain seeks it out, pulls it in, and readily digests it. As an endogenous psychedelic, DMT may be involved in naturally occurring psychedelic states that have nothing to do with taking drugs, but whose similarities to drug-induced conditions are striking. While these states certainly can include psychosis, we must also include in our discussion conditions outside of mental illness. It may be upon endogenous DMT's wings that we experience other life-changing states of mind associated with birth, death, and near-death, entity or alien contact experiences, and mystical/spiritual consciousness. These we will explore in much greater detail later.

In this chapter, we've learned the "what" about DMT. We now need to turn our attention to the "how" and "where." We have prepared the groundwork into which we may now introduce the mysterious pineal gland. In its role as a potential "spirit gland," or producer of endogenous DMT, the pineal is the topic of our next two chapters. We'll also start investigating the circumstances under which our bodies might make psychedelic amounts of DMT.

The Pineal:
Meet the Spirit Gland

One of my deepest motivations behind the DMT research was the search for a biological basis of spiritual experience. Much of what I had learned over the years made me wonder if the pineal gland produced DMT during mystical states and other naturally occurring, psychedelic-like experiences. These are ideas I developed before performing the New Mexico research. In chapter 21, I enlarge these hypotheses to incorporate what we discovered during the experiments themselves.

In this chapter I will review what we know about the pineal gland. In the next, I will elaborate upon these data to suggest conditions in which the pineal, in its role as a possible spirit gland, might make mind-altering amounts of endogenous DMT.

As a Stanford University undergraduate in the early 1970s I performed laboratory research on the development of the fetal chicken nervous system. I was curious about how a single fertilized cell could result in a fully grown and functioning organism. This was an exciting research field, and I wanted to see how I liked laboratory science. Less nobly, I also believed a research elective would help my chances of getting into medical school.

Despite the passion I had for this research, I felt guilty about killing fetal chicks. I had nightmares of chickens chasing me through vague and menacing landscapes. In these dreams, I escaped by lifting myself onto my mother's washing machine!

It also did not seem as if laboratory science would provide me the opportunity to study the topics with which I was increasingly fascinated. While at Stanford, I took classes on sleep and dreams, hypnosis, the psychology of consciousness, physiological psychology, and Buddhism—all cutting-edge material in California universities in those days.

Wanting to sort things out, I went to the student health service and talked with one of their psychiatrists. He recommended I meet James Fadiman, Ph.D., a psychologist who worked at Stanford's School of Engineering.

I called Jim's secretary, set up an appointment to meet him, and got the confusing directions to the "engineering corner" of the university. After finding my way out of a few wrong turns and blind alleys, I found Jim's office. He sat with his back to the window, the sun streaming in. I couldn't see him very clearly due to the glare. The halo effect around his head added to my already moderate anxiety. I knew this would be an important meeting.

To deal with my own nervousness, I began the conversation and asked him what he, a psychologist, was doing in the engineering department. He chuckled and replied, "I teach engineers how to think. They're smart, no doubt about that, but can they really solve problems imaginatively? How do they approach the creative process? I help them look at situations from different perspectives."

Little did I know that Jim had worked with Willis Harman, who was administering psychedelic drugs in an attempt to enhance creativity, at a nearby research institute. The published results of this work, over thirty years old, remains the only such data in the literature and showed great potential for stimulating the creative process. I wonder how many of the

Stanford engineering students he supervised were in those studies![1]

Jim leaned forward, and the blinding glare from the sun worsened. He asked, "And what are you doing here?"

I told him. My ideas were poorly formed. I was fascinated by psychedelics. I had just started practicing Transcendental Meditation. My coursework was leading me into some very interesting fields. There seemed to be a thread running through it all, but what was it? Where could I look for a unifying factor?

Jim sat back and looked thoughtful, or so it seemed—his face was nearly invisible because of the sun's rays behind him. "You ought to look into the pineal gland," he said at last. "My wife Dorothy is making a film about the experience of inner light described by mystics. The pineal gland is drawing her in as the metaphysical source of this light, the crowning achievement of many traditions. Maybe it really does generate that light inside our heads."

"How do you spell 'pineal'?" I asked, taking notes.

We chatted a little more about my plans after graduation. Our brief meeting ended.

Building upon Jim's advice, I began investigating what was known about the pineal gland, a tiny organ situated in the middle of the brain. I wrote several papers for classes that school year that began to lay out the broad framework for the theories I later developed.[2]

Western and Eastern mystical traditions are replete with descriptions of a blinding bright white light accompanying deep spiritual realization. This "enlightenment" usually is the result of a progression of consciousness through various levels of spiritual, psychological, and ethical development. All mystical traditions describe the process and its stages.

In Judaism, for example, consciousness moves through the *sefirot*, or Kabbalistic centers of spiritual development, the highest being *Keter*, or Crown. In the Eastern Ayurvedic tradition, these centers are called *chakras*, and particular experiences likewise accompany the movement of energy through them. The highest *chakra* is also called the Crown, or the Thousand-Petaled Lotus. In both traditions, the location of this Crown *sefira* or *chakra* is the center and top of the skull, anatomically corresponding to the human pineal gland.[3]

We first read about the physical pineal gland in the writings of Herophilus, a third-century B.C. Greek physician from the time of Alexander the Great. Its name comes from the Latin *pineus*, relating to the pine, *pinus*. This little organ is thus *piniform*, or shaped like a pinecone, no bigger than the nail of your pinkie finger.

The pineal gland is unique in its solitary status within the brain. All other brain sites are paired, meaning that they have left and right counterparts; for example, there are left and right frontal lobes and left and right temporal lobes. As the only unpaired organ deep within the brain, the pineal gland remained an anatomical curiosity for nearly two thousand years. No one in the West had any idea what its function was.

Interest in the pineal accelerated after it attracted Rene Descartes's attention. This seventeenth-century French philosopher and mathematician, who said, "I think, therefore I am," needed a source for those thoughts. Introspection showed him that it was possible to think only one thought at a time. From where in the brain might these unpaired, solitary thoughts arise? Descartes proposed that the pineal, the only singleton organ of the brain, generated thoughts. In addition, Descartes believed the pineal's location, directly above one of the crucial byways for the cerebrospinal fluid, made this function even more likely.

The ventricles, hollow cavities deep within the brain, produce cerebrospinal fluid. This clear, salty, protein-rich fluid provides cushioning for the brain, protecting it from sudden jolts and bumps. It also carries nutrients to, and waste products away from, deep brain tissue.

In Descartes's time, the ebb and flow of the cerebrospinal fluid through the ventricles seemed perfectly suited for the corresponding movement of thoughts. If the pineal gland "secreted" thoughts into the cerebrospinal fluid, what better means for the "stream of consciousness" to make its way to the rest of the brain?[4]

Descartes also had a deeply spiritual side. He believed that thinking, or the human imagination, was basically a spiritual phenomenon made possible by our divine nature, what we share with God. That is, our thoughts are expressions of, and proof for the existence of, our soul. Descartes believed that the pineal gland played an essential role in the expression of the soul:

> Although the soul is joined with the entire body, there is one part of the body [the pineal] in which it exercises its function more than elsewhere. . . . [The pineal] is so suspended between the passages containing the animal spirits [guiding reason and carrying sensation and movement] that it can be moved by them . . . ; and it carries this motion on to the soul. . . . Then conversely, the bodily machine is so constituted that whenever the gland is moved in one way or another by the soul, or for that matter by any other cause, it pushes the animal spirits which surround it to the pores of the brain.[5]

Descartes thus proposed that the pineal gland somehow was the "seat of the soul," the intermediary between the spiritual and physical. The body and the spirit met there, each affecting the other, and the repercussions extended in both directions.

How close to the truth was Descartes? What do we know now about the biology of the pineal gland? Can we relate this biology to the nature of spirit?

The pineal gland of evolutionarily older animals, such as lizards and amphibians, is also called the "third" eye. Just like the two seeing eyes, the third eye possesses a lens, cornea, and retina. It is light-sensitive and helps regulate body temperature and skin coloration—two basic survival functions intimately related to environmental light. Melatonin, the primary pineal hormone, is present in primitive pineal glands.

As animals climbed the evolutionary ladder, the pineal moved inward, deeper into the brain, more hidden and removed from outside influences. While the bird pineal no longer sits on top of the skull, it remains sensitive to outside light because of the paper-thin surrounding bones. The mammalian, including human, pineal is buried even deeper in the brain's recesses and is not directly sensitive to light, at least in adults. [6] It is interesting to speculate that as the pineal assumes a more "spiritual" role, it needs the greater protection from the environment afforded by such deep placement in the skull.

The human pineal gland becomes visible in the developing fetus at seven weeks, or forty-nine days, after conception. Of great interest to me was finding out that this is nearly exactly the moment in which one can clearly see the first indication of male or female gender. Before this time, the sex of the fetus is indeterminate, or unknown. Thus, the pineal gland and the most important differentiation of humanity, male and female gender, appear at the same time.

The human pineal gland is not actually part of the brain. Rather, it develops from specialized tissues in the roof of the fetal mouth. From there it migrates to the center of the brain, where it seems to have the best seat in the house.

We have already noted the pineal's proximity to cerebrospinal fluid channels, which allows its secretions easy access to the brain's deepest recesses. Additionally, it sits in strategic closeness to the crucial emotional and sensory brain centers.

These sensory or perceptual hubs are called the visual and auditory *colliculi*, little mounds of specialized brain tissue. They are relay stations for the transmission of sense data to brain sites involved in their registration and interpretation. That is, electrical and chemical impulses that begin in the eyes and ears must pass through the colliculi before we experience them in our minds as sights and sounds. The pineal gland hangs directly over these colliculi, separated by only a narrow channel of cerebrospinal fluid. Anything secreted by the pineal into that fluid would settle onto the colliculi in a moment.

In addition, the limbic, or "emotional," brain surrounds the tiny pineal. The limbic "system" is a collection of brain structures intimately involved in the experience of feelings, such as joy, rage, fear, anxiety, and pleasure. Therefore, the pineal also has direct access to the brain's emotional centers.

For many years physiologists considered the mammalian pineal gland the equivalent of the "brain's appendix." It was a residual, vestigial organ, a throwback to our early reptilian days, with no known role. That changed when American dermatologist Aaron Lerner discovered melatonin in 1958. This and related findings began what might be called the era of the "melatonin hypothesis of pineal function."

Lerner was interested in *vitiligo,* a skin disorder in which there are depigmented, or lightened, patches of skin throughout the body. A 1917 study observed that cow pineal gland extract lightened frog skin. Lerner thought that a pineal factor therefore was involved in vitiligo. He ground up over twelve thousand cow pineals and finally found the skin-lightening compound. He named it *melatonin* because it lightened skin by contracting the black pigment in special cells: *melas,* black; and *tonin,* contract or squeeze. (Despite all of Lerner's work, there is little evidence today that melatonin plays a role in vitiligo.)[7]

At the same time, scientists were manipulating light and dark cycles in order to better understand the effect of light on reproduction, no small issue when one considers the economic value of well-timed animal breeding for the livestock industry. They found that constant darkness blocked reproductive function and shrank the sexual organs; it also stimulated pineal growth and the production of melatonin. On the other hand, constant light shrank the pineal, reduced melatonin levels, and turned on sexual function. Using these experimental results, scientists concluded that melatonin was the crucial pineal factor in whose presence reproductive function flagged, and in whose absence reproductive function flourished. Put simply, melatonin possessed powerful anti-reproductive effects.[8]

Now that the pineal gland had lost some of its mystery, how did melatonin relate to the alleged *spiritual* properties of the gland? I firmly believed that there was a spirit molecule somewhere in the brain, initiating or supporting mystical and other naturally occurring altered states of consciousness. My first best guess was that pineal melatonin was this "spirit molecule," the chemical interpreter through which the body and spirit met and communicated. If melatonin had profound psychedelic properties, my search for the vehicle by which the pineal affected our spiritual lives was over.

Melatonin's full name is N-acetyl-5-methoxy-tryptamine. We can tell by its name and structure that, like DMT and 5-methoxy-DMT, melatonin is a tryptamine.

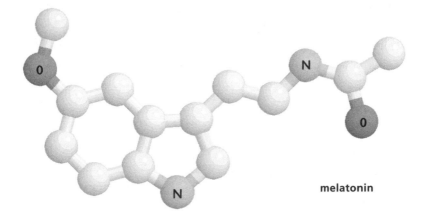

melatonin

We have a good understanding of how the body regulates melatonin production. It is the "hormone of darkness." Light turns off melatonin production, both during daylight hours and in the presence of artificial light during nighttime hours. The longer the nighttime dark hours, the more melatonin. The greater the daylight hours, the less melatonin. Besides indicating whether it is day or night, the patterns of melatonin production also inform the animal about the time of year. These longer-term melatonin effects help prepare for the appropriate seasonal responses—pregnancy in spring or fall, hibernation during the winter, or fat loss in summer.

Noradrenaline and adrenaline (or norepinephrine and epinephrine) are the two neurotransmitters that turn on melatonin synthesis in the pineal. They are released directly onto the pineal gland by nerve cells that almost touch it. The neurotransmitters attach to specialized receptors, which then begin the chemical process of melatonin formation.

The adrenal glands also make adrenaline and noradrenaline, releasing them into the bloodstream in response to stress. They are crucial factors in the body's reaction to danger: the "fight-or-flight" response. However, only adrenaline and noradrenaline released by nearby pineal nerve endings, not by the adrenal glands, have any effect on pineal function.

This is not what we would expect. Since the pineal gland does not originate from brain tissue, it exists outside the blood-brain barrier and ought to be responsive to blood-borne chemicals and drugs. Nevertheless, the body protects the pineal gland with a fierce tenacity. The stress-related surges of adrenal-gland adrenaline and noradrenaline secreted into the blood never get to the pineal. The pineal security system, made up of "vacuuming" nerve cells, simply cleans up the blood-borne adrenaline and noradrenaline in an incredibly efficient manner. Not surprisingly, this barrier makes it nearly impossible to stimulate the pineal gland to produce melatonin during the day.

Tiny blood vessels surround the pineal, so once it makes melatonin, the hormone quickly enters the bloodstream and spreads throughout the body. The pineal also secretes melatonin directly into the cerebrospinal fluid, where it can affect the brain even more quickly.

The function of melatonin in humans is uncertain, despite major advances in our understanding of its effects in other animals. There is great interest in determining whether melatonin has the same effects on reproductive function in humans as it does in other mammals. Melatonin levels fall dramatically at human puberty. Some investigators think this may allow the sexual apparatus to free itself from pineal restraint and thus begin functioning in an adult manner. Conclusive evidence remains elusive. Neither is it scientifically established that melatonin plays a role in jet lag, winter depression, sleep, cancer, or aging.[9]

For any chemical to qualify as a spirit molecule, it must at least possess psychedelic effects. Does melatonin's striking chemical similarity to DMT and 5-methoxy-DMT mean that it also is profoundly psychoactive?

Some early studies suggested that melatonin has mind-altering properties. For example, administering high doses before bedtime seemed to induce vivid dreams. However, it is difficult to interpret those older studies. They were not looking for, nor did they measure, psychedelic effects of melatonin. There was only one way for me to find out if melatonin was psychedelic, and that was to administer it to my own human volunteers.

After completing my psychiatric residency, I spent a year in Fairbanks, Alaska, working at the local community mental health center. My experience in the Arctic introduced me to the new field of "winter depression." This syndrome revitalized interest in the human biology of the pineal gland and melatonin. Research into their role in winter depression held promise for helping us understand and treat a wide range of seasonal human syndromes. This astonishing coincidence provided me a context for beginning to probe the pineal's mysteries. However, I knew little about human research, so I sought ways to further my training.

I moved to San Diego to take up a year-long fellowship in clinical psychopharmacology research at the University of California. I learned how to write scientific proposals and grants, design experiments, and administer research drugs in a clinical environment. I gave and scored rating scales, collected blood and other biological samples, and analyzed and wrote up data.

Following a San Diego colleague, Jonathan Lisansky, M.D., to Albuquerque, I began working under the guidance of Glenn Peake, M.D., a pediatric endocrinologist. Glenn was the Scientific Director of the University of New Mexico's General Clinical Research Center, an outstanding research site funded by the U.S. National Institutes of Health. Glenn, Jonathan, and I performed a comprehensive three-year study of melatonin effects in normal human volunteers. Out of this emerged the first, and so far only, documented role for melatonin in human physiology: melatonin contributes to the early morning drop in body temperature.

There is a daily rhythm in many biological functions in humans. One of the most robust is body temperature, in which there is a sharp dip at 3 A.M. This also is when melatonin levels are highest.

We studied nineteen male volunteers who stayed awake all night in light that was bright enough to prevent any melatonin formation. The drop in body temperature was not nearly as deep as normal in these melatonin-deprived men, and we wondered if the lack of melatonin was responsible.

Administering melatonin back to the volunteers caused body temperature to fall in a typical manner. From these results, we proposed that melatonin plays a major role in the early morning temperature drop found in all of us.[10]

Most important to me were results from several rating scales that measured the psychological properties of melatonin. My reading led me to hope for some profound mind-altering effects of this pineal product. However, we found that melatonin produced little more than sedation and relaxation.

I was disappointed by the lack of significant mind-altering effects of melatonin. So, toward the end of this project, when I got a call late one night from the research unit telling me that one of our volunteers accidentally received about ten times the normal dose of melatonin, it was difficult to mask my excitement. This might be very interesting. If low doses of melatonin had such timid effects, this accident might breathe some life into my pursuit of its psychological properties.

I listened carefully to the research nurse's description of how the staff miscalculated the delivery rate of melatonin. It seemed an honest mistake. In addition, the volunteer's heart rate and blood pressure were holding up fine. It was his state of mind, however, that drew most of my concern.

"How's he doing?" I asked.

"Well," she yawned, "I'm having an awfully hard time keeping him awake to fill out his rating scales. He can't keep his eyes open."

"He's not hallucinating or anything?" I offered hopefully.

"No such luck for you, Dr. Strassman," she laughed in reply.

"No, no, I'm glad he's fine," I said, quickly returning to a more professional tone.

This event, more than any other, convinced me that melatonin was not psychedelic. However, my reading continued to persuade me that the pineal gland was the prime site in which to search for a spirit molecule. Let's turn to that information, and the ideas that developed while pondering it. In doing so, we'll begin to consider a DMT-forming function for the pineal gland.

4

The Psychedelic Pineal

Even before I began the melatonin study, my review of the literature indicated it might not be the spirit molecule. I wondered if the pineal gland made other compounds with psychedelic properties. However, while still in the early stages of my career, and well before I began outlining my DMT project, I quickly discovered how controversial these ideas could be.

In 1982 I undertook a year of clinical psychopharmacology research training at the University of California in San Diego. While I concentrated mostly on the relationship between the thyroid gland and mood, I also learned everything I could about the pineal gland.

One of my teachers was Dr. K., an authority on biological rhythms, melatonin, and sleep. Halfway through my fellowship training, I decided to share with him some of my nascent ideas about a psychedelic role for the pineal. We were walking along one of the innumerable halls of the San Diego Veterans' Administration Hospital. Our conversation was rambling and wide-ranging. There was a pause, and I took the chance.

"Do you think," I offered, "that the pineal might produce psychedelic compounds? It seems to have the right ingredients. Maybe it somehow mediates spontaneous psychedelic types of states—psychosis for example." I was hesitant to get much deeper than this and avoided mentioning my more controversial ideas about the pineal—that it played a role in more exotic states, such as near-death or mystical experiences.

Dr. K. stopped in his tracks and turned on his heels. His brow furrowed and he peered at me intently through his glasses. A palpable menace glinted from his eyes. "Oops," I thought.

"Let me tell you this, Rick," he said very slowly and firmly. "*The pineal has nothing to do with psychedelic drugs.*"

That was the last time that year I said the words *pineal* and *psychedelic* in the same breath to anyone.

Nevertheless, I continued examining the literature and began developing some of the theories that inform this book. Further study of other scientists' work, and the results of my own later melatonin research, added to the body of evidence upon which I drew in formulating the following proposals.

These hypotheses are not proven, but they derive from scientifically valid data combined with spiritual and religious observations and teachings. Many of these ideas are testable using available tools and methods. The implications of these theories are profound and disturbing but also create a context of hope and promise.

The most general hypothesis is that the pineal gland produces psychedelic amounts of DMT at extraordinary times in our lives. Pineal DMT production is the physical representation of non-material, or energetic, processes. It provides us with the vehicle to consciously experience the movement of our life-force in its most extreme manifestations. Specific examples of this phenomenon are the following:

When our individual life force enters our fetal body, the moment in which we become truly human, it passes through the pineal and triggers the first primordial flood of DMT.

Later, at birth, the pineal releases more DMT.

In some of us, pineal DMT mediates the pivotal experiences of deep meditation, psychosis, and near-death experiences.

As we die, the life-force leaves the body through the pineal gland, releasing another flood of this psychedelic spirit molecule.

The pineal gland contains the necessary building blocks to make DMT. For example, it possesses the highest levels of serotonin anywhere in the body, and serotonin is a crucial precursor for pineal melatonin. The pineal also has the ability to convert serotonin to tryptamine, a critical step in DMT formation.

The unique enzymes that convert serotonin, melatonin, or tryptamine into psychedelic compounds also are present in extraordinarily high concentrations in the pineal. These enzymes, the *methyltransferases*, attach a methyl group—that is, one carbon and three hydrogens—onto other molecules, thus *methylating* them. Simply methylate tryptamine twice, and we have di-methyl-tryptamine, or DMT. Because it possesses the high levels of the necessary enzymes and precursors, the pineal gland is the most reasonable place for DMT formation to occur. Surprisingly, no one has looked for DMT in the pineal.

The pineal gland also makes other potentially mind-altering substances, the beta-carbolines. These compounds inhibit the breakdown of DMT by the body's monoamine oxidases (MAO). One of the most striking examples of how beta-carbolines work is *ayahuasca*. Certain plants that contain beta-carbolines are combined with other plants that contain DMT to make this psychedelic Amazonian brew, which allows the DMT to become orally active. If it weren't for the beta-carbolines, MAO in the gut would rapidly destroy this swallowed DMT, and it would have no effect on our minds.

It is uncertain whether beta-carbolines by themselves are psychedelic. However, they do markedly enhance the effects of DMT. Thus, the pineal gland may produce both DMT and chemicals that magnify and prolong its effects.

Under what circumstances might the pineal gland make DMT instead of the minimally psychoactive melatonin? For this to happen, there needs to be an overriding of one or more of the following constraints normally preventing pineal DMT production:

- The *cellular security system* around the pineal gland;
- The presence of an *anti-DMT compound* in the pineal gland;
- The low activity of the *methyltransferase enzymes* that produce DMT; and
- The efficiency of the *monoamine oxidase enzymes'* breakdown of DMT.

The guiding principle of the first wave of human DMT research was to compare DMT and schizophrenic states. Therefore, this was the context in which scientists studied these four different elements of the human DMT system. From these psychosis studies, we can extract data supporting my hypotheses about how the pineal may make DMT.

My emphasis on the relationship between DMT and psychosis, therefore, is not because I believe that this is the only role for endogenous DMT. Rather, psychosis is the only naturally occurring altered state of consciousness for which we have any real data. I believe that other "spontaneous psychedelic" conditions, such as near-death and spiritual experiences, also share a similar relationship with endogenous DMT. Those studies, however, have yet to be performed.[1]

Most likely, the primary factor inhibiting excessive pineal DMT production is the supremely efficient pineal security system discussed in the last chapter. The best-known example of this defense is the difficulty we encounter when trying to stimulate daytime melatonin production.

Adrenaline and noradrenaline, the neurotransmitters that stimulate nighttime melatonin formation, collectively are called *catecholamines*. Nerve cells nearly touching the pineal gland release these catecholamines, which activate specific receptors on pineal tissue and thus initiate melatonin synthesis.

The adrenal glands also produce adrenaline and noradrenaline, releasing them into the bloodstream in response to stress. However, when blood-borne adrenal catecholamines approach the pineal, the nerve cells around the pineal immediately take up and dispose of them. Therefore, circumstances in which adrenal catecholamine release occurs, such as in times of stress or during exercise, don't stimulate daytime melatonin formation.

We performed a research study that demonstrated this quite clearly. Elite athletes ran a high-altitude marathon, spending much of it above 10,000 feet. We measured melatonin before and after the race. For many of the runners, this was "nearly" a near-death experience. Yet melatonin levels in these athletes rose only to those observed at night during normal sleep—hardly an explosion of brain chemistry! Nevertheless, we did see that it *is* possible to override the pineal's defense shield if the stress is great enough.[2]

Neuroscientists believe this barrier to pineal activation exists because it would be problematic for an animal to experience its environment as "dark" during daylight hours. Since the pineal normally releases melatonin only at night, daytime melatonin release would "feel" as if it were dark at the "wrong" time, and the animal would be disoriented.

However, this explanation is weak. Daytime melatonin secretion is hardly "dangerous" enough to merit such a complex and efficient security system. Melatonin effects are not immediate, but rather take hours to days to materialize. In addition, daylight almost instantly suppresses melatonin production to near zero, returning the system to baseline before any internal disruptions occur.

However, consider what might happen if stress easily triggered the pineal to produce DMT, rather than melatonin. DMT is physically immobilizing and produces a flood of unexpected and overwhelming visual and emotional imagery. Certainly, frequent bursts of DMT release would be much more dangerous for an animal than would be those of melatonin.

It may be that melatonin is so hard to make during the day because *any* breach in the pineal security system is intolerable. The pineal erects a barrier to inordinate stress that protects equally everything behind it. So, one set of circumstances in which pineal DMT may form is when stress-induced catecholamine output is just too great for the pineal shield to withstand.

It also is possible that the pineal security system does not function normally in psychotic individuals. There are strong indirect data supporting this idea. Stress worsens hallucinations and delusions in psychotic patients. DMT levels in those patients are related to the degree of psychosis—the more intense the symptoms, the higher the levels of DMT. We know that DMT also rises in animals exposed to stress. More common levels of stress-induced catecholamines may overwhelm inadequate pineal defenses in psychosis, thus producing too much DMT. This DMT then brings on or worsens symptoms in psychotic patients.[3]

Another factor normally protecting the body from pineal production of psychedelic amounts of DMT resides within the pineal gland itself. A particular kind of small protein, first discovered in blood, has been shown to interfere with the activity of the DMT-forming enzymes. The pineal has quite high levels of this protein, a sort of "anti-DMT." If this inhibitor itself were blocked, DMT formation is more likely. Where better to provide an anti-DMT for preventing potentially dangerous excessive DMT formation than where it is made—in the pineal gland?

Data from psychosis research also support this contention. Individuals with schizophrenia received pineal gland extracts as an experimental treatment in the 1960s. Their symptoms improved markedly. The explanation for this finding was that the pineal extracts provided patients with an additional dose of the anti-DMT that their own pineal glands lacked. Thus, they were better able to combat pathologically high levels of DMT, and their psychotic symptoms improved.[4]

Two other possible brakes on DMT production in the pineal relate to enzymes: those that produce and those that break down the spirit molecule within the body.

Researchers have found that the methyltransferase enzymes that form DMT are more active in schizophrenia than in normal conditions. This would raise production of DMT. Scientists looked at many human tissues for the source of this abnormal enzyme function, but unfortunately did not study the pineal gland.[5]

Finally, if the MAO system normally destroying DMT were defective, more DMT might linger and produce "psychedelic"/psychotic symptoms. MAO is less efficient in schizophrenics than in healthy volunteers, and it may be that schizophrenics do not clear DMT quickly enough from their systems. This also would result in DMT levels too high for normal mental function. While researchers examined MAO activity in several human tissues, they unfortunately did not assess *pineal* MAO activity in schizophrenia.

Let's now consider less pathological, but also relatively common and naturally occurring, altered states of awareness in which pineal DMT may play a role. Dream consciousness is one of these.

The most likely time for us to dream is also the time at which melatonin levels are highest, that is, around 3 A.M. Since melatonin itself has such mild psychological effects, it suggests a role for another pineal compound whose levels parallel those of melatonin. DMT is a likely prospect for such a substance. However, no one has looked at 24-hour DMT rhythms in normal volunteers in an attempt to relate DMT levels to dream intensity or frequency.

Jace Callaway, Ph.D., has suggested that pineal derived beta-carbolines may mediate dreams. While the uncertain psychological effects of the beta-carbolines shed some doubt on this hypothesis, pineal beta-carbolines certainly could, by virtue of their DMT-boosting effects, indirectly stimulate dream production.[6]

Meditation or prayer also may elicit deeply altered states of consciousness. Pineal DMT production could underlie these mystical or spiritual experiences.

All spiritual disciplines describe quite psychedelic accounts of the transformative experiences, whose attainment motivate their practice. Blinding white light, encounters with demonic and angelic entities, ecstatic emotions, timelessness, heavenly sounds, feelings of having died and being reborn, contacting a powerful and loving presence underlying all of reality—these experiences cut across all denominations. They also are characteristic of a fully psychedelic DMT experience.

How might meditation evoke the pineal DMT response?

Several meditative disciplines bring about an intense fine-tuning of attention and awareness; for example, one-pointed focus on the breath. The brain's electrical activity, as measured by the electroencephalogram, reflects this synchronization, or bringing together, of brain activity. Many studies have reported that experienced meditators produce brain wave patterns that are slower and better organized than those found in everyday awareness. The "deeper" the meditation, the slower and stronger the waves.

Other techniques supplement these attentional practices with methods like chanting. Chants, using words from ancient languages with supposedly unique spiritual properties, may cause profound psychological effects. Visualization practices, in which one builds up increasingly complex and dynamic images in the mind's eye, also can lead to blissful and sublime states of mind.

In these conditions there is a dynamic yet unmoving quality to the experience, like a standing wave in a river. It looks as if the wave is not moving at all, while water rushes along on all sides of it. In fact, it is the rushing water that produces the wave. And those waves create a unique note, or sound.

Such wave phenomena, by their production of a particular note or sound associated with their frequency, establish wide-ranging and diffuse fields of influence. Objects within those fields vibrate sympathetically, or with the same frequency, a phenomenon called *resonance*.

An example of the powerful effects of resonance is when a particular note shatters a glass, even though the sound is not especially loud. The glass vibrates sympathetically, or resonates, at the same frequency as that of surrounding sound. Certain notes can create intolerable stress within the unique structure of the glass, and it bursts.

In a similar way, meditative techniques using sound, sight, or the mind may generate particular wave patterns whose fields induce resonance in the brain. Millennia of human trial and error have determined that certain "sacred" words, visual images, and mental exercises exert uniquely desired effects. Such effects may occur because of the specific fields they generate within the brain. These fields cause multiple systems to vibrate and pulse at certain frequencies. We can feel our minds and bodies resonate with these spiritual exercises. Of course, the pineal gland also is buzzing at these same frequencies.

A resonance process may occur in the pineal similar to that of the shattering glass, although not quite as destructive. The pineal begins to "vibrate" at frequencies that weaken its multiple barriers to DMT formation: the pineal cellular shield, enzyme levels, and quantities of anti-DMT. The end result is a psychedelic surge of the pineal spirit molecule, resulting in the subjective states of mystical consciousness.[7]

So far, we have looked at non-life-threatening situations: psychosis and spiritual experiences. Now we may turn to more dramatic instances that also are nearly always accompanied by psychedelic subjective realities: birth, near-death, and death experiences.

It is no exaggeration to say that birth, near-death, and death are extraordinarily "stressful" events. The life-force is doing all it can to sustain its struggling residence. Tremendous outpourings of stress-related hormones occur at these times, including the pineal-stimulating catecholamines adrenaline and noradrenaline.

Let's start with the birth process. The birth experience is highly psychedelic for the unanesthetized mother. How much more so for the newborn! We know that DMT is present in newborn laboratory animals. There's no reason to believe it's not also present in newborn humans. However, no one has yet looked for DMT in human newborns or their mothers during delivery.

Normal vaginal delivery produces an enormous outpouring of catecholamine release. The massive flooding of these stress hormones over the mother's and fetus's pineal glands may be enough to override the pineal defense system and set in motion DMT release. If the mother is anesthetized, catecholamine production is less, and the least occurs when the baby is delivered by Cesarean section. Therefore, these latter two situations may result in less robust, if any, DMT release by mother's and baby's pineals.

High levels of DMT at birth provide an explanation for a particular piece of conventional wisdom from psychedelic psychotherapy. According to Stanislav Grof, M.D., an LSD psychotherapist with unparalleled experience, much of what takes place during psychedelic therapy sessions is a reenactment of the birth process. He has found that those born by Cesarean section are less able to "let go" in psychedelic therapy than those born vaginally. The presence of psychedelic levels of DMT at normal birth, and inadequate levels during Cesarean births due to too little stress-hormone-induced DMT output, may explain this finding.[8]

Perhaps in order to fully "let go" into any powerful emotional experience as adults we need a baseline of a safe and secure resolution to our first naturally occurring "high-dose DMT session," which accompanies the birth process. Otherwise, later, as an adult, exposure to such unusual and unexpected states throws us into a completely unfamiliar set of experiences, disorienting and frightening us. We lack a reliable history of such experiences ending successfully.

Massive surges of stress hormones also mark the near-death experience, or NDE. Much of the literature on the NDE describes this as a mystical, psychedelic, overwhelming psychological experience. It also may be a time when the protective mechanisms of the pineal are flooded and otherwise inactive pathways to DMT production turn on.

We know very little about the physiology of death itself. What happens to our bodies, our brains, and our minds when we die? How long is the process? Does it end when we stop breathing? Or is there a reason many traditions counsel us about when to move or bury the dead? Why are they concerned about not wanting to disturb residual consciousness? Thus, we also must consider decomposing pineal tissue's effects upon our consciousness, both near and after death.

Pineal tissue in the dying or recently dead may produce DMT for a few hours, and perhaps longer, and could affect our lingering consciousness. While our "dead" brain wave readings are "flat," who knows about our inner mental state at this time?

To begin testing the hypothesis that decomposing pineal tissue produces psychedelic compounds, many years ago I collected pineal glands from about ten human cadavers to which I had access at a local morgue. I sent them to another laboratory to measure DMT. Unfortunately, the brains were not "fresh frozen," or removed immediately at the time of death and placed into liquid nitrogen. This instant deep freeze stops all breakdown of tissues from that point onward. We found no DMT in these pineal glands. If there were any, it is possible the long delay in processing the tissue, several days in some cases, resulted in its loss before analysis.

Finally, psychedelic drugs may affect the pineal gland, and thereby use it and DMT formation as an intermediary in their action.

There are LSD receptors on the pineal gland, and mescaline raises serotonin levels in the pineal. Beta-carbolines accelerate melatonin formation, in addition to their previously described property of magnifying and prolonging DMT effects. And DMT is the most potent of several psychedelics that stimulate pineal melatonin production.

DMT promoting the formation of its own possible building blocks is similar to the kindling process, in which a tiny match can start a huge bonfire. The match begins by burning paper, which then lights larger twigs. Burning twigs ignite branches until ultimately, a raging blaze ensues. Similarly, the various circumstances we've discussed that are conducive to endogenous DMT production may begin with just a little bit of newly formed material. These conditions could begin a process of making even more by raising levels of necessary precursors. Finally, there is a "flash point" for a full psychedelic burst of pineal DMT. The psychedelic "fire" burns itself out after it has run its course and exhausted the supply of raw materials.

This "DMT hypothesis of pineal function" allows us to tie up several loose ends left by the melatonin hypothesis of pineal function.

One of these questions I have already discussed is why the pineal gland possesses such a potent defense system against stress. The melatonin hypothesis does not adequately answer this. The DMT hypothesis, however, provides a much more satisfactory explanation. That is, the body so ruthlessly defends the pineal gland so that we are not disabled by everyday levels of stress releasing psychedelic levels of DMT.

Another mystery unsolved by the melatonin hypothesis relates to the pineal gland's unique location. The pineal gland is not even made of brain tissue. Rather, it comes from specialized cells originating in the roof of the fetal mouth. Why does it migrate in every one of us to the middle of the brain?

From its unique perch, the pineal nearly touches visual and auditory sensory relay stations. The emotional centers of the limbic system surround it, and its position allows for instant delivery of its products directly into the cerebrospinal fluid.

Traditionally, we believe that the placement of the pineal is such that it can respond best to lighting conditions. However, the route from the eyes to the pineal is curiously tortuous. Nerves from the eyes to the pineal actually exit the head and detour through the neck before returning to the pineal deep within the skull. It would be just as efficient for the gland to stay in the neck or upper spinal cord and release melatonin directly into the bloodstream as a way of notifying its host animal of lighting conditions.

It may be the pineal's placement is necessary so that melatonin may best affect nearby important brain centers, such as the pituitary gland, which regulates reproductive function. But this requirement really does not demand a deep brain location for the pineal. Melatonin carried by the blood from somewhere else could do just as good a job, as is the case with ovary and adrenal gland hormones.

Perhaps melatonin needs immediate access to cerebrospinal fluid, and that's why it hangs from the roof of a fluid-containing ventricle. However, the pineal gland releases melatonin in a steady stream lasting for many hours, and its effects develop over days and weeks. A hormone with melatonin's characteristics has no need for access to cerebrospinal fluid.

Finally, melatonin's psychological properties are rather insignificant. These minor mind-altering effects do not justify immediate access to the colliculi and limbic system, the deep brain structures that regulate perceptions and emotions.

Thus, the pineal does not need to be in the middle of the brain if this location were to support melatonin's role in our lives.

If the pineal gland were producing DMT, however, that would certainly warrant its strategic location. A DMT release directly onto the visual, auditory, and emotional centers the pineal nearly touches would profoundly affect our inner experience. We would see, hear, feel, and think things in a way unimaginable to consider for melatonin.

Because of its extraordinarily short life span of just a few minutes, DMT would also benefit from the small distances, only millimeters wide, between the pineal and important brain structures. It could diffuse directly onto these brain sites by way of the cerebrospinal fluid, without first having to enter the blood circulation. If DMT first entered the blood, MAO enzymes would destroy it long before it returned to the brain to exert its profound mental effects.

These considerations also effectively dispense with one of the major objections to the DMT theory of psychosis: the lack of differences between DMT blood levels in normal volunteers and in patients with psychosis. We now see that DMT concentrations in forearm vein blood may have little to do with its effects at discrete brain sites, sites at which DMT is broken down nearly as quickly as it is produced.

This reasoning further develops the idea that decomposing pineal tissue affects residual awareness after death. If this postmortem DMT emptied directly into the spinal fluid, simple diffusion is all it would take for it to attach to those sensory and emotional centers. A pumping heart would not be necessary.

Now that we've discussed two theories of pineal gland function in humans, the melatonin model and the DMT model, it is time to venture into analyzing the implications of these opposing paradigms.

In the last chapter, I described how the pineal gland, by way of melatonin, inhibits reproductive function. In this chapter, I hypothesize that pineal DMT opens our senses to profound psychedelic experiences. It is as if within the pineal gland there is a powerful dynamic or tension between the two roles it may play—one spiritual and the other sexual.

It's fascinating to note that many religious disciplines believe celibacy is necessary to attain the highest spiritual states. The explanation for this idea is that sexual activity diverts the energy required for full spiritual development. One chooses either the life of the flesh or the life of the spirit. Nevertheless, celibacy isn't consistent with reproduction, and there is a conflict between the continuity of the species and the anti-sexual attainment of reaching the greatest flowering of the individual spirit.

This conflict may be played out biologically in the pineal gland. Valuable resources may go to the formation of either the reproductively important melatonin or the spiritually indispensable DMT, the hormone of darkness or the chemical of inner light.

However, this opposition may be more apparent than real. Consider the possibility that pineal DMT release mediates sexual ecstasy, resulting from the strenuous exertion, hyperventilation, and intense emotions of the sex act. Psychedelic features do emerge at orgasm. In fact, the highly pleasurable effects of sexually activated DMT production may be one of the major factors motivating reproductive behavior.

Practitioners of Tantra attempt to achieve the best of both these worlds. This spiritual discipline recognizes that sexual excitation and orgasm produce highly ecstatic states, and therefore uses sexual intercourse as a meditative technique. By combining sex and meditation, Tantric practitioners access states of consciousness not available with either practice alone. Pineal DMT release, stimulated by both deep meditation and intense sexual activity, may then result in especially pronounced psychedelic effects.

There is a third element that ties together reproduction and higher consciousness, the energetic matrix within which is played out these competing pineal priorities. This is *spirit*, or *life-force*.

It is difficult to introduce the concept of "spirit" into any discussion of science in general, or biology in particular. However, it is even more difficult *not* to do so when the phenomena beg for it. In order to deal directly and deeply with the issues raised by the material I have presented, we must address this issue.

How do we define the spirit?

Compare life and death: the state of being alive to that of being dead. One moment we are thinking, moving, and feeling. Cells are dividing, replacing dying ones with fresh recruits for the liver, lung, skin, and heart. The next moment we are no longer breathing; our heart has pumped its last beat. What is the difference? What's gone that was just there?

There is something that "enlivens" us when joined with our body. When present in matter, it shows itself by way of movement and heat. In the brain, it provides the power to receive, and transform into awareness, our thoughts, feelings, and perceptions. When it is gone, the light is extinguished and the engine stops. Whatever it is, the presence of this enlivening force provides us the opportunity to interact with this time and place.

While not "personal," this spirit or life-force has a "history" associated with our particular collection of animated matter. It has experienced things with us, while being essentially unchanged by those events. Its movements have created unique fields of influence by the notes or sounds it has generated by our body's mental and physical activities. When the body is too weak to contain it, it leaves. Some goes to other matter, and some joins the ambient background of fields. The unique fields produced by its cleaving to our body, however, remain for a while before dissipating. The stronger the field, or the louder the note, the more time it takes to fade.

One of the most powerful reasons for my fascination with the pineal gland relates to its function in the life of the spirit. The importance and potential of this was brought home to me when, as a medical student in the mid-1970s, I learned of a startling coincidence involving the pineal gland and Buddhist beliefs about reincarnation. I cannot overemphasize how strong an impression this discovery made on me, and how it strengthened my search for a spiritual role for the pineal gland and, within it, the spirit molecule.

I already knew that the Tibetan Buddhist *Book of the Dead* teaches that it takes forty-nine days for the soul of the recently dead to "reincarnate." That is, seven weeks from the time of death of one person elapses until the life-force's "rebirth" into its next body. I remember very clearly, several years later, feeling the chill along my spine when, reading my textbook of human fetal development, I discovered this same forty-nine-day interval marking two landmark events in human embryo formation. It takes forty-nine days from conception for the first signs of the human pineal to appear. Forty-nine days is also when the fetus differentiates into male or female gender. Thus the soul's rebirth, the pineal, and the sexual organs all require forty-nine days before they manifest.

I unearthed this synchronicity when I was in my early twenties. I didn't know exactly how to make sense of it at the time. I still do not. In fact, conjectures relating far-flung phenomena based upon similarities in time may be as much wishful thinking as the old herbal "doctrine of signatures," which suggested that an herb's properties depended upon how it looked. If a plant looked like a heart, it must be good for heart disease.

What I'm proposing is almost a "doctrine of elapsed time." If Buddhist texts and human embryology reveal that different developments require forty-nine days, the events must be related. This association is perhaps logically shaky, but also intuitively appealing.

How might the anatomical emergence of the pineal and the reproductive organs forty-nine days after conception involve the spiritual or life force?

As we die, if near-death experiences are any indication, there is a profound shift in consciousness away from identification with the body. Pineal DMT makes available those particular non-embodied contents of consciousness. All the factors previously described combine for one final burst of DMT production: catecholamine release; decreased breakdown and increased formation of DMT; reduced anti-DMT; and decomposing pineal tissue. Therefore, it may be that the pineal is the most active organ in the body at the time of death. Might we say that the life-force therefore exits the body through the pineal?

The consequence of this flood of DMT upon our dying brain-based mind is a pulling back of the veils normally hiding what Tibetan Buddhists call the *bardo*, or intermediary states between this life and the next. DMT opens our inner senses to these betwixt states with their myriad visions, thoughts, sounds, and feelings. As the body becomes totally inert, consciousness has completely left the body and now exists as a field among many fields of manifest things.

The spirit molecule has outlived its usefulness as a scout for these realms. It has led us to the other shore, and we are on our own. During the next forty-nine days, we use our will, or intent, to process our unique life's signature, the accumulated experiences, memories, habits, tendencies, and feelings of the life that has ended. This conscious contending with our personal histories, where complete, results in a joining of those fields with ambient ones. It is as if a bell has been rung; the sound, loud at first, joins background noise, then gradually fades away.

What is left over settles onto the next physical life-form that seems most appropriate for subsequent processing of unresolved issues. There is a resonance, a sympathetic vibration, of similar fields: C-minor gravitates to C-minor, animal traits to animals, plant qualities to plants, human issues to humans.

In the case of human beings, these unmetabolized tendencies, this unfinished business, can enter the fetus only when it is "ready." This readiness may require forty-nine days, too, and may take the form of a pineal gland able to synthesize DMT. The pineal could act as an antenna or lightning rod for the soul. And sexual differentiation into male or female, occurring at exactly the same moment, provides the biological framework through which the life-force now may assert itself.

The movement of this energy, the residual life-force of the past into the present, through the pineal and into the fetus, might be the first and most primordial DMT flash. This is the dawning of consciousness, of mind, of awareness as a distinct biological and sexual entity. The blinding light of pineal DMT, secreted within the developing brain, marks the passage through this threshold.

Until this forty-nine-day watershed, the fetus may be only a physical, rather than a physical-spiritual, being. Therefore, is forty-nine days when we truly can consider a fetus to be an individual sentient, and therefore spiritual, entity?

This chapter suggests that naturally occurring altered states of consciousness result from high levels of pineal DMT production. However, what might happen if someone does not have a pineal gland, due to pineal cancer or a stroke destroying it? Would he or she have the same access to conscious experiences from endogenous DMT as someone with an intact pineal?

The enzymes and precursors in the pineal gland are not unique to it, but the high concentrations of these compounds, and the gland's remarkably convenient location, make it an ideal source of the spirit molecule. Lung, liver, blood, eye, and brain all possess the appropriate raw materials for DMT production. In fact, for some years researchers jokingly referred to schizophrenia as a lung disease because of the high concentrations of DMT-forming enzymes within the lung! These other organs may produce DMT when the same sets of circumstances exist as those that would stimulate the pineal to do so.

As radical as these theories were, I believed they could be tested using the traditional scientific method: designing experiments, analyzing data, and redefining the theories based upon results of this step-by-step research. So, the next step in this hypothesis-building process was to determine if DMT given to people reproduced the features of those experiences. If outside-administered DMT elicited effects similar to those presumably resulting from inner-produced DMT, such as near-death and mystical states, my hypotheses would be much stronger. Therefore, I needed to find some way to perform a human research study with DMT.

However, I was studying melatonin, and this pineal hormone's effects scarcely resembled those of DMT. Further studies into melatonin's physiology seemed futile.

A paper I wrote in San Diego on adverse reactions to psychedelics, published while I was performing the melatonin project, drew the attention of Rick Doblin, a tireless fund- and consciousness-raiser for psychedelic drug research. He invited me to a conference in 1985, where I met the major figures of the psychedelic research and therapy field. Representatives from a wide variety of disciplines joined together for wide-ranging, far-reaching discussions about what to make of, and do with, the psychedelic experience. These new colleagues provided support, inspiration, valuable experience, and crucial information. They made it much easier to begin conceptualizing how a psychedelic research project actually might look.

In 1987 my University of New Mexico mentor, Glenn Peake, died suddenly on a snowy Christmas day while returning from his morning run. Saddened and grieving, I saw my research trajectory waver. There had been a split between the research I believed was "respectable" and what I personally felt most inclined to study. There was my melatonin research, and then there was my interest in psychedelics. Glenn's premature death hastened the closing of that gap. During his memorial service, I remembered some of his most direct advice: "Do what you really want in research. Who cares what other people think?"

I decided to stop my melatonin research and attempt a DMT project. I talked these ideas over with the chairmen, directors, and heads of the university divisions supporting my melatonin experiments. They all believed a change in fields involved a real but reasonable risk. However, all were supportive of a psychedelic research project, "if that's what you really want to do."

The years of preparation were over. It was now or never. It was 1988.

Part II

Conception
and
Birth

89-001

There were two separate but overlapping fields upon which I would work out my attempt to perform a human DMT study. One was the clinical research realm; the other was regulatory. In this chapter I will focus on the science of the study: the actual research proposal. The next chapter will describe the labyrinth of boards and agencies through which the protocol passed.

The Human Research Ethics Committee at the University of New Mexico reviews any project intending to study humans. This committee stamps all such proposals with a number. The first two digits correspond to the year, and the next three digits reflect the order in which the protocol arrives. I submitted the DMT proposal in late 1988. It was the committee's first study up for review at their January meeting. Thus, it became *89-001*.

The first sentence, which I'd spent hours writing and rewriting the month before, trying to find the perfect opening line, read:

"This project will begin a reexamination of the human psychobiology of the tryptamine hallucinogen of abuse, N,N-dimethyltryptamine (DMT), which is also an endogenous hallucinogen."

It was nearly two years later, on November 15, 1990, before the U.S. Food and Drug Administration wrote to me, stating:

"We have completed our review . . . and have concluded that it is reasonably safe to proceed with your proposed study."

I already had some experience with the difficulties involved in giving an abusable, mind-altering drug to humans. This was from submitting a protocol to the Food and Drug Administration (FDA) several years before deciding to attempt a DMT study. The drug in this case was MDMA, popularly known as Ecstasy, a stimulant drug with mild psychedelic properties.

In the early 1980s, a loose-knit network of therapists was giving this drug to their patients as an aid to psychotherapy. It was not illegal, and these psychiatrists and psychologists found that its effects were more reliable and easier to use than those of LSD. To their dismay, this "wonder drug," like LSD decades before, soon became widely abused across college campuses. In addition, scientific papers began reporting that MDMA caused brain damage in laboratory animals. The U.S. Drug Enforcement Administration (DEA) placed MDMA into the most restrictive legal category for drugs, Schedule I, in 1985.

Nearly all the therapists using MDMA tried to make the DEA reverse its opinion. I went a different route and requested permission to give MDMA within its new legal status.

I submitted an application to the FDA in 1986. I proposed to give MDMA to human volunteers and measure its psychological and physical effects. When they sent me their standard "you may proceed if you don't hear from us in 30 days" letter, I thought to myself, "Great! I'll be able to start the research within a month!" However, like clockwork, the FDA called after twenty-nine days and said I couldn't begin yet. Soon a letter came detailing their concerns about the neurotoxic effects of MDMA. They didn't know when there would be enough information to allow me to go ahead. It might be quite a while.

My MDMA application languished in the FDA files and never amounted to much. However, I did learn that the FDA was a large and rather conservative organization. They had to be. This was made clear to me during an informal conversation with Dr. L., the director of the FDA division responsible for reviewing my MDMA proposal.

Dr. L. and I were attending a scientific meeting in 1987. We happened to be standing near each other during a coffee break. Introducing myself, I asked him if he would consider allowing me to study MDMA in the terminally ill, since he had concerns about long-term brain damage in normal volunteers. In what now seems a somewhat cavalier and callous manner, I told him that these issues wouldn't be as much of a problem in those with a six-month life expectancy. In addition, I added gamely, it would be an opening into some psychotherapy work with the terminally ill.

Dr. L. replied matter-of-factly, "Even the terminally ill have rights, and you don't want to waste their death. And besides, sometimes the diagnosis of terminal is wrong." He wrote me later to reaffirm his opposition to any MDMA studies involving dying patients.

Years later, halfway through the DMT study, the FDA sent me a letter asking if I'd like to cancel the request for an MDMA permit. It seemed like a good idea, so I agreed.

As my melatonin project began revealing the unmistakably timid psychological effects of this pineal hormone, I decided to visit a close friend and colleague, one whose opinions I valued regarding these matters. Sitting up in the loft of his northern California home in August 1988, we spent a day sorting through a wide range of approaches with which to frame a human psychedelic research project. By sunset, we arrived at two relatively simple but solid conclusions.

First, DMT clearly was the drug to study. It was incredibly interesting, and we all had some circulating in our bodies. Second, any psychedelic research project must not conflict with, and in fact must be consistent with, the current concerns about drug abuse. The U.S. government was spending billions of dollars contending with the problems associated with out-of-control substance use. Surely some of that money could fund a human DMT study. Rather than fighting against the government by trying to remove legal restrictions, it made more sense to appeal directly to the scientific thinking that ultimately drives research. We all wanted to know what drugs like DMT did, and how they did it.

My psychedelic colleagues weren't especially optimistic about a DMT project's chances for success. The MDMA affair had demoralized many. "You know what?" one predicted. "The only paper you'll ever write is how you couldn't do it. Look at how your MDMA protocol fared." However, I had been working alone in my MDMA project. For the DMT study I had the support and advice of Daniel X. Freedman, M.D.

I met Danny Freedman in 1987 at one of the many scientific meetings I was beginning to attend. Such conferences, and the networking occurring at them, is part of the ritual of establishing a successful research career. A diminutive, gnomelike man, Dr. Freedman was arguably the most powerful individual in American psychiatry at the time. He began his career in the psychiatry department at Yale University studying LSD in laboratory animals. He later moved on to become chairman of the psychiatry department at the University of Chicago. By the time I met him, he had moved again and was professor and vice-chairman of psychiatry at the University of California in Los Angeles.

He had been president of the American Psychiatric Association as well as of every major biological psychiatry organization. Rather than take a government health position, he chose to wield his power as the editor of psychiatry's most influential academic journal, the *Archives of General Psychiatry*. He routinely made and dashed careers by accepting or rejecting any one of the thousands of papers aspiring researchers endlessly submitted to him.

Freedman trained dozens of topflight researchers in academics and industry. He made late-night calls to anyone he liked to discuss the latest research ideas or political developments. He possessed unlimited energy and seemed to require almost no sleep. He chain-smoked cigarettes and drank endless quantities of frighteningly strong coffee. Seductive and charming, he could also lash out unpredictably if you aroused his ire.

His 1968 paper "On the Use and Abuse of LSD" was a seminal article in my thinking.[1] I admired his no-nonsense but openminded approach to clinical psychedelic research. While he had worked with schizophrenic patients under the influence of LSD in the 1950s, he nearly exclusively performed animal studies. His early animal pharmacology papers on LSD established the groundwork for future laboratories' approaches to assessing the role of serotonin in psychedelic drugs' effects. He also testified in front of the 1966 U.S. Senate committee, chaired by Senator Robert Kennedy, that sealed the fate of psychedelic drugs' placement into their restricted legal category.

Freedman had serious doubts about the possibility of performing good human psychedelic research. He believed volunteers had too many expectations of drug effects. He also was worried about the risk of "unreliable personnel," a euphemistic reference to drug-taking by members of a research team. This latter concern unerringly predicted some of the problems our own group would encounter in New Mexico.

In our meetings and correspondence, Freedman predicated any help he would provide me upon the premise that my DMT research would focus solely on pharmacology. He thought psychotherapy research would result in irrational enthusiasm, questionable results, and scientific controversy. It was safer and more practical first to confirm and extend the wealth of data coming from animal laboratories. While his logic was unassailable, our adherence to this biomedical model did set the stage for certain problems that developed later on in our research.

With Dr. Freedman's guidance, I wrote up a DMT study, the "dose-response" project. It was simple, levelheaded, and achievable, containing four specific goals:

- Recruit "well-functioning, experienced hallucinogen users" for volunteers;
- Develop a method to measure DMT in blood;
- Create a new rating scale by which we could assess DMT's psychological effects; and
- Characterize psychological and physical responses to several doses of DMT.

After briefly summarizing the history of psychedelics within academic psychiatry, I pointed out that while animal studies continued, human experiments lagged far behind. Psychedelics continued to be popular drugs of abuse, and understanding what they did, and how they did it, would address real public health concerns.

I also reviewed previously published animal and human data on DMT and listed the qualities that made it an ideal candidate with which to resume human psychedelic drug research. I noted that one of the best reasons for choosing DMT was that very few people had heard of it. When the media discovered my research, it would draw much less attention than would an LSD project.

Next I exhumed the endogenous psychotomimetic argument, arguing that scientists had yet to find any better candidate for a naturally occurring schizotoxin. Researchers were developing new antipsychotic drugs that blocked the same serotonin receptors that psychedelics activated. Thus, the more we knew about DMT, the more we might learn about psychotic disorders. If we could block the effects of DMT in normal individuals, perhaps we would have a new weapon in our armamentarium against schizophrenia.

I also proposed that DMT's short duration of effects would make it easier to use than longer-acting drugs, especially in the potentially negative setting of a hospital environment.

Finally, DMT had a track record of safe use in previously published human research, especially that of Dr. Szára.

This introduction led to the theoretical underpinnings for studying DMT: the biomedical model. Psychopharmacologists had firmly established that psychedelics, including DMT, activated many of the same brain receptors as did serotonin. Laboratory animal research, continuing for decades after human studies ended, revealed the specific types of serotonin receptors involved. I was to build upon this animal data and determine if it also applied to humans.

The most important biological variables were to be *neuroendocrine* in nature. Neuroendocrinology is the study of how drugs influence hormones by first stimulating certain brain sites. For example, activation of specific serotonin receptors in the brain causes a rise in blood levels of particular pituitary hormones, such as growth hormone, prolactin, and beta-endorphin. The hormones that change in response to drugs reflect which brain receptors those drugs affect.

Serotonin receptors also regulate heart rate, blood pressure, body temperature, and pupil diameter. I would measure these, too, in an attempt to thoroughly catalog other signs of serotonin receptor activation by DMT. These were objective, numerical data.

I would recruit only experienced psychedelic users for the study. Experienced volunteers would be better able to report drug effects than those with no idea what to expect. In addition, seasoned research subjects were less likely to panic under the influence of the extremely powerful effects of DMT, which potentially would be more disorienting in the stark clinical research center environment. Finally, there were unpleasant, but real, liability issues. I had to protect myself from any lawsuits that might result if people claimed they began using psychedelics because of their participation in the study. If they had used psychedelics in the past, it would be more difficult for them to claim the study had introduced them to these drugs.

Volunteers also would be required to be functioning at a relatively high level, working or in school, and in stable relationships. This would help assure me that they were grounded enough in everyday reality to handle what would be a rigorous and demanding study. I wanted them to have support from sources other than the research team to whom they could turn if they needed help outside of the sessions.

There would be careful medical and psychological screening of the volunteers. Women must neither be pregnant nor likely to become pregnant, and we would test urine for recreational drugs before every study day.[2]

In reviewing the techniques for measuring psychedelics' psychological effects, I concluded that all previous questionnaires presumed their effects to be unpleasant and psychotic. A newer scale with less of a bias, based on responses in people who liked psychedelics, might provide a broader perspective on their effects. I proposed interviewing as many recreational DMT users as I could for this purpose. These individuals would provide a broad overview of DMT's effects, which would form the basis of a new rating scale. As the research progressed, I could appropriately modify the questionnaire.

It also was necessary to develop an assay, or method of measuring, for DMT in blood. There were several older assays from which to choose, and we would try our hand at whichever seemed easiest and most sensitive. The most likely method was one used by researchers at the National Institute of Mental Health, the same group that had written the "decent burial" paper on DMT.

Based upon a 1976 study describing hormone effects of DMT in humans, we calculated that twelve volunteers were enough to show statistically significant differences between doses of DMT and an inactive saltwater placebo. Most dose-response studies of any new drug give volunteers one "high" dose, one "low" dose, and one or two "medium" doses in order to describe the entire spectrum of effects. I wanted to give as much DMT as possible, so I decided that each volunteer in the study would receive a placebo and four doses of DMT—one high, one low, and two medium.

Volunteers would receive the different DMT doses in a randomized and double-blind manner. *Randomized* means that the sequence of doses is in no particular order, as if a roll of the dice determined which day would involve any particular dose. Clifford Qualls, Ph.D., the University of New Mexico General Clinical Research Center's biostatistician, generated a random sequence of the required doses on his computer, sealed it in an envelope, and delivered it to the pharmacy for their use. *Double-blind* means that neither the volunteers nor I would know which dose any volunteer was to receive on any particular day. Only the pharmacist possessed the list detailing the unique ordering of doses for each person.

The purpose of randomized double-blind studies is to reduce the role of expectation in affecting results. In chapter 1 I referred to the classic study demonstrating the power of expectation in determining drug effects. Similarly, if volunteers knew when they were going to get a low dose of DMT, their responses might be biased. They might react in a way consistent with what they expected a low dose to be like, rather than what actually happened, be it in reality placebo or a medium dose they received that day.

In addition, before entering into a complicated double-blind study, we thought it best to begin a volunteer's involvement in the research by first giving them two "non-blind" doses of DMT. An introductory low dose of 0.05 mg/kg would let people settle in to the research setting without having an effect so strong that it might disorient them. A subsequent high dose, 0.4 mg/kg, would let volunteers experience the greatest level of intoxication they would ever reach on any subsequent double-blind day. We called this the "calibration dose." If someone received their first high dose in the middle of the full study but didn't know it was the most they'd ever get, they might drop out for fear of getting even more of an effect on another dose. With a non-blind high dose, volunteers had the option of dropping out of the study right away, before we had begun collecting a lot of data on them. So subjects actually would receive six doses of DMT— two non-blind and four double-blind.

Tests of new drugs always include a placebo, and our study would, too. Placebo-controlled studies further help tease apart the effects of anticipation from those of the drug. *Placebo* comes from the Latin, meaning *I shall please,* or to paraphrase, *I shall meet your expectations.* Most of us think of a placebo as an inert substance, what we refer to as *inactive placebo*. Sugar pills are the best-known example of inactive placebos. In our DMT studies, the inert placebo was sterile saltwater, or saline.

Practically speaking, it is extraordinarily difficult to keep double-blind, placebo-controlled studies "double-blind." Effects of active drugs are usually much more obvious than those of inactive saltwater or sugar, and both research subjects and staff almost always can tell the difference.

However, in this first dose-response DMT project, we wanted to use a placebo to see if volunteers and we could distinguish between the lowest dose of drug and none at all. In that capacity, the placebo day served a valuable function.[3]

There were drawbacks to this design. Volunteers usually felt substantial anxiety before getting their first double-blind dose. Was today going to be another shattering high dose? Or could they relax? If it was apparent that the first few double-blind sessions did not involve the large dose, anxiety also built up before later sessions in a way that didn't for those who got the high dose out of the way on an earlier day. While the randomized order in which all volunteers received their full complement of doses probably statistically "evened out" this factor, at a human level there was a price to pay.

I also addressed how we would manage psychological and physical adverse effects. The first line of response to a panic reaction would be talking people down using reassurance and support. If this didn't work, we would use a minor tranquilizer, such as injectable Valium; we would use a injection of a major tranquilizer, like Thorazine, if anyone got completely out of control. For allergic reactions, such as wheezing or a severe rash, an intravenous antihistamine was available. If blood pressure went up too high, nitroglycerin tablets under the tongue, much like the way people with angina heart pain use them, would be effective.

I attached a list of several dozen references supporting the ideas I had laid out. These included papers from the first wave of human psychedelic research. There were articles describing what we knew about psychedelics' effects on animals and on serotonin receptors. Anticipating concerns about safety, I pointed to my previously published review of adverse effects of psychedelics. In it, I suggested that if people were mentally healthy, well prepared, and closely supervised before, during, and after the experience, the chances of serious and prolonged psychiatric side effects were extremely low.

Copies of the proposal went to all the boards that had control over human drug abuse research, including the Human Research Ethics Committee at the University of New Mexico, the U.S. Food and Drug Administration, and the U.S. Drug Enforcement Administration. The study would occur at the University of New Mexico Hospital's General Clinical Research Center, so I sent a copy of the proposal there as well. The Research Center might cover the costs of measuring the large number of blood samples for DMT and hormone levels, so I also submitted a budget to their laboratory.

Now for the hard part: Getting everyone responsible for overseeing and funding this project to agree it was safe, was worth doing, and deserved money.

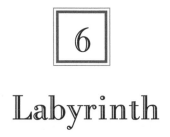

Labyrinth

In the United States, the Controlled Substances Act of 1970 exists to protect the public from potentially harmful drugs. This law also is a barrier preventing access to those drugs by the clinical research community. It is the labyrinth through which anyone who wishes to perform human research with psychedelic drugs must pass.

The Controlled Substances Act placed all drugs into "schedules," depending on their "abuse potential," "currently accepted medical use," and "safety of use under medical supervision." Schedule I drugs, the most restricted, are "highly abusable, lack medical utility, and are unsafe under medical supervision." Over the objections of dozens of high-level psychiatric researchers, including Dr. Daniel Freedman, Congress placed LSD and all the other psychedelic drugs into Schedule I.

Schedule II includes drugs like methamphetamine and cocaine. They possess high abuse potential but some medical utility—cocaine as a local anesthetic for eye surgery, and methamphetamine for the treatment of hyperactive children, for example. Codeine is in Schedule III, because this commonly used painkiller has abuse potential "less than" Schedule I and II drugs, as well as fewer and less severe adverse consequences when used under medical supervision. Schedule IV drugs like Xanax and Valium possess abuse potential "less than" Schedule III and have "limited" problems associated with their medical use.

In the case of the psychedelics, the high abuse potential that lawmakers noted was not the compulsive, out-of-control use commonly seen with drugs like heroin and cocaine. Psychedelics don't cause craving or withdrawal. In fact, one of their hallmarks is that they produce almost no effects after three or four daily doses, and abruptly stopping them causes no withdrawal. Rather, it was their *acute* effects that were so profoundly disruptive and at times disabling. Because of those highly destabilizing effects, Congress decided psychedelics must be tightly regulated.

Clinical research scientists in the 1950s and 1960s recognized and usually took into account the unique dangers of LSD and other psychedelics. By doing so, they could successfully prevent or quickly deal with any adverse psychological reactions to these drugs. However, uncontrolled public use, and media-intensive breaches in research protocols by Leary and his colleagues at Harvard, brought the expected responses. These drugs *were* causing highly publicized problems, and the door had to be shut for damage control.

In order to turn this tide of abuse, Congress emphasized psychedelics' negative properties at the expense of their positive or neutral ones. What one day was "safety under medical supervision" became "lack of safety under medical supervision" the next. "Medical utility" as research and training tools and aids to psychotherapy quickly changed into "no currently acceptable medical use."

It was into this black hole I peered as I prepared to shepherd the DMT protocol through the regulatory system.

The process began in December 1988. I kept a log during the next two years of every phone call, letter, meeting, fax, and discussion related to 89-001, the DMT protocol. From my notes, I summarized and extracted the most relevant information obtained from these interactions and wrote them up in 1990, immediately after getting permission to begin the study. I referred to this article as the "what if I'm run over by a bus?" paper. It was important that other people knew how to wind their way through this maze. It was possible, and there was a route through it. If nothing else came of the DMT project, I wanted to leave behind this map for success.[1]

The initial guardians of the regulatory realms were two University of New Mexico School of Medicine committees: the Research Center's Scientific Advisory Committee and the Human Research Ethics Committee.

The General Clinical Research Center Scientific Advisory Committee dealt with the science behind my proposal. Fellow researchers on the panel looked at the scientific merit of the study and offered remedial suggestions. They also decided whether to allow its performance at the Research Center, and whether to pay for the many blood tests I requested. Because I had spent the last two years running the human melatonin project at the Research Center, I was a member of this committee at the time.

The Human Research Ethics Committee dealt with the safety of my proposed study. Its duties were to make sure the project had an acceptable safety profile, and that the informed consent document clearly spelled out the nature of the study and its risks.

It was incredibly fortunate that the chairman of the crucial ethics committee was a firm believer in libertarianism; that is, that the individual takes precedence over the state. He believed that educated people could make up their own minds. His motto, as head of one of the first and most important review panels, was great encouragement: "We're not here to play God."

The informed consent document is a crucial element of human research. In it, the researcher describes the objectives of the protocol, and why he or she is performing it. The consent states exactly, and in mind-numbing detail, what to expect from participating. It lists the potential risks and benefits associated with volunteering, details how the research team will manage risks, and notes that volunteers will receive all necessary treatment for adverse effects free of charge. The consent reminds the potential research subject that participation is totally voluntary and ongoing. He or she may withdraw at any time, for any reason, with no penalty or withholding of necessary care. In case a volunteer feels unfairly treated, the informed consent document provides names and phone numbers of people he or she can contact in order to complain.

While negotiating with the university committees, I also began working with the two United States federal agencies that formed the final, and more formidable, regulatory barriers. They held in their hands the ultimate decisions.

The first was the U.S. Drug Enforcement Administration (DEA). They had a local Albuquerque office, but their headquarters were in Washington, D.C. The DEA would decide if I would be allowed to possess DMT. If granted, this permission would take the form of a *Schedule I permit*.

The other federal regulatory agency was the U.S. Food and Drug Administration (FDA), which also is based in Washington, D.C. The FDA would decide if it was safe and worthwhile to give DMT to human research volunteers in my study. If granted, the FDA's permission would take the form of an *Investigational New Drug (IND) permit*.

When submitting the protocol to the university committees, I told them the study would not begin until the FDA and DEA both gave their permission to administer DMT. However, these federal agencies first required local approval.

The informed consent document would be a major hurdle, and I was direct with the ethics committee about the expected effects of DMT. I did not want to lull volunteers into thinking it would be an easy day, but I also did not want to scare them away by emphasizing potential negative effects. On page two of the consent, this is what the volunteer read:

> I understand that the primary effects of this drug are psychological. Visual and/or auditory hallucinations or other perceptual distortions may occur. My sense of time may be altered (short lengths of time passing slowly or vice versa). I may experience very powerful emotions, pleasurable or unpleasant. Opposite feelings or thoughts may be experienced at the same time. I may be extremely sensitive

and aware of the environment; on the other hand, I may not notice anything at all in the environment. It may feel like my body and mind have separated. Feelings of impending or actual death or confusion may occur. Euphoria is very common. The onset of the experience is rapid, the experience being very intense with the higher doses within 30 seconds. It peaks within 2 to 5 minutes and is usually felt as only a mild intoxication within 20 to 30 minutes. I will quite likely feel like my normal self within an hour after the injection.

Regarding risks, the consent form was brief, but honest:

The main effects of DMT are psychological and have been described above. These usually last less than 1 hour. Rarely, emotional reactions to these effects may last longer (i.e., 24 to 48 hours). I can stay at the Research Center as long as necessary to regain my equilibrium, including overnight if desired. . . . DMT is physically safe. Mild to moderate brief increases in blood pressure and heart rate occur.

It would have been premature and inappropriate to suggest in the informed consent that participation in the DMT study offered any potential benefits. While I knew volunteers probably would enjoy their DMT experiences, this was different from suggesting that I was providing treatment for a diagnosable condition. Thus, the consent went on to say:

There are no benefits to me personally as a result of participating in this research. However, the potential benefits are a greater understanding of the mechanism of action of hallucinogenic agents.

Within a week of submitting the DMT study, the ethics committee asked me to include the phrase "no currently accepted medical use" in the informed consent's introductory paragraph. I replied by suggesting this phrase would unnecessarily frighten off prospective volunteers. In addition, if I ever did get permission to run the study, the phrase would no longer, strictly speaking, be true. It then would have currently accepted medical use; in this case, as a clinical research tool. They accepted this answer.

Confidentiality and anonymity were important issues I had to work out with the ethics committee, the Research Center, and the university hospital administration. Nearly all the DMT volunteers had jobs and families, neither of which they cared to endanger by admitting to the use of illegal drugs. Confession to having broken the law was a prerequisite for enrolling in the study, since only experienced psychedelic drug users could participate. I met with staff from the hospital's medical records department and admitting offices, the head nurse and administrator of the Research Center, and the hospital's attorney. Together we worked out a complicated but effective arrangement.

Records of the medical screening performed in the outpatient clinic of the Research Center would hold important medical information. This might be extraordinarily helpful if the volunteer at some future date developed health problems for which the treating physician needed baseline values, for example, regarding heart function. Therefore, we placed the volunteer's real name on the chart containing results of the physical examination and screening laboratory tests. In this chart was no mention of drug use, nor a linking of the volunteer to my drug studies.

The signed informed consent document, which was usually attached to the chart, required the volunteer's real name on the signature line. To protect confidentiality, I kept all signed informed consents under lock and key in my home office. All that was necessary for the "real name" chart was the comment: "Consent signed. Held by Principal Investigator."

Each volunteer then received a code number, such as DMT-3. From that point on, this anonymous identification was the only one they possessed, and I was the only person who knew the key. They each received a new hospital chart labeled only with their DMT number. The first time we used the code number was for the psychiatric examination detailing their history of drug use and emotional problems.

There was one final concern. This related to outside agencies looking at charts in order to assess long-term effects of exposure to experimental drugs. In my melatonin studies, I included a phrase in the informed consent stating that the manufacturer of melatonin and the FDA might review patient files in order to investigate any risks or problems associated with receiving melatonin. When I included this comment in the DMT consent, prospective volunteers objected. Nevertheless, there had to be some mechanism by which legitimate investigation into possible long-term health risks resulting from DMT could occur. However, it must be voluntary.

The compromise we developed was that if the FDA or the DMT manufacturer wanted to interview research volunteers or look at their medical records, they first had to go through me. I would check with the individual volunteers to see who was interested. Research records certainly could be subpoenaed, but without the key to the code numbers they would be of limited use. I would refuse to divulge the key on the grounds of patient-doctor privilege. It would be a mess, but it was worth it.

As it turns out, in five years of studies with over sixty DMT volunteers, not one breach of confidentiality or anonymity ever occurred. Neither have there been, five years since the studies' completion, any requests by the authorities to review volunteers' charts.

The Research Center's Scientific Advisory Committee acknowledged that the science of the DMT protocol was relatively direct and uncomplicated. They realized the primary obstacles were ethical, political, and administrative, areas in which they had less authority and responsibility than the ethics committee.

There were security and liability concerns, however. The Research Center asked me to keep volunteers in the hospital overnight, to make sure they were watched by the nursing staff for a full day after their participation. I replied that this would cut down on the number of prospective volunteers. Previous DMT studies had sent their volunteers home in the afternoon, following morning studies, with good safety results. They accepted this.

The Research Center scientists also wanted to establish the best time of day to give DMT. Was there a daily rhythm in DMT sensitivity? Were responses greater in the morning or evening? I answered that I didn't know, but that by giving DMT to everyone at the same time of day, in the morning, we would standardize that factor. We could investigate possible changes in sensitivity throughout the day in a different study.

My research colleagues also requested more justification from the animal literature for drawing blood levels of the various hormones I wanted to measure. These references were easy to provide. Finally, they wanted volunteers to submit urine samples for testing for drugs of abuse.

Within a month, on February 19, 1989, the Research Center approved the DMT protocol. They also agreed to fund my request for testing hormone levels and for developing a method of measuring DMT in human blood.

Three days later, the Human Research Ethics Committee also approved the study.

I then began looking for a source of DMT. At the same time, I had to make sure it was legal for me to possess it once I found it. The simpler of these two tasks was possession, and this depended on the DEA providing me a Schedule I permit.

In April 1989 I met with the university hospital pharmacy about the security requirements the DEA would request for storing a Schedule I drug. Since the pharmacists previously had worked on a marijuana study, they believed their safeguards were adequate.

I sent in my DEA Schedule I permit application. It stated that the permit was necessary to possess laboratory-grade DMT so we could begin developing a way to measure DMT in human blood. Later, the permit would need to cover the human-grade DMT volunteers would receive. This human-grade DMT needed to be purer than that required for laboratory work. Giving people DMT would not begin until the FDA approved the study and the purity of the human-grade drug.

One section of the DEA application asked for DMT's "drug number." I called the DEA office in Washington, D.C., and a staff person looked up DMT on the list of national drug codes. This number went into the appropriate box.

I called the DEA two weeks later, but they had no record of receiving my application. The person with whom I spoke said, "We're moving into a new office, and everything's in boxes."

Another two weeks passed—still no record of my request. In a few days, though, I received the entire application back. They needed the correct drug number for DMT. *This* number was on a sheet of paper they enclosed with the returned application. The person with whom I had spoken earlier had given me the wrong number. I entered the correct number and mailed back the "revised" application that day.

The DEA also wanted a New Mexico Board of Pharmacy Schedule I permit; I applied for and received this certificate within a few weeks. "It's all up to the DEA," the staff at the New Mexico Board said.

The DEA then told me they would approve the request for laboratory-grade DMT if the hospital pharmacy and staff passed necessary security checks. The paperwork went from Washington to Denver, and from Denver to Albuquerque.

The local Albuquerque DEA field officer, Agent D., came to the university to meet me and look over the pharmacy in early June of 1989. She asked for the names of all those pharmacy staff who might have contact with the DMT, as well as our addresses, phone numbers, and social security numbers. She found several breaches in security and asked us to get a locked freezer. That freezer was to be placed in the locked narcotics vault. She said I could not have a copy of the freezer key—only the hospital pharmacists should. If any of the drug ended up missing, they didn't want to suspect me of stealing it.

She had the unsettling habit of joking, every so often, "Well, that won't land you in jail." And, "Don't worry—we won't take you away in handcuffs for that."

I tried to laugh with her.

When we said good-bye that day, she summed it up: "It's your ass on the line. If anything goes wrong—theft, loss, bad record keeping—we look to you for explanations."

As anxious as her visit made me feel, Agent D.'s last words were the most troubling: "By the way, where will you get the DMT you'll give to your volunteers?"

Later that month, the DEA approved in principle my request for permission to possess laboratory-grade DMT. I promised not to give this lower-grade drug to volunteers and would await FDA approval on human-grade DMT before starting the study. The DEA still held control over whether I could possess human-grade DMT, because this was to be a different batch of drug.

In March 1989, within a week of obtaining university approvals for the DMT study and just after mailing in my forms to the DEA, I called Sigma Laboratories in St. Louis, Missouri. Sigma was the chemical supply house that had provided melatonin for my human pineal project. There was a listing for DMT in their catalog, and I asked if they would sell some to me. I requested laboratory-grade DMT for our efforts to measure DMT in body fluids. I also asked for clinical-grade drug for human use. Sigma told me that there was no problem in purchasing laboratory-grade DMT—the only requirement was a Schedule I permit from the DEA.

Obtaining human-grade DMT was going to be more complicated, as it called for Sigma putting together specific documentation for the FDA, a "drug master file." Sigma recommended contacting the investigators who administered DMT to humans in previous studies to find out who had supplied them. Sigma then would know how much detail to provide the FDA. If there were problems finding out who used to have those files, they recommended utilizing the U.S. Freedom of Information Act. This law allows citizens to request privileged information as long as it does not threaten American national security interests.

I obtained a list of all the currently active investigational drug permits in the country so that I could contact anyone who possessed one for DMT. Unfortunately, there weren't any. My request to find out about the existence of old permits, using the Freedom of Information Act, was not successful. There were no records or files at the FDA for previous DMT permits.

My application to give DMT to humans went in to the FDA in late April. I asked for a reactivation of the old DMT permits that the first generation of researchers had used, hoping the FDA itself might be able to find those old hidden files. One of the scientists who had given humans DMT, a co-author of the "decent burial" paper, agreed to let the FDA look at his old records on my behalf. However, in later correspondence, he discovered he had no information about the drug and couldn't remember who had been his supplier. He wished me good luck.

In early May the FDA sent their first letter, signed by Ms. P., advising that if they didn't get in touch within a month, the study could proceed. Of course, I had no DMT. However, they now had the application, and my request received a file number. Sigma now agreed to discuss with the FDA putting together a drug master file for me.

In June, Ms. P. at the FDA said Sigma was not providing them enough information about how their DMT was made. Sigma replied that their European DMT supplier refused to release any such information—it was a trade secret. Sigma also was concerned that the FDA was asking for more information about DMT than they did for other drugs Sigma previously had provided for human studies. Sigma gave me the name of the FDA chemist assigned to my application: Ms. R. She and I were to carry on dozens of conversations over the next year and a half.

I asked Ms. R. why the FDA was requiring more information about DMT than they did about melatonin for my previous research.

She replied, "It's case by case."

Sigma complained that the FDA was being unreasonable. The FDA wouldn't move forward until they had more information. When I asked Ms. R. if she knew who was Sigma's supplier, saying that I wished to contact them directly myself, she offered their name. When I asked Sigma to confirm this, they were upset by what they felt was a breach of confidence. Nevertheless, they agreed to send the FDA all the information they possessed about their DMT.

I asked Ms. R., "If Sigma's DMT doesn't have all the necessary manufacturing data, could I purify it so it meets your requirements?"

She doubted it. The director of the division within the FDA where she worked before was the fellow who told me, at the brain science meeting some years back, "the dying have rights, too." He had blocked all requests by previous researchers to purify laboratory-grade drugs in order to give them to humans.

"Maybe it's different now," she said. "This is a new division, with new directors."

This was true. The rising tide of AIDS and drug abuse brought into focus the delays in the drug approval process at the FDA. A new division formed to provide expedited review of new drugs for these problems. Fortunately, my DMT request went to this new division rather than Dr. L.'s, where my MDMA proposal never made any progress.

Several months passed, and Ms. R. never did receive any information from Sigma. Sigma felt that the FDA had broken confidentiality, and they probably did not want to get any deeper into what they knew would be a long and complicated process. What was in it for them? I gave up hoping to obtain Sigma's DMT for human use.

A densely worded letter arrived from the FDA in August 1989, spelling out twenty separate requirements the human-grade DMT must meet. There were no questions about general toxicity, which would require complicated and expensive animal testing. Nor were there concerns about the study's scientific merit. On those counts, in any event, I was encouraged.

I called the chemist colleague who previously had offered his dire prediction about my only publication being one on the failure to obtain permission to run the study. I asked him directly, "Will you make me some DMT?"

He declined. He did not believe his current laboratory would meet the requirements to qualify as a "manufacturer." It would be too expensive and time-consuming to try.

I also asked David Nichols, Ph.D., a chemist and pharmacologist at Purdue University in Indiana. He recommended Dr. K. at the National Institute of Mental Health, who directed a program that made hard-to-find research drugs. Dr. K. said his contract prohibited use of his compounds in humans, although perhaps in the future he might request to synthesize human-grade drugs. Dr. K. recommended calling Lou G., an old colleague at a chemical supply house in Chicago.

As it turned out, Lou, who stayed on after another firm bought his company, had provided much of the DMT for American human studies. However, his Chicago firm did not give those researchers any manufacturing or animal toxicity data.

Lou laughed on the phone as he said, "We just told them it was pure—'95 percent, more or less.' Things were a lot looser then."

I wrote to the National Institute on Drug Abuse (NIDA), asking if they had some human-grade DMT. When a month elapsed, I wrote again. Mr. W. replied and said NIDA drugs usually came from a laboratory in North Carolina. Dr. C. directed this group.

I called Dr. C., who told me they could not make human-grade drugs. When reminded of a recently published study in which his laboratory did so for another research project, he said he'd look into it. Even if he did agree to make the drug, he wouldn't put the drug master file together for the FDA.

He said, "I don't want the liability. I don't have insurance for human use. It's not in my contract."

Dr. C. recommended getting some DMT from NIDA and purifying it to the required 99.5 percent purity. He thought they might have 5 grams or so "on the shelf."

When asked about this, Mr. W. answered, "Our DMT is too old. And we don't have any manufacturing data."

He continued, "We've got a contract with Dr. C. They make what we ask them. There's another laboratory that prepares their drugs for human use. I think the bigger issue is that there's not a lot of movement on DMT these days. It wouldn't be very cost-effective for us to use much money from our contract for such an obscure drug. Let me see what I can find out."

A few weeks later Mr. W. called back, saying Dr. C. could make DMT, but I would have to pay for it. Dr. C. agreed to calculate an estimate, but repeated that he would not put together the required drug file for FDA. "It's too much work."

This seemed minimally promising. When I asked Ms. R. at the FDA about putting together my own drug file on Dr. C.'s DMT, she said she'd get back to me.

"If Dr. C. made the DMT, could I really use it?"

"I'll check with the drug abuse staff here," she answered.

"Why wouldn't I be able to?"

She answered, "I don't know. Maybe our director, Dr. H., will call you."

Dr. C.'s estimate of the cost was over $50,000.

"Well," I said, "thanks for looking into it."

Another door closed.

I called Ms. R.: "I'm not having much luck. What do you suggest?"

"I'll go to the Federal Archives Building and see if I can find the previous DMT researchers' files."

In July 1989 Ms. R. found the files for these old studies. "The data in them are terrible," she said. "There's nothing—no animal data, no chemistry data. We closed it. They never responded to our requests for progress reports. It won't help you."

"How did you ever approve that study?"

"I don't know. I didn't work here then." She tried sounding hopeful. "I'll send the information you need to set up your own drug file."

The information she sent was designed for a large drug company such as Lilly, Merck, or Pfizer. It had nothing to do with an individual investigator.

I called Ms. R. "I need help. Why aren't you helping me?"

"Our director's name is Dr. H. Here's his phone number. Insist on speaking with him."

I called Dr. H.'s office. Dr. H.'s secretary said, "You'll need to speak to Dr. W."

Before I could protest, he transferred the call to Dr. W.

"This is Dr. W.!," boomed the friendly but commanding voice on the other end of the line. "I'm the only physician on the drug abuse staff in this new division. I know what you've been going through. We're here to help. Don't despair."

"How can I get human-grade DMT?" I asked.

"Find someone to make it for you."

"How about Dave Nichols at Purdue?"

He replied, "That's possible."

"Could you and Dave talk with each other?"

"Have Dr. Nichols write to the director, Dr. H. Here's his address. The name of the staff working on your request is Ms. M. Call her in two weeks."

I felt something shift with that phone conversation.

I called Dave Nichols. He quoted me a price of $300—just the cost of supplies.

While all these calls were taking place, I knew that funding from outside the University was crucial for the project to gain all the legitimacy it needed. Additional financial support also would free up my time to find human-grade DMT and help the Research Center pay for some of the work I requested. This, in turn, would increase the Research Center's backing of the protocol.

In looking over some of the old DMT and schizophrenia research, it appeared that the Scottish Rite Foundation, a branch of the Freemasons, had funded some of it through their Schizophrenia Research program. I asked this program to send an application for funding. My DMT proposal already discussed the importance of understanding DMT's effects in its possible role as an endogenous schizotoxin. Therefore, it took little work to modify the grant to emphasize these issues more clearly.

I wrote Dr. Freedman, telling him of my grant submission to the Scottish Rite Foundation. He replied that he was on their scientific review committee, and "maybe" they would fund a year's support. Within a month, in September 1989, a notification of award arrived announcing a one-year grant for the project.

I again wrote Dr. Freedman, updating him on the search for human-grade DMT. He scribbled a note on my letter and sent a copy of it to the Director of the National Institute on Drug Abuse, one of his former students. His telegraphic missive ended: "Strassman needs someone at NIDA responsive. Any suggestions??"

In September I called Mr. W. at NIDA. He had just returned from a meeting with Dr. C. They were discussing how to get Schedule I drugs to researchers.

"We want to help," he said. "Call Ms. B. at the DEA and see if she can tell you how to get approval for Dr. Nichols to make a small batch for you. If the amount is too large, he'll need to be a legally designated manufacturer and will never be able to afford the required security."

I called Ms. B.

"Can Dave Nichols make some human-grade DMT for my project?"

She began, "Well, if Dr. Nichols is going to be a manufacturer, he needs to meet rather stringent security requirements. Is there a DEA office near his university? They could drop over and tell him what he needs to do. Then Dr. Nichols could decide if he's able to meet their recommendations."

I heard the edge start creeping into my voice. I was alarmed at how close I felt to losing it.

"I've looked everywhere for human-grade DMT: Sigma and another chemical supply house, the National Institute on Drug Abuse, the National Institute of Mental Health, former investigators, Dr. C. in North Carolina. Dave Nichols is willing to make some for me, incredibly cheap. He needs your okay. I've got an outside grant, and the Research Center at the university is behind this project. I'm losing my mind. I'm pulling out my hair. My gums are bleeding. I'm getting on my wife's nerves."

There was a pause. I heard what sounded like her pushing her chair away from the desk.

"Oh," she said, sounding genuinely concerned. "Let me see here. . . Yes, there's a 'coincidental activities' clause in the regulations. Dr. Nichols can make a small batch if you're collaborating. This won't require any additional security for his laboratory."

I heard her pull a large book out from somewhere: "It's acceptable for him to make it . . ." and she started reading some text, "'. . . if and to the extent set forth . . .'"

She spoke too quickly for me to write down the information.

Ms. B. finished: "Have Dr. Nichols write me. Here's my address. He'll need to amend his current permits, saying how much DMT he'll make. I'll check with our pharmacist to be certain it's a reasonable amount."

"Okay," I said. "That sounds great. I really appreciate your help."

I called Dr. W. He confided that "off the record," my project was pointing out a flaw in the drug laws: How do researchers study drugs of abuse?

He then described exactly how to respond to the twenty requirements the FDA had written about in the four-page letter that had arrived from them several months earlier. These steps would provide the FDA the information they needed to determine if the DMT was "safe for human use."

The UNM Department of Psychiatry agreed to pay Dave Nichols three hundred dollars for the DMT. However, they would not write the check until the DEA issued the Schedule I permit.

The DEA would approve neither Dave's request to make DMT nor my Schedule I permit to possess it until the FDA approved the protocol. The FDA couldn't give me permission until I possessed the drug and tested it for safety. The DEA also required verification from the FDA that Dave could go ahead and make the drug.

Four months later, in January 1990, Dave finally received DEA approval to make the DMT. He ordered the precursors immediately and began working on it.

In the meantime, I had gotten laboratory-quality DMT from Sigma and put it into the special locked freezer in the narcotics vault in the hospital pharmacy. One hundred milligrams, a tenth of a gram, in a little vial. The Research Center began developing a method to measure DMT in human blood.

In addition, I received a high score from NIDA for a grant application to actually run the DMT study, and it was likely to be funded. Two grants approved, but no drug! It was bizarre. Everyone wanted the study done, but no one knew how to get me the drug necessary to perform it.

By February the DEA had obtained enough information from the FDA to know that the protocol was sound enough for the FDA to approve "in principle." The DEA agreed to give me the Schedule I permit. However, my contact there, Ms. L., called with some bad news.

"Diversion Control blocked the permit."

"Who's Diversion Control?" I asked.

"I'll try and get your request exempted. I'll call you next week."

The next day, Ms. B. from the DEA, the woman who had broken the logjam, called to say that Dave was indeed a manufacturer and would need additional security requirements. I didn't know what to say.

I told her, "I don't know what to say."

"Here's the name and phone number of the DEA agent in Indianapolis, near Purdue University. He's responsible for that area. He'll tell Dr. Nichols what he needs to do."

She called back that day. "I'm sorry. Dr. Nichols is making another drug, and we mixed up that one with your DMT request. My error. You may go ahead as you were planning."

Dave called later that week, saying the lawyers at Purdue were advising him not to make the DMT because of liability issues. I called Mr. W. at NIDA and asked him if there were ever any malpractice claims resulting from studies using their Schedule I drugs.

He offered some encouraging news: "We've never been sued for providing marijuana, a Schedule I drug, for human research. Just make sure you've got an airtight informed consent document."

He called back that day and put the NIDA attorney on the phone.

The attorney said, "You'd be sued first, then your university, then maybe the FDA, and last and most remotely Dr. Nichols. All he's doing is making it according to FDA regulations. He's not deciding who gives what dose to whom—that's your responsibility."

I told Dave this, and he replied, "I hope you know what you're doing. This is a real leap of faith for me and our lawyers."

May and June involved finding laboratories to run the FDA-required tests on the DMT once it arrived. One test required the DMT to be sent out, and the first two laboratories I contacted refused to work with a Schedule I drug. Finally a third company agreed to do the testing.

By July 1990, Dave had made the drug and was running all the tests on it that the FDA needed to determine its identity and purity. It was nearly 100 percent pure.

In early July he sent five grams of DMT to my clinic by overnight courier. I kept it in my office that day and drove to the hospital pharmacy to deliver it before going home.

I called Dr. W. to tell him that the DMT had arrived and that it might take a few months to get all the tests performed and collect the results.

He said, "Get everything together, and send it to Ms. R. the chemist and Ms. P. Call them a week later. They'll say they never saw your letter. Then call me in two weeks if you don't hear anything after that. Some poor guy got his approval and waited a month before we found someone to type the letter to him."

The pharmacy prepared a solution of DMT dissolved in saltwater. This was the form in which I would give DMT to the volunteers. The pharmacist divided it into one hundred separate glass vials. The samples for the FDA's tests would come from them. I had a few last-minute questions and called Ms. R. in September. We hadn't talked for a few months. "I need to refresh my memory about your case," she said. After a few additional phone calls, she provided the necessary information.

By late October all the tests were complete, and the DMT passed every one. I put together my package and sent it to the FDA by overnight mail. I started calling within a week. No one replied to the dozen messages I left with the secretary. I phoned Dr. W.

"What's the matter?" he asked. "You usually call when things aren't going well."

"May I begin the DMT study?"

"I'll just toodle on over there and find out what I can."

I called back in early November. The secretary told me their division had changed offices, but that they came by every half-hour to check for messages.

On November 5, 1990, Ms. M., my project officer, called at the end of the day. "Your hold has been removed."

"Is a verbal okay all I need?"

"Yes."

"The university won't accept that. Would you fax a letter?" I asked.

"I'll fax one tomorrow."

November in the mountains of New Mexico is cold and dry, windy and harsh. I made many of these phone calls from my house in the Manzano Mountains southeast of Albuquerque. I sometimes joked to friends that my applications had to be approved because my view was nicer than anyone's in D.C.

My former wife's weaving studio was in a separate building about fifteen yards from the main house. Hanging up the phone after that last conversation with Ms. M., I braced myself against the cold wind and slowly walked along the crunchy gravel path to the outbuilding to share the news.

"They said I could start." I lay down on the cold cement floor, staring up at the ceiling.

"That's great, dear," she replied, leaning down to ground level to kiss my cheek.

I called every day for the next ten days, asking for the fax. It arrived on November 15. At the bottom of the handwritten fax, Ms. M. wrote, "Have a Happy Thanksgiving!"

That day, the university laboratory called to tell me the DMT in the glass vials had decomposed by 30 percent; it was too weak to use. I called the laboratory technician.

"How did you calculate the concentration?"

He answered, "By using the weight of free base DMT."

"It's not free base. It's a salt."[2]

"Oh, I didn't know that. Hmm, let's see. That's right. It's the correct concentration after all. Sorry about that."

Four days later, I gave Philip the first dose of DMT.

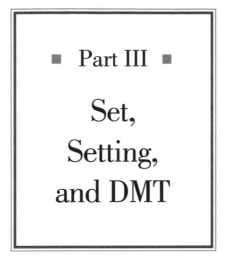

■ Part III ■

Set,
Setting,
and DMT

7

Being a Volunteer

I obtained approval for the DMT research in late 1990 and soon, with Philip and Nils as my human guinea pigs, determined the best doses and manner of administering the drug. It now was time to begin recruiting volunteers. While I found many volunteers among my longtime friends, I needed to enlarge the pool of research subjects beyond personal acquaintances.

I was reluctant to advertise. Such an announcement might have resulted in a flood of calls, and I did not have the time to speak to everyone with a casual interest. A public call for research subjects also might find its way to the local media and would draw unwanted attention.

Upon considering recruiting UNM students, I remembered the trouble that Leary and his associates encountered at Harvard when they included undergraduates into their program. If I were to canvas the university for volunteers, they would need to be graduate students, rather than the younger and less mature undergraduates. I also wanted to include no more than one representative from any department. Leary's research at

Harvard had created cliques of drug-taking graduate students. These students developed an "us" versus "them" mentality that contributed to intense conflicts within departments between those participating in psychedelic research and those who were not. Such envious and competitive ill will at Harvard was a significant factor in the ultimate expulsion of Leary's group.

Several volunteers in this new group were social or professional acquaintances. Two were academic colleagues in the psychiatry department, one was a friend of my former wife, and seven belonged to a social group to which I was introduced several years after the research began. The nearly three dozen remaining people found out about the study by word of mouth; they were friends of volunteers, received psychedelic newsletters describing the Albuquerque research, or just happened to be in a conversation during which the studies were discussed.

For the sake of convenience, I will invent a hypothetical volunteer named Alex, a thirty-two-year-old married male who worked as a software programmer outside of Santa Fe. Since most of our research subjects were men, I hope no one is put off by making our generic volunteer male.

Alex's first step was to make a phone call to my office, which was fielded by the psychiatry department secretary and subsequently answered by a member of the research team. After a brief conversation regarding age, previous psychedelic experience, and medical and psychiatric health, Alex and I made an appointment to meet in my department office.

Before this meeting took place, I sent him a packet of files, including a copy of the informed consent document for his particular study, several popular articles about DMT, and a paper I wrote some years before about the pineal gland, DMT, and consciousness. Later, when the project was well underway, I included papers describing the results of our own work.

This meeting took at least an hour. I needed to learn enough about Alex to decide whether to include him in the study. In a comparable manner, Alex needed to know I was someone he could trust to supervise his deeply psychedelic DMT experiences.

An important issue was how stable his life was at the time. If it seemed in chaos, I would be reluctant to include him. If he was in a transitional stage, he might decide to leave the area halfway through the study. If his ability to sustain relationships appeared tenuous, he might not be able to bear up in the face of the powerfully destabilizing effects of DMT. He might have problems trusting us in the hospital under the influence, or he might not be able to find enough support between sessions if his experiences were especially upsetting.

If Alex were using drugs or alcohol, he'd need to limit or stop taking them. This was especially the case if they were ones like cocaine or psychedelics, which might affect his responses to DMT.

Information about previous psychedelic drug use and experiences was crucial. The number of his experiences was not as important as their having been fully psychedelic. Because his high-dose DMT sessions probably would propel him further into psychedelic space than he had ever gone before, I wanted to be reasonably certain Alex was at least familiar with the terrain.

"What's the furthest out you've ever been on a psychedelic?" I asked Alex. "Have you thought you died? What about losing all connection to your body and the outside world?"

Just as critical was finding out if Alex was steady and responsible under the influence. In a way, I was more interested in hearing about bad trips than I was the beautiful ones, because I knew our setting would tend toward producing some unpleasant moments.

The nature of psychedelic research ideally is highly collaborative. In addition to my comfort level with Alex, he had the right, and the responsibility to himself, to know how he'd feel about my giving him DMT. Alex asked about my motivations for the research, what I hoped to find, and how we supervised sessions. He wondered if I had a religious practice, and about my own experience with psychedelics. The way I handled his concerns and questions provided him with important emotional information.

A week later, we met on 5-East, the research wing of the University of New Mexico Hospital, for his medical screening. We drew blood for basic medical tests and obtained an electrocardiogram, or ECG, to assess his heart's health.

We all gathered around to watch Alex's veins bulge under his skin after the nurse placed the tourniquet above his elbow. Good veins were an important element of a volunteer's successful participation because we drew so much blood. If Alex's veins collapsed or clotted easily, it would cause a lot of stress on study days.

I went over a painstakingly detailed medical history and performed a physical examination. The results of the medical tests were important, but equally so was the continuation of our building a close, basic relationship before giving and receiving any DMT. Asking Alex sometimes embarrassing health questions, touching, and otherwise relating at a fundamental and physical level helped establish a foundation of trust and familiarity upon which I hoped we could rely when he was in the throes of powerful, disorienting, and potentially regressive DMT sessions.

Alex's laboratory values and ECG were normal, so we scheduled the psychiatric examination. This formal psychiatric interview followed a ninety-page form and could take several hours. Laura, our research nurse, performed all these interviews; it was their first opportunity to get to know each other. Laura then sent Alex off with one more pile of questionnaires and rating scales.

After he returned them to us, we scheduled Alex's first non-blind, screening DMT sessions: a low dose of 0.05 mg/kg, followed by a high dose of 0.4 mg/kg the following day. For Alex and the other men, the first sessions could occur whenever our schedules permitted. In women's cases, we needed to standardize when in the menstrual cycle we studied them. We arranged for the women's first two doses, and all subsequent ones, to occur during the first ten days after their menstrual bleeding stopped.

On the morning of his admission, Alex left his car across the street in the monolithic parking structure facing the south side of the hospital. He told the guard he was coming in for "a research study" and got his appropriate sticker. Walking across the footbridge over busy Lomas Boulevard, he found the hospital's Admitting Office, where clerical staff checked him in as DMT-22. They directed Alex upstairs to the fifth-floor Research Center. He walked past the outpatient clinic and entered the ward through a set of double doors.

Alex signed in at the nursing desk, where one of the regular ward nurses greeted him.

"Hi, DMT-22," she said. "How are you doing?"

"Fine, although it's weird being called DMT-22."

"Oh, don't worry. We're used to it. Here, let me put your ID band on you."

She attached this identification to his wrist, then walked Alex down to Room 531.

At first, we used whatever room happened to be available in the Research Center. It was best to have a quiet one—far from the nurses' station, away from the bustling kitchen, but not too close to the double doors leading onto 5-East.

Some days we had little choice about which room we could use, and the setting could be grim. For example, occasionally we had to use a lead-lined room at the very end of the ward designed for patients who were receiving radioactive implants for cancer. Other days we might need to use the "traction room," where patients stayed who suffered from multiple trauma and fractured bones. A "cage" over the bed provided several convenient access points from which to attach ropes, pulleys, and cables for suspending casted broken limbs. A few volunteers professed that they didn't mind the cage, but I found it intimidating and disconcerting. After one or two sessions maneuvering around it, I made certain to disassemble this structure before we got started.

Another room on the same end of the ward was the bone marrow transplant room. Absolutely sanitized, with a ceiling full of high-powered fans and two sets of double doors partitioning off an anteroom, it was a germ-free environment where these highly infection-prone patients could remain in relative safety. Thankfully, there were switches with which I could turn off the fans.

We needed a nicer room. I requested to remodel a room on the ward over which we would have scheduling priority. The budget in my grant from the National Institute on Drug Abuse included funds for this renovation. We chose Room 531.

This room was square, about fifteen feet to a side, and relatively quiet, being the last one on the north side of the hall. At the end of the hall was the door to a hospital stairwell, and across it, but nearer the stairway, was the lead-lined room. Directly across from Room 531 was the entrance to the bone marrow transplant room, but from our doorway, it was hard to see what was in it.

We met with the hospital's clinical engineering department and made several modifications to the room. Carpenters built a cover over the tubes and hoses emerging from the panel behind the bed and a little closet below the sink to hide its pipes. Extra insulation on the top and bottom of the door more efficiently sealed the room from hallway sounds. And, after one particularly unnerving session in which the public address system blared repeatedly from the speaker in the ceiling, the electrician designed a switch, controlled at the nurses' station, that turned off the room's speaker.

We could do little about the bed, because it needed to be a regulation unit, and specially built hospital beds are outrageously expensive. A wooden headboard and footboard added a somewhat more pleasant touch. However, nicer furniture made a big difference: a rocking chair and foot-rest for me, a comfortable oversized chair for Laura or other research nurses, and two visitors' chairs.

My former wife, a tapestry artist, and I pored over dozens of swatches of material for the chairs before finding one that met all our needs. The design needed to be relatively soothing, but not so dull as to dampen or depress the volunteers' mood and perceptions upon opening their eyes. Another requirement was that it be consistent with the particular type of visual effects wrought by DMT, but not so stimulating that volunteers would be startled or disoriented looking at the furniture in their highly altered state. The best fit was a pleasing blue, subtly multicolored, with speckles, flecks, and patterns embedded within it. A solid light blue carpet and soothing pale blue paint covering the formerly bright white walls were the final pieces of the refurbishing effort.

These changes to Room 531 nevertheless left several minor, but insurmountable, problems. Because the room now had become almost soundproofed from the outside hall, the ceiling fan seemed louder than ever. Many volunteers paid this no heed, but for others it was an irritant. In addition, the bathroom shared a wall with the shower between our room and the next. When someone used the shower, we could hear it quite well. If that person happened to be ill, their coughs, groans, and cries were audible through the wall.

Another factor over which we had no control was noise from outside of the hospital. The busy Albuquerque International Airport and a major U.S. Air Force base were only five miles south of the hospital. While flight patterns usually were concentrated south of town, away from the hospital, weather occasionally forced jets to fly overhead. The noise, although buffered by double-paned windows, could be jarring. Sounds from the hospital grounds also could be grating, especially those arising from the trash compactor located right below Room 531's window.

Once Alex settled himself into Room 531, the ward nurse who walked him down the hall checked his heart rate, blood pressure, weight, and temperature. Someone from the research kitchen staff came by and asked Alex what he'd like to eat after the study: a snack, late breakfast, early lunch, vegetarian or meat, what to drink. We rarely received complaints about the food!

Laura was the research nurse working with us that day. She arrived and began the preparations for the low dose. She placed a blue, plastic-lined cloth, about fourteen inches square, under Alex's arm. This cloth protects the bed linens from the antiseptic iodine solution. The cloth also absorbs any blood that might drip out of the intravenous line before she can cap it. She began scrubbing his forearm skin over the vein in which she was to insert the intravenous line with the antiseptic. She placed the blood pressure cuff on the other arm and took another heart rate and blood pressure reading.

On these first non-blind DMT test days, we drew no blood. Rather, a single small needle was all we needed for administering DMT. However, if we were going to take blood samples, Laura would insert another more complicated apparatus into the other arm. This setup consisted of several extra pieces of plastic "plumbing" that permitted drawing blood into syringes, while at the same time providing a steady drip of sterile saltwater into the vein. After drawing blood, Laura would squirt a little bit of heparin, a blood-thinning drug, into the line to reduce the likelihood of any clots. Clogging of that needle made for a very difficult day, since we were so dependent upon measuring levels of various substances in the blood.

On blood-drawing days, we had to keep the samples chilled, and for this purpose we would keep a basin filled with ice chips next to the bed. Test tubes waited for transferring blood collected from the syringes. It was best to remove the tops from these vacuum tubes before the study began; otherwise, they made a loud distracting "pop" when opened.

Finally, there was the rectal probe, or "thermistor." We wanted to measure temperature several times before, during, and after DMT administration. The least trouble was to have the thermometer in place throughout the session, rather than requiring Alex to actively interact with yet one more piece of equipment. And the most accurate temperature readings are from the rectum. All these factors added up to a rectal probe. Laura inserted it a half-hour before the study, and it stayed in place until we were done. The probe was about an eighth of an inch in diameter; it was made out of rubber-coated wire and was quite flexible. It went in about four to six inches and rarely caused any discomfort, except in those with hemorrhoids. Despite being taped in place, it sometimes slipped out if a volunteer was especially restless during the session. Only Nils refused the rectal probe.

The thermistor attached to a small portable computer that recorded temperature every minute. We clipped this to the handrail of the bed, and after the session was complete, I downloaded the data directly onto the Research Center's computers.

By the time all of these preparations were complete, even for a double-blind blood-drawing day, Alex had been in the room for no more than 20 minutes. We were efficient.

I usually arrived on the ward about 30 to 40 minutes before hoping to give the DMT. Asking the admitting nurse at the front desk how Alex seemed gave me the first sense of what the morning might be like. In Room 531, Alex and I exchanged a few pleasantries before I went to pick up the DMT.

Walking down six flights to the basement, I turned right, making my way down the container-strewn hall. The solid metal pharmacy door was to the left. In bold letters, a sign commanded, "DON'T RING MORE THAN ONCE. PUSH GENTLY AND QUICKLY AFTER THE DOOR UN-LOCKS." I pushed the intercom buzzer. A closed-circuit camera stared down at me.

There were days when, despite my better judgement, I did buzz more than once—I could wait in the hallway only so long. There also were days when I wasn't quick enough to push open the door when the lock released, and I had to ring again.

Inside, a waist-high countertop ran along the length of a narrow antechamber. From it rose a four-foot-high wall of thick glass, probably bullet-proof. Behind the glass stood several busy pharmacists, and beyond them was the storage site for all the hospital's medications, including the narcotics vault.

The research pharmacist unlocked the narcotics room, went behind another set of doors, and unlocked the little freezer containing our drugs. He had filled the syringe with the prearranged dose of DMT the previous night. He only capped the syringe, because attaching a needle was cumbersome and potentially dangerous—he might accidentally inject himself with DMT. The drug solution in the syringe was frozen, and I put it in my breast pocket so that it could begin to thaw while I signed various forms.

Returning to the ward, I told the nurses at the front desk that the injection would take place in about 15 minutes. My warning was intended to help lend a slightly quieter air to the usually very busy ward. They had heard enough strange stories from the volunteers, and sometimes even yells and cries from the study room, to know that something serious was about to begin. They switched off the public address system to Room 531 and awaited my return an hour or so later. I went to the medication room and prepared a syringe full of sterile saltwater for the flush that followed the DMT injection. I fastened a needle to the top of the DMT-containing syringe. Finally, I stuffed a few alcohol swabs into my pocket for use in wiping off the end of the IV tube into which I'd inject Alex's DMT.

I reentered Alex's room and placed the "Session in Progress. Do Not

Disturb" sign on the outside of the door. Sometimes even this didn't work. Once or twice housekeeping staff, accustomed to entering hospital rooms at will, noisily intruded upon sessions. Unexpected phone calls also were not welcome. Making certain the phone was unplugged from the outlet in the wall, I walked around Alex's bed and took my seat.

"Here's the DMT," I said, pulling out the little syringe from my shirt pocket and placing it on the bed next to Alex's leg.

We spent a few minutes catching up on any important news and preparing for the session. While we were talking, I opened up the top drawer of the nightstand near his bed and took out another vial of sterile saltwater. Inserting the needle into the vial, I drew back enough saline to nearly fill the DMT-containing syringe. This additional volume in the syringe made it easier to control the rate of injection. The nurses wanted me to keep the saline vials for this purpose separate from the ones they used. They were afraid that if a drop or two of DMT leaked into one of their vials, it might cause an unwelcome and unexpected "trip" in one of the ward's other residents.

Initiating my own ritual while talking and listening, I placed my yellow notepad in a clipboard and wrote down Alex's DMT number, the date, the protocol number, and the dose. In the left-hand margin, I scribbled a column of minutes at which I would measure blood pressure and heart rate: -30, -1, 2, 5, 10, 15, 30.

I asked, "Did you have any dreams last night?"

A volunteer's dreams the night before a study might give us insights into fears, hopes, and wishes about the upcoming session, or about previous ones. Alex couldn't recall any.

I pulled the saltwater-flush syringe and the alcohol swabs out of my pocket, placing them all on the bed next to the DMT solution.

"Did you take any medications this morning or last night?"

"No."

"What are you doing after today's session?"

"I've got a few hours of work to do. Then, not too much. Relax, think about tomorrow. Get a good night's sleep."

Sometimes these little visits took the form of brief counseling or therapy sessions. Relationship problems, career or school concerns, spiritual or religious issues raised by participation in this research—all these were important to air before beginning such deep and profound journeying through the DMT realms.

I started telling Alex what to expect.

"Today's DMT dose is small. You might not notice too much from it. But don't be too blasé. It's better to be too prepared than caught off-guard. We won't do much after the DMT's in you. We'll sit quietly, be alert, pay attention to you, be available, hold good thoughts and feelings for you. If you need human contact, just put out your hand and someone will take it. If you lose control, we're here to help. Otherwise, this is your experience, not ours. You're pretty much on your own."

In the first series of DMT studies, I recommended that volunteers close their eyes to start, and open them as effects began fading. Sometimes, however, the shock of the first minute or two of the high-dose DMT experience would cause an almost reflex opening of the eyes in an attempt to orient. This almost always made things worse. The room, already rather forbidding, could take on even more troubling overtones, and the research nurse and I, our visages hopelessly transfigured, did not look much more appealing. Now we placed black eyeshades on all the volunteers at this point in the session. The eyeshades were the soft satin ones airline travelers use, or those who need to sleep during daylight hours. It was difficult finding any at the local drugstores.

Once this orientation was done, I said, "Spend as much time as you like getting ready. It might help to focus on your breath, how your body feels on the bed. That will start the process of letting go.

"When you're ready, let me know. I'll tell you when it's about 5 to 10 seconds before the beginning of the injection. I like to start giving the drug when the second hand of my watch is in an easy-to-read position.

"I'll now clean off the tubing with a little alcohol swab. Like this. The alcohol will quickly evaporate, so the smell won't distract you. I'll now insert the needle into the tubing, but I won't empty out the DMT. It's easier for me to have the needle in place beforehand. That way I won't fumble around trying to fit it in right as the injection should begin.

"I'll tell you when I start. It might feel cold, or tingly. Maybe it will burn slightly, or feel a little bubbly; some people describe those sensations. The DMT goes in over 30 seconds. Once it's all in, I'll tell you. Then there will be 15 seconds of saltwater flush of the tubing, to make sure all of the DMT gets into you and there's none left in the line. I'll tell you when I start and finish the flush, too. Any questions so far?"

"That's pretty straightforward."

The ebb and flow of tension in the room at this point was always fascinating. Only one of our many volunteers had ever used a recreational drug intravenously before, and no one had taken a psychedelic that way. The novelty of this element itself was sufficient to get all our nerve endings more alert than usual.

As I described the process to Alex and prepared this small dose, I was thinking ahead to how Alex would negotiate tomorrow's high dose. However, there was no guarantee that this minor dose might not have some major effects. Several people did drop out after this first session. Others we had to excuse because their blood pressure surpassed our predetermined cutoff point.

I continued: "Alex, it starts fast. Perhaps even before the injection is done. It can be a little frightening. Do your best to remain alert and relaxed, poised but passive. The effects will peak in a couple of minutes. Then relax and wait a while until you decide to start talking. It's tempting to speak right away, but you'll miss some of the subtle coming-down effects if you don't wait at least 10 or 15 minutes, even today. So, let's get started. Are you ready?"

Alex answered, "Sure, I'm ready."

For the deep letting go and relaxing necessary to successfully experience the full effects of DMT, it was best if the volunteers were lying down for the injection. Otherwise, there might be a lot of fussing involved with maneuvering Alex into a more comfortable position as he was losing normal awareness of his body and the rush of psychedelic effects began.

We adjusted his bed. Some volunteers liked their head a little elevated. A few preferred to have their knees slightly bent, for which we raised that part of the bed or placed a pillow under the knees. We made sure the eyeshades fit loosely but securely.

A few deep breaths, some adjusting of clothes, arms, legs, feet, and then Alex's words:

"Go ahead."

"Good. Let's start in about 5 seconds here. . . . Okay, I'll start right now."

Gently pressing on the plunger of the syringe, I hoped there would be no obstruction, which would indicate a clot or that the needle had worked its way loose out of the vein.

The syringe was empty at 30 seconds. I pulled it out of the line.

"The DMT's in."

Using my teeth, I pulled off the cap covering the needle attached to the saltwater syringe. Inserting that needle, I said, "Here's the flush now."

Fifteen seconds later, pulling out that needle: "All right, I'm all done."

In addition to familiarizing Alex with the technical details of getting IV DMT on this low-dose day, it was an excellent time to instruct him in filling out the questionnaire. We might spend an hour going over any questions he had about what particular terms or phrases meant. After a few sessions, Alex could complete the questionnaire in 10 minutes.

Before wrapping up this session, I said to him, "Don't eat or drink too much tonight. Get a good night's sleep. Remember to skip breakfast. If you must have coffee, make sure you drink it at least two hours before you come in."

This was commonsense advice. If the DMT brought on intense nausea, it was best to have an empty stomach. However, it wasn't worth bringing on a coffee-withdrawal headache.

I dated the note in DMT-22's chart and wrote: "Low dose tolerated without incident. Patient sent home on overnight pass from the hospital. Will return tomorrow a.m. for high dose."

Alex returned the next morning. We followed the same preliminary routine until it was time for the injection. I looked over at Laura, on the other side of the bed, and noted that there was a vomit basin close enough for her to pick up, just in case. Tossing the used alcohol swabs and their wrappers into the nearby wastebasket, I began, "It comes on just as fast, but it's a lot stronger. It may startle you. Don't bother trying to resist, because it's usually impossible."

"Okay." Alex smiled thinly but determinedly.

"What do you normally do when you find yourself overwhelmed in a psychedelic experience?"

"I usually breath deeply and slowly. That's something I learned from my years of meditation. Or I may touch these," he said, fingering his necklace of Tibetan prayer beads.

Other volunteers might hold a fetish, a rock or piece of wood. Some might hum, sing, or chant. A few evoked the image of a teacher, friend, or loved one. Those with a deep and sustained meditation practice started meditating before the DMT went in and tried to maintain that mental balance throughout the session.

I said, "Sometimes people think they've died, or are dying, or that we've overdosed them. So far, no one's been injured. This is a physically safe dose, although your blood pressure and heart rate will probably take a nice jump. We can respond if there are problems.

"If you think you've died, there's two ways I tell people they can deal with it. One is 'Man, I'm dying, and I'm going to kick and scream and try and stop it.' The other is 'Okay, I'm dying, now let's see what this is like. Very interesting.' Easier said than done, of course."

"I know what you're talking about."

"You probably won't notice the first blood pressure reading at 2 minutes. You'll most likely be down enough at 5 minutes to feel that one."

I was done marking my notepad: DMT-22, date, protocol number, dose. Blood pressure and heart rate columns.

When all was said and done, we three—Alex, Laura, and myself—looked at each other. If a plane were flying overhead, we paused, waiting for it to pass. As the time for the injection approached, the air in the room and on the ward took on a certain density. There was little more to say.

Alex put on the eyeshades, and we lowered the head of the bed. I prepared all the syringes and moved my chair closer. Laura warmed up her hands, getting ready to hold Alex's if he needed a loving touch.

"Are you ready?" I asked.

"Yes." Barely audible.

Laura said, "Good luck. We'll be here waiting."

I watched the second hand of my watch as it approached the 9. I said, "I'll start in about 5 to10 seconds."

Then, as the second hand hit the 12, I told him quietly, "I'm beginning the injection now. . . ."

Ten, 20, 30 seconds, slowly emptying the drug into Alex's vein. My feelings at this point were always intense and contradictory: jealousy of his impending fantastic experience, sadness for any pain he might undergo, doubt mixed with certainty regarding the wisdom of what I was doing.

"The DMT's in."

Time was speeding up and slowing down at the same time. My movements felt quick, but also leaden. Was Alex going to be all right? Could he manage his trip? I felt my heart beating in my chest. Could *we* manage his trip?

There was no turning back.

"Here's the flush. . . ."

Before I could finish my sentence, Alex murmured,

Here it comes. . . .

He took in an enormous breath, then sighed it out loudly, just as I finished saying, "The flush is done."

I knew he probably had not heard the end of my sentence. Nor would he likely remember his loud exhalation.

Leaning back into my chair, I sighed, too, although silently, looking over at my nurse colleague, then gazing down at Alex, his body motionless. One minute. Ninety seconds. It was almost time for the first blood pressure check. He would be peaking and wouldn't feel the iron grip of the cuff.

His words echoed in my head and my heart.

Here it comes. . . .

8

Getting DMT

Twelve subjects participated in the original dose-response study, which took most of 1991 to perform. They each received non-blind low and high doses of DMT and subsequently got the same doses double-blind. Two intermediate doses and a saline placebo completed this series of injections.

Once we had thoroughly characterized DMT's effects in the dose-response study, the first follow-up project investigated whether it was possible to develop tolerance to repeated injections of DMT.

Tolerance occurs when the same dose of a drug produces smaller effects when taken repeatedly. LSD, psilocybin, and mescaline all produce rapid and nearly complete tolerance after three or four daily doses. In other words, an amount that had quite profound psychedelic effects on the first day, given every day, would be barely noticeable on the fourth.

DMT appeared unique in that tolerance was quite difficult to demonstrate, even in animals given full doses every two hours around the clock for twenty-one days in a row. The only published human study couldn't elicit tolerance when researchers gave full intramuscular doses twice a day for five days.[1]

"Field" reports among recreational DMT users were inconsistent. Some believed they could smoke DMT all night with no diminishing effects, while others described being able to use it only three or four times in a row before they seemed immune to it. However, an important factor in these field stories is fatigue—it's difficult to inhale large volumes of DMT vapor time and time again at one sitting. Maybe this "tolerance" was the result of not getting enough DMT into the lungs after the second or third trip.

DMT's lack of tolerance development also was one of the factors making it a likely naturally occurring schizotoxin. If tolerance to endogenous DMT did develop, psychotic symptoms of schizophrenia, for example, would last only as long as it took for tolerance to build up. Since psychotic symptoms are usually chronic and constant, demonstrating that DMT could not elicit tolerance would be powerful evidence that it could play a role in these disorders.

There were other reasons a tolerance study intrigued me. The brevity of DMT's action seemed to limit its usefulness as a tool for any inner psychological or spiritual work. All one could do was hold on tight through the rush. By the time volunteers got their bearings, they were already coming down. Repeated entrance into the DMT state might provide better conditions for applying its incredibly profound psychedelic properties.

Another less clearly articulated reason for performing this study right after the dose-response one was that it was a "pure" DMT study. Protocols following up the tolerance project would start investigating mechanisms of action by modifying brain serotonin and other receptors using various drugs in combination with DMT. Something in me knew that these studies, which attempted to replicate animal laboratory experiments in humans, would be difficult. In retrospect, I think that I wanted to delay getting on with those types of projects as long as possible.

I proposed that DMT's short duration was the reason previous studies failed to demonstrate tolerance. LSD, psilocybin, and mescaline tolerance experiments all used once-daily doses. However, their effects last 6 to 12 hours, while those of DMT were much shorter. This suggested the need to give DMT at much shorter intervals, every 30 to 60 minutes, in order to demonstrate reduced responses over time.

The other option was a continuous intravenous infusion, a "drip" of DMT into volunteers' veins. However, I liked the idea of people "coming down" after each injection so we could hear what had happened. With a continuous drip, communication would be problematic.

After two months of trial and error, I determined that the best regime was four injections of 0.3 mg/kg DMT given at 30-minute intervals. This dose, while highly psychedelic, was just below our highest, 0.4 mg/kg. One man, Cal, was able to manage four 0.4 mg/kg injections at half-hour intervals. However, his wife, Linda, was completely spent after three doses and refused the fourth and final one during this preliminary work. Remembering the harrowing nature of giving too much DMT to Philip and Nils, I backed off without argument and settled for one notch less. Better safe than sorry.

We enrolled thirteen volunteers in the tolerance study, many of whom had already participated in the dose-response project. New research subjects went through the same screening and received their non-blind low and high doses.

While the tolerance experiment was double-blind and saline-placebo-controlled, the "blind" became apparent within a few seconds of the first injection. It was either a big dose of DMT or saline. And, if it was DMT, there would be three more big trips before the morning was over.

We drew blood samples similar to those for the dose-response project and gave a shortened version of the rating scale that took only about five minutes to fill out. The timing was split-second but worked perfectly. Volunteers began talking at about 10 to 15 minutes, and then filled out the rating scale. We'd have a chance to process their trip and get ready for the next one over the ensuing 5 to 10 minutes. If it were four injections of saltwater, we spent the morning in more casual conversation.

This study showed that there was no tolerance to the psychological effects of repeated DMT injections. The experience was as intensely psychedelic the fourth time as it was the first. Because of this, and as I had hoped, subjects were much more able to process and do something with the repeated high dose than with a single isolated experience. Many of the most moving tales from DMT volunteers in the following chapters derive from this study.[2]

After demonstrating what DMT *did*, the biomedical model requires determining *how* those effects occur. These are *mechanism-of-action* studies. As our research was pharmacologically based, these follow-up experiments would attempt to establish which brain receptors mediated DMT's effects.

The first of these was the pindolol project. Pindolol is a drug used in medical practice to lower high blood pressure. It does this by blocking certain adrenaline receptors. Another property of pindolol is that it obstructs one particular type of serotonin receptor in the brain, the serotonin "1A" site. Since DMT attaches firmly to 1A receptors in animal brains, this site might be involved in DMT's effects. If, for example, blocking the 1A site with pindolol made for a "less emotional" experience relative to DMT alone, we would propose that the 1A site regulated the emotional responses brought on by DMT. As it turned out, pindolol markedly *enhanced* the psychological and blood pressure effects of DMT.

Eleven volunteers participated in the pindolol study, several of whom were veterans of the dose-response and tolerance ones. This protocol yielded less dramatic examples of inner work than did the tolerance study, although there were remarkably powerful single experiences.

The next serotonin receptor blockade study used cyproheptadine, an antihistamine drug with additional anti-serotonin properties. In this case, cyproheptadine prevents drugs from attaching to the serotonin "2" site, the receptor researchers believe is the most important in controlling how psychedelics work.

This protocol was identical in design to that of the pindolol study in that volunteers received cyproheptadine several hours before DMT. Eight volunteers completed this study. Most were new recruits.

There appeared to be some suppression of effects, so we gave the high dose, 0.4 mg/kg, with and without the serotonin blocker. Because cyproheptadine clearly did not magnify DMT's effects, we hoped that using this large dose would give us the best chance of establishing a significant level of DMT suppression. However, the sedating properties of the drug were so pronounced that they complicated interpretation of the data. It was difficult to tell how much was specific DMT blockade, and how much was general tranquilization.

At this juncture, it was becoming difficult to bring in first-time research subjects, or to induce experienced ones to return. Who wanted to take a drug that would suppress the effects of DMT? I could draw people in to this study by emphasizing that they would get two unadulterated high doses: one on the first screening day, and the other in combination with placebo-cyproheptadine. However, I heard myself sounding apologetic for this project, a bit like a used-car salesman.

I initiated several other experiments that received university and FDA approval. However, they did not receive enough funding to perform full-scale investigations.

One of these, the naltrexone study, continued with mechanism-of-action experiments designed to determine brain receptors regulating DMT effects. In this case, naltrexone blocks opiate receptors, and for that purpose it is helpful in treating heroin addiction. Animal data showed some interaction between opiates and psychedelics, and naltrexone might help us find out more about that relationship in humans.

We began preliminary work in three volunteers for this project. However, one fellow felt so bad on naltrexone alone that he dropped out after his first session. In the other two men, we saw little effect one way or the other, and so we went no further.

Another pilot project was to assess if the phase of the menstrual cycle in women affected the DMT response. Many women report cyclical variations in their sensitivity to psychedelics. In addition, animal studies clearly indicated that sex hormones influenced responses to psychedelic and other serotonin-active drugs.

We divided the cycle into early, middle, and late in one woman, Willow, who usually had quite deep and insightful DMT experiences. In this sole volunteer, no obvious differences in psychological effects emerged. Since we didn't have funding to pursue this fascinating line of DMT research, we brought in no more volunteers for it.

We also turned some high technology onto the DMT state. Three men received 0.4 mg/kg DMT doses at the Research Center while we recorded their brain waves using an EEG, or electroencephalogram. We hoped this would show us which brain areas were more or less active during the DMT intoxication.

These were difficult studies, as the EEG machine was extraordinarily bulky and noisy and required constant adjustments. As well, there were eighteen electrodes firmly attached to volunteers' scalps, glued in place by some of the strongest-smelling contact cement I have ever encountered. While all three subjects had "full" responses to DMT, the setting was terribly unpleasant. I recruited no more volunteers than these three, wanting first to be sure the data were so impressive as to justify the discomfort. The results were not especially striking, and we ran no more EEG experiments.

Finally, I took advantage of some state-of-the-art brain-imaging research taking place at the University of New Mexico. This was "functional magnetic resonance imaging," a modified MRI head scan that measures brain metabolism, rather than just its structure. For example, we might be able to show that the brain areas involved in vision were using more sugar after a visual DMT experience.

To an even greater extent than the EEG equipment, the MRI equipment absolutely dominated the setting. This scanner, support equipment, and staff required their own building on the other side of campus. These were the only DMT studies ever performed outside the Research Center.

The MRI machine generates intensely high energy magnetic fields, and there can be no metal anywhere in the room, or in the person's body. Otherwise, that metal gets instantly and irresistibly pulled into the machine. To accommodate the scanner, the room is cavernous, and it is kept quite cool because this reduces the power necessary to maintain the magnetic fields.

The space into which we slid volunteers for their scans was a very narrow shiny metallic tube. I knew many people suffered their first panic attack during an MRI scan because of the cramped quarters into which one has to fit for the procedure. I now saw why.

Worst of all was the noise. The machine contains a massive coil that swings back and forth, much like a washing machine, only ten times as fast and hundreds of times as loud. The "BANG-BANG-BANG-BANG-BANG-BANG-BANG" of the coil reminded me of a jackhammer. Anyone in the scanner, or the room, had to wear earplugs. Even so, the tumult set one's teeth on edge.

Nevertheless, some of our research subjects were unbelievably robust. They liked DMT, they wanted to help with the experiments, and they were interested in knowing what the scans would show. I was alone with them in the MRI room while four or five other researchers sat on the opposite side of a thick "soundproof" window, in front of the instrument panels, adjusting dials, flipping switches, and keeping in contact through the intercom system. The scan began; I injected the DMT and stayed in the room throughout the session, checking blood pressure and providing moral support. During the trip, my colleagues took scans every few minutes.

For all of the effort, stress, and expectations, these data, too, were not especially revealing. The MRI team believed that major and expensive modifications to the scanner might have helped in increasing its ability to reveal DMT-induced brain changes. However, I didn't like the machine, and I didn't want to expose any more volunteers, or myself, to its deafening sound, claustrophobic quarters, and powerful magnetic fields.

While it may sound as if I had lost all modesty, or common sense, regarding what sort of studies I enrolled volunteers in, I did draw the line at radioactivity. Positron emission tomography (PET) scans provide very nice color photographic images of brain activity using what I thought were negligible amounts of radioactivity. I located some colleagues who were interested in a DMT PET scan study. PET scans would most certainly provide a more refined analysis of where DMT was acting in the brain. However, after learning about the amount of radiation involved, I decided against it.

This chapter and the last have described the set and setting of our studies: who volunteers were, and in what circumstances and studies they received DMT. Earlier chapters reviewed what we know about the drug itself. Now that the tripod of set, setting, and drug is complete, we can begin following the spirit molecule to where it leads.

9

Under the Influence

Describing what it's like in the DMT realms is about as easy as giving words to scaling a mountain peak, sexual orgasm, undersea diving, and other nonverbal but breathtakingly profound experiences. However, since most of us will never participate in a DMT research project, I will try to provide a general overview of what happens after receiving various doses of intravenous DMT.[1]

In our volunteers, a full dose of IV DMT almost instantly elicited intense psychedelic visions, a feeling that the mind had separated from the body, and overpowering emotions. These effects completely replaced whatever had occupied their minds just before drug administration. For most people, psychedelic doses of DMT were 0.2, 0.3 and 0.4 mg/kg.

Effects began within seconds of finishing the 30-second DMT infusion, and people were fully involved in the psychedelic worlds by the time I finished clearing the intravenous line with sterile saline 15 seconds later. The peak of the DMT response occurred by 2 minutes, and volunteers felt as if they were coming down at 5 minutes. Most were able

to talk about 12 to 15 minutes after drug injection, even though they remained moderately intoxicated. Nearly everyone felt relatively normal at
the 30-minute point.

We measured levels of DMT in the blood frequently after injecting it
and verified that the time course of psychological effects and DMT blood
levels overlapped exactly. That is, blood levels of DMT reached their peak
at 2 minutes and were nearly undetectable at 30. Since the brain actively
transports DMT across the blood-brain barrier into its confines, it's reasonably certain brain levels of DMT rose as quickly as blood levels.

Lower doses of DMT, 0.1 and 0.05 mg/kg, generally were not psychedelic, but certainly produced some psychological effects. These were
primarily emotional and physical, although some particularly sensitive
people had significant psychedelic and physical responses to even these
low doses. In fact, some volunteers dropped out because they didn't like
the intensity of 0.05 mg/kg. We also excused other subjects after this
small dose because their blood pressure response made us worry about
how their hearts would hold up after eight times that amount the next day.

While the profound psychological effects of DMT were progressing, the
physical self followed suit with its own constellation of responses. The
body initially reacted to a high dose of DMT with a typical "fight-or-flight"
stress reaction. Heart rate and blood pressure jumped radically, their time
course closely following the psychological responses. After a while we
could almost predict how intense a volunteer's session was by the rise in
their blood pressure.

On average, heart rate, or pulse, bolted from about 70 beats per minute
up to 100. The range, however, was wide. Some subjects' pulse climbed
up to 150, while others' got no higher than 95. Blood pressure also jumped
from values of about 110/70 to an average of 145/100. Heart rate and
blood pressure fell as rapidly as they rose, already beginning to taper off
between the 2- and 5-minute recordings.

Every pituitary gland hormone we measured increased rapidly. For
example, blood levels of the endogenous morphine-like chemical beta-
endorphin begin a steep ascent at 2 minutes following DMT administration

and reached their peak at 5 minutes. DMT also stimulated sharp spikes in the release of vasopressin, prolactin, growth hormone, and corticotropin. The last is a hormone responsible for stimulating the adrenal glands, which then release cortisol, a powerful, all-purpose stress steroid similar to cortisone. The elevations of these hormones may have exerted some psychological effects—I'll discuss this in chapter 21.

Pupil diameter doubled, from 4 millimeters to nearly 8, with a high dose of DMT, with biggest responses at 2 minutes. Body temperature took longer to rise, beginning at 15 minutes and continuing to climb by the time we removed the rectal temperature monitor at 60 minutes.

Of all the biological factors we measured, the only one that did not increase was the pineal gland hormone melatonin. This was startling, and again brought home to me the incredibly mysterious nature of this potential spirit gland.

It may be that outside-administered DMT was not a powerful-enough stimulus to overcome the pineal defense mechanism we've discussed previously. While it's clear that stress hormones rose in response to the spirit molecule, they may not have gotten high enough to stimulate daytime melatonin production.

Another possibility is that exogenous DMT actually did stimulate the pineal to make more of its own *endogenous* DMT. However, our method of measuring DMT in the blood would not have been able to distinguish between the two sources of the spirit molecule.

Volunteers, of course, did not feel the rise in prolactin or experience in their consciousness their elevated blood pressure. Rather, it was in their minds that the images, feelings, and thoughts defined the essence of the spirit molecule's effects.

The initial moments of the first non-blind high dose of DMT overwhelmed almost everyone. There was an intense, rapidly developing, and at least temporarily anxiety-provoking "rush" throughout the body and mind. This rush began even before I had finished the saline flush.

It is difficult to do justice in describing the rush. My dictionary uses such terms as "a sudden turbulent movement, drive, or onset; a feeling of urgency or haste; a swift or violent movement." Almost without thinking, several volunteers blurted out, as effects began, "Here we go!" Some compared this feeling to a "freight train," "ground zero," or a "nuclear cannon." Several people reported that the "breath caught in my throat" or "the wind was knocked out of me." Those who previously had smoked DMT were at an advantage in being able to anticipate its disorienting onset. However, they believed the rush of IV DMT was more rapid and powerful than that of the smoked method.

Nearly everyone remarked on the "vibrations" brought on by DMT, the sense of powerful energy pulsing through them at a very rapid and high frequency. Typical comments were: "I was worried that the vibration would blow my head up," "The colors and vibration were so intense I thought I would pop," "I didn't think I would stay in my skin."

This tidal wave of DMT effects quickly led to losing awareness of the body, causing some volunteers to think they had died. This dissociation of body and mind paralleled the development of peak visual effects. We typically heard phrases like: "I no longer had a body," "My body dissolved—I was pure awareness." There seemed to be a clearly identifiable sense of movement of consciousness away from the body, such as "falling," "lifting up," "flying," a feeling of weightlessness, or rapid movement.

Some male volunteers, but no females, experienced localized sensations in their genitals. While sometimes these were pleasurable, for others they were emotionally neutral or bland. No one ejaculated.

The rush of early effects almost inevitably caused some fear and anxiety. However, most volunteers quickly settled in to the experience within 15 to 30 seconds by deep breathing, physical relaxation, or whatever else they knew would help them to deeply let go. Perhaps because of their previous psychedelic experience, they frequently could separate their emotions from their body's physical reaction without panicking.

Visual images were the predominant sensory effects of a full dose of DMT. Usually there was little difference between what volunteers "saw" with their eyes opened or closed. However, opening the eyes often caused the visions to overlay what was in the room. This had a disorienting effect, and it was less confusing to keep their eyes closed. That's one of the reasons we decided to place black silk eyeshades on all the volunteers before we gave any DMT.

Subjects saw all sorts of imaginable and unimaginable things. The least complex were kaleidoscopic geometric patterns, which sometimes partook of "Mayan," "Islamic," or "Aztec" qualities. For example, "beautiful, colorful pink cobwebs; an elongation of light," "tremendously intricate tiny geometric colors, like being one inch from a color television."

The colors of this imagery were brighter, more intense, and deeper than those of normal awareness or dreams: "It was like the blue of a desert sky, but on another planet. The colors were a hundred times deeper." Background and foreground distinctions might merge so that countless images would occupy a volunteer's visual field. It was impossible to tell what was "in front" and what was "behind." Many used the term "four-dimensional" or "beyond dimensionality" to describe this effect.

There were more formed, specific visual images, too. These included "a fantastic bird," "a tree of life and knowledge," and "a ballroom with crystal chandeliers." There were "tunnels," "stairways," "ducts," and "a spinning golden disc." Others saw the "inner workings" of machines or bodies: "inside a computer's boards," "DNA double helices," and "the pulsating diaphragm around my heart."

Even more impressive was the apprehension of human and "alien" figures that seemed to be aware of and interacting with the volunteers. Non-human entities might be recognizable: "spiders," "mantises," "reptiles," and "something like a saguaro cactus."

Visual effects lingered as volunteers' bodies rapidly metabolized the DMT. The room was uncomfortably bright when they removed the eyeshades or opened their eyes. Objects in the room took on a wavy, undulating motion, radiating with their own inner light. Subjects commented on an exaggerated depth perception, sometimes being mesmerized by the patterns in the wooden bathroom door.

A few participants told us of a peculiar breakdown in the normal fluidity of their vision: "Your movements were not your own, they were no longer smooth and coordinated," and "You guys looked robotic; moving jerkier, more mechanical, geometric."

About half the volunteers experienced auditory effects: sounds were different, or they heard things that we did not. These were most pronounced during the DMT rush. Sometimes this was little more than intensification of normal hearing. Others became functionally deaf and did not hear the grinding motor of the blood pressure machine or any other outside sounds.

However, it was quite rare for volunteers to hear formed voices or music. Rather, there were simply sounds, variously described as "high-pitched," "whining and whirring," "chattering," "crinkling and crunching." Many remarked on the similarity of DMT auditory effects to those of nitrous oxide, where there is a "wah-wah," oscillating, wavering distortion of sounds. Occasionally there were the sorts of things one hears in cartoons: comical "sproing, boing" noises.

Sometimes volunteers did lose their bearings and forgot that they were in a hospital or involved in a research study. Bespeaking their mental strength and agility, some retained their perspective even in this condition: "My mind was definitely in a different place, but it was commenting on the state as it was going on." Nevertheless, there were sessions when the confusion of the initial rush stayed with the volunteer until drug effects began wearing off.

Most people found the high dose of DMT exciting, euphoric, and extraordinarily pleasurable. Sometimes this ecstasy related to the visions. The elation also might come from new insights gained during the session: "I feel great, like I had a revelation." Often, it was pure bliss without any particular object.

For others the fear and anxiety were nearly unbearable. Comments such as "I hated it. I've never been so frightened," "menacing," "incredible torture; I thought it would never end" refer to these feelings.

While many research subjects experienced powerful feelings on DMT, both negative and positive, some commented on how unemotional their high-dose sessions were: "I tried to get myself worked up over what I was seeing, but I just wasn't able to respond emotionally."

Once DMT effects established themselves, the drug had surprisingly little effect on volunteers' ability to think and reason. "My intellect wasn't altered at all. I was just alert to what was unfolding during the experience"; "As I started coming down a little, I got journalistic. I became an observer."

Others, however, sensed their thinking was abnormal and, in fact, even wondered if DMT might cause psychotic thought processes. "Everything looked right, but just a little off. It seemed as if the clock was just starting to move every time I looked at it. The colors in the room were malevolent." Another said, "You know how schizophrenics talk about different meanings to things? A leaf on the ground takes on great significance? That kind of thing."

One common effect was a loss of normal time perception. For example, nearly everyone was surprised at how late in the session it was by the time they found out the time, believing only a few minutes had passed. Nevertheless, there was a sense of timelessness in the peak DMT state: they experienced an enormous amount in those first few minutes.

Volunteers usually found the high dose caused an almost complete loss of control. They felt utterly helpless, incapacitated, unable to function or interact in the "real" world: "I felt like an infant, helpless, unable to do anything." DMT volunteers decided, at this point, they were happy to be in the hospital! Beyond their own loss of control, some volunteers felt another "intelligence" or "force" directing their minds in an interactive manner. This was especially common in cases of contact with "beings."

Almost every research subject believed their first non-blind high dose of DMT brought them "higher than they had ever been." However, this first session usually was more anxiety-ridden than any other high doses they received subsequently. Once volunteers were prepared to lose control, it was easier for them to do so. They understood that the drug experience was essentially safe, that they would live through it and not suffer any psychological or physical damage. What also helped was their growing confidence in our ability to support their regressed condition as our work together progressed.

While the most stunning effects came from the high doses of DMT, smaller ones also produced a variety of responses, many of which volunteers found pleasurable and interesting.

The tolerance study dose, 0.3 mg/kg, was fully psychedelic, and for some was their "dose of choice," causing the full spectrum of mind-altering effects with slightly less anxiety.

The next lower dose, 0.2 mg/kg, was the threshold at which typical psychedelic effects reliably emerged. Nearly everyone had relatively intense visual imagery, but auditory effects were rare. Some particularly sensitive volunteers preferred 0.2 over 0.3 or 0.4 mg/kg.

The 0.1 mg/kg dose was the least popular. The vibratory energizing effects predominated, but there never was a breakthrough into a full psychedelic experience. Volunteers felt "left hanging," uncomfortably tense, both physically and mentally. "My body feels like pepper tastes," one said. "This dose has all the negative physical effects without any of the positive mental ones."

The lowest dose of DMT, 0.05 mg/kg, was pleasant, and almost all volunteers said they felt like smiling or laughing after receiving it. One volunteer who previously had used heroin thought this dose felt something like that drug: "There was a warm cotton batting sensation." A few people experienced relatively intense effects from this little bit of DMT we gave on the first day. This warned us that the next day's large dose might be especially powerful.

For readers familiar with other psychedelics, the effects of DMT must sound more or less typical. While its properties are similar in many ways to those of LSD, mescaline, and psilocybin, there is something peerless about the spirit molecule. I don't know if this is because it works so quickly or because it possesses a unique chemical structure. Maybe it's because the brain is familiar with, and actively seeks out, this endogenous psychedelic. Whatever the reasons, at the further limits of the spirit molecule's reach, volunteers returned with tales of encounters neither they nor I knew were possible. It is to these stories we'll now turn our attention.

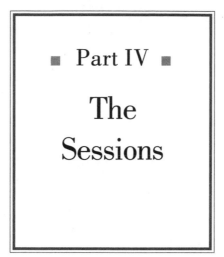

■ Part IV ■

The
Sessions

Introduction
to the Case Reports

During each DMT session, I took detailed notes of every aspect of that day's events: what volunteers said and did; how they looked, sounded, and felt to me; the state of the research ward, weather, and world politics; the behavior and emotional tone of others in the room with us, including the research nurse, family or friends of the volunteer, and visitors; and my own thoughts and feelings.

After I got back to my office, I dictated these notes, and my secretary transcribed the dictation into a word-processor file. When printed, these records occupy more than one thousand pages of single-spaced text.

Upon completing a particular DMT experiment, I sent the volunteer a copy of these notes to review. I asked him or her to edit for clarity, accuracy, and completeness, as well as to add anything that may have come to mind since finishing the study. Some volunteers supplemented my records with journal entries, letters, art, and poetry related to their encounters with the spirit molecule.

While most sessions involved psychedelic amounts of DMT, there also were many low-dose and placebo days. These were more relaxed and gave us an opportunity to discuss and work through earlier high-dose sessions. It was quite helpful for volunteers to do this in a less altered, or even completely normal, state of mind. The shock waves elicited by a big DMT experience extended far beyond a single session, continuing to reverberate in all aspects of someone's life for days, months, or years.

DMT does a lot to our consciousness, but not everything. If we can limit the number of types of experiences DMT produces, we can start focusing on a manageable number of hypotheses to help understand them. Developing coherent and reasonable groupings helps us make sense of the amazingly wide array of stories we're about to hear.

Another reason to categorize these experiences is to support the hypothesis that outside-administered DMT elicits altered states of consciousness similar to those that people report during spontaneous psychedelic experiences: near-death and mystical states and the phenomenon we call alien abduction. If drug-induced and naturally occurring conditions appear to have sufficient overlap, it supports a role for endogenous DMT in the production of these spontaneous psychedelic experiences. This would then open a wide range of possibilities for us to study, understand, and apply these findings beneficially.

Three major groupings capture nearly all the various experiences within these reports. While most people's actual drug sessions partook of at least two of these types, one particular category usually predominated.[1]

These three categories are *personal*, *invisible*, and *transpersonal* experiences.

Personal DMT experiences were limited to the volunteer's own mental and physical processes. DMT helped open avenues to his or her personal psychology and relationship to the body. Chapter 11, "Feeling and Thinking," presents several examples of this type of response. Once volunteers began approaching the furthest boundaries of this category, near-death and spiritual themes began to emerge. The personal then became *transpersonal*.

The hallmark of the *invisible* category is an encounter with seemingly solid and freestanding realities coexisting with this one. When these planes of existence were inhabited, contact by our research subjects with these "beings" made for the most disturbing and unexpected type of DMT session. I cover these bizarre stories in chapters 13 and 14.

The most sought-after and highly prized sessions were the *transpersonal* ones. These involved near-death and spiritual-mystical experiences. I describe these in chapter 15, "Death and Dying," and chapter 16, "Mystical States," respectively.

The last chapter of case reports, "Pain and Fear," discusses the negative, frightening, and potentially damaging effects of DMT on our volunteers. Here we encounter the negative aspects of all three types of experiences: personal, invisible, and transpersonal.

This introduction is a good place to begin addressing how we responded to what people said and did during their DMT sessions. In chapter 7 I described how, after administering the DMT, the research nurse and I sat quietly on either side of the person's bed. We allowed the volunteer to have his or her own experience, with no more than the barest minimum of "coaching." However, we could not maintain absolutely neutral and passive stances when someone began talking about confusing or anxiety-ridden experiences. If a volunteer needed our help and support, we provided it.

There is a fine line between supporting a person and telling him or her what sort of experience he or she has just undergone. After a big dose of DMT, volunteers were extraordinarily suggestible, open, and vulnerable. These factors demanded exquisite sensitivity to the interpersonal field existing in the room at the time. Reflection, support, education, advice, and interpretation are quite different from criticism, argument, persuasion, and brainwashing.

11

Feeling and Thinking

For the most part, *personal* experiences with DMT stay within the confines of one's own body and mind—the realms of feeling and thinking. As such, the phenomena we encounter are not very different from the sorts of things any psychotherapist hears in the office: body-based feelings and mind-based thoughts.

Most of our volunteers more or less consciously hoped for a spiritual breakthrough with the aid of DMT—a final resolution to questions regarding why they were born, or a union with the Divine in which all conflict ended and an unshakeable certainty prevailed. However, DMT, as a true spirit molecule, gave our volunteers the trip they needed, rather than the one they wanted.

Some research subjects resolved difficult personal problems during their sessions. Afterward, they realized they had worked something through in a positive way and felt better. The basic processes of psychotherapy seemed to be at work: thinking, recollecting, feeling, connecting emotions with ideas. For most of us, facing painful feelings is difficult, and DMT can make those feelings easier to confront. Stan's DMT sessions, for example, helped him contact feelings too raw to touch in everyday consciousness.

Dreams are a basic tool for any personal growth and understanding, and DMT may generate highly symbolic dreamlike images. Marsha's high-dose sessions are a beautiful example of how the spirit molecule can show us what we need to know using this particular facet of its power.

For many of us, traumatic experiences set the stage for painfully blind reenactments of situations in which we face those same feelings over and over again. A high dose of DMT shares many features with physical and psychological trauma. We'll see how it is possible to turn these aspects to good use in Cassandra's story.

I expected to see many volunteers working through emotional and psychological conflicts during these studies. Sessions of this nature might help prepare the way for psychedelic-drug-assisted psychotherapy in patients. We would note how DMT affected volunteers in potentially beneficial ways, then build those effects into any subsequent psychological treatment protocols.

The first generation of psychedelic scientists made such therapy projects the mainstay of many centers' research activities. We would essentially be doing little more than retracing their steps in anticipation of renewing their work in a contemporary context.

I was ready for these types of sessions. I believed it was possible for the volunteers to reach some valuable insights into personal conflicts, difficulties, and psychosomatic symptoms by using psychedelics. In addition, many years of undergoing, practicing, and teaching psychoanalytic psychotherapy prepared me for dealing with the painful emotions I thought would emerge during some DMT sessions.

Stan was forty-two years old when we met and he began participating in the DMT studies. His wife of fourteen years was a respiratory therapist who worked with many medical patients at the Research Center. She thought he'd be interested in the project, and he gave me a call.

He was one of the most experienced psychedelic drug users of anyone in our studies, having taken LSD "over four hundred times." "They don't call it 'acid' for nothing," he laughed during our first meeting. He took LSD or mushrooms every few months, using them with several close friends with whom he shared a strong belief in their beneficial effects.

Stan was married, had a young daughter, and held a highly responsible position in the local government. He was of medium height and build, good-looking and attentive to his appearance. He was rather disinclined to talk about his inner experience, and he stated his interest in the DMT studies in a typically concise manner: "To further legitimate studies and for personal exploration."

Stan's low screening dose of DMT, 0.05 mg/kg, was uneventful. Like many others, he felt an urge to smile early on in the session.

The next day was Stan's high-dose session. Carrying my varied assortment of needles, syringes, and disinfectant swabs, I entered his room and found Stan sitting in cross-legged position on a meditation cushion with the back of the bed raised as close to a right angle as possible. He was one of the few people who felt better sitting up than lying down.

Stan didn't say a lot about that morning's high-dose experience. Mostly, he was impressed with the power of the onset of effects. In fact, he thought he might even have liked a dose slightly higher than 0.4 mg/kg.

He wasn't sure if DMT had any beneficial effects, either.

It's not as useful as LSD or psilocybin. It's too much too fast. You can't really work with it. You're totally out of control. It wasn't a spiritual experience. There was very little emotional flavor to it at all.

Regarding what he actually saw, all Stan ventured was that there were "lots of kaleidoscopic blues and purples."

Stan went through the dose-response study successfully, but without it making a particularly deep impression on him. However, he enjoyed participating in the research and wanted to be notified when the tolerance study began.

About a year later, Stan signed on for the DMT tolerance project. A lot had happened. His wife had experienced a recurrence of her serious psychiatric illness and was filing for divorce. A very difficult child custody battle was developing, and their eight-year-old daughter was living with him.

I wondered if the DMT sessions might provide him with some emotional clarity for these trying times. While the goals of the research remained unchanged, Stan was a fellow human being undergoing a major loss, and if we could help him within the project's context, all the better.

As it turned out, his first "double-blind" day was active drug—four consecutive high-dose DMT injections. The first two doses helped him clarify the stress under which he'd been laboring.

Mmm. There were the usual colors. I guess I'll do the next several doses, in spite of the anxiety.

Gently teasing him, appealing to his "psychedelic machismo," but also encouraging him to go a little deeper, I said, "I didn't think you'd have it any other way."

He lay quietly with his eyeshades on.

I like the eyeshades.

"They've turned out to be quite helpful. . . . Did you have any thoughts or feelings?"

I had some anxiety, more or less. I don't remember that from before.

I offered this suggestion: "There's a lot more going on in your life now. I wonder if the anxiety is related to the uncertainty and loss of control in your life right now. This is a drug that causes loss of control. That might be uncomfortable."

At 5 minutes after the third injection:

There is a very slight nausea.

I've noticed that nausea in an altered state of consciousness often is a way for the body to distract us from anxiety and sadness. During meditation or hypnosis, or on psychedelic drugs or even marijuana, it's somehow easier to feel sick than sad.

I'm not going to throw up. Don't worry. Maybe it's the combination of anxiety and my sinuses. Part of my anxiety relates to my daughter's school next year. She's in fifth grade. I need to decide this morning. She's having a hard time with the divorce, especially having difficulties with her mom. It's hard on me but it's harder on my daughter.

"I'm sure it's hard on your wife, too. It's a terrible situation."

Yes. I wish it were a higher dose in a way. I could blast through it.

"Blow it out of the water?"

Yes, blow it out of the water.[1]

"How do you feel about two more doses?"

He smiled.

I have two very opposite emotions: fear and anticipation of pleasure.

Perhaps lying down, Stan might feel safer to give up some control, to "throw up," if he really needed to expel his inner emotional toxins. I asked, "Do you want your head down?"

I'm not sure it will make any different but okay, I'll try it. If I have to vomit do you have something I can throw up into?

"Yes, we have a wastebasket. It's not pretty but it has a wide mouth and we can catch it all."

After the third dose was in he took one of Laura's hands with his right hand and one of mine in his left.

I'm not sure about the fourth dose. I don't know if I can do another one.

"It's only been 3 minutes. Let's see how you feel in a little while."

At 5 minutes he said in a humorous tone,

I will do a fourth for you, Rick.

"The third dose seems to be the hardest."

You're just saying that.

"Not really. People look bad after the third dose and they look good after the fourth."

I guess I have a lot of unresolved feelings.

"That makes sense."

That's easy for you to say.

"I know. I'm sorry if I sound glib. Why do you think these things are unresolved?"

The emotions are intense. They're there, but I think I'm shielding myself from them to get through the divorce. It's not entirely pleasant. That's an understatement, I guess. The emotional intensity builds each time, but I feel most at peace now. That unresolved feeling is gone. Maybe something's been done. Maybe 15 minutes from now I won't be saying this.

At 10 minutes after his fourth and last injection, Stan blew through his pursed lips, then said,

It's a much nicer ride this time. It's like three waves you catch bodysurfing. They knock you down getting ready for the fourth, which is great. I want to do it again!

We all laughed, relieved he was feeling better. In this man who kept so much to himself, his earlier admission of anxiety must have indicated intensely powerful feelings.

He spent the next several minutes lying quietly, relaxing and basking in his newly found inner peace.

Stan seemed refreshed and in good spirits after the fourth dose. He ate lunch and left quickly after finishing.

Stan and I talked by phone a couple days later.

He said, "I'm feeling fine. I felt some mild euphoria yesterday and today, probably related to the experience. I wasn't sure about continuing with all four doses. Something finally clicked and got resolved. Maybe it was surrendering. It really put me through some changes. The first one was mixed emotions. The second and third ones were overwhelming. Just a lot of unresolved anxiety. The fourth one really did it."

I asked, "Was there any content to your sessions?"

"Very little. It's like a roto-rooter for your nervous system. It clears some things free. It was purely energetic. There are cumulative effects. Something happened, something changed between the third and fourth doses. After the third, I just gave up."

Stan kept his feelings at bay. Like many of our volunteers, he enjoyed psychedelics because of their emotional intensity. He could feel *something* on high doses of LSD—perhaps not pleasant or enjoyable feelings, but at least more than nothing. Any time we find ourselves stuck in life, it usually is because we can't connect with the feelings that come with that situation. While in Stan's case there certainly seemed to be a "roto-rooter" gradually wearing down his psychological resistance, there was a conscious processing that helped, too. He was anxious and uncertain. Although he "knew" what it was about at one level, the inner emotional contact just wasn't there. His "free-floating" anxiety was anything but nameless. His life was in turmoil and simply making that interpretation helped him to start a process. The emotional power of DMT then drew it to some resolution.

Stan's joking about taking his last dose of DMT for me, rather than for himself, pointed out an interesting conflict: We needed data, but we were also concerned with the volunteers' own needs. If Stan were having a clearly traumatic experience and seemed to be decompensating, we would have called off the study. But he seemed willing, on his own part, to continue, and we never seriously thought about stopping early. Nevertheless, his comment did have a ring of truth about it.

The visual images volunteers encountered on DMT sometimes reminded them of dreams. And, as Freud said, dreams are "the royal road to the unconscious." Looking at, thinking about, and discussing dreams may help us understand hidden emotions known only by the distressing symptoms they cause during ordinary wakefulness.

Let's imagine that someone develops paralysis in his right hand, and multiple medical examinations reveal no physical problem. He's sent to a psychiatrist, who asks him to remember his dreams. That night our theoretical patient dreams of beating up his boss at work. The psychiatrist suggests that his paralyzed hand represents deep anger at the boss, rage that he didn't know he had. Maybe these are emotions he's afraid to feel because he doesn't know what might happen if he did so. A light goes on in the patient's mind, and he regains function of his hand!

While such an example smacks of a Saturday morning cartoon program, it captures the essential process by which dreamwork can be personally helpful. Symptoms are not often as obvious as paralysis; they commonly include anxiety, depression, or relationship problems.

The approach we took to supervising DMT sessions was as clinically neutral as possible, but ignoring psychological issues emerging from volunteers' experiences would have been negligent. Sometimes I had to decide quickly whether or not to take up the personal psychological thread a research subject had begun, whether to push that volunteer forward just enough to see some resolution to his or her confusion or uncertainty. I also had to take into account the risk that such comments or interpretations might cause some destabilizing effects in his or her life. In Marsha's case, for example, she was struggling with her marriage.

Upon entry into the DMT study, Marsha was forty-five years old, had been divorced twice, and had been with her current husband for six years. She was of African-American descent, while her husband was white. Marsha possessed a delightful sense of humor and frankness. Her mood was significantly better this past year than it had been for some time. She felt a great sense of relief after dropping out of a graduate school program she found dehumanizing and unsupportive of her racial and ethnic background. Continued problems at home, however, revolved around her husband "being more depressed than I was," and she had been thinking of leaving him.

Marsha had taken psychedelic drugs perhaps thirty times in her life, and she found them "very mind-opening." She volunteered for our research "to help out my friends," "to experience this drug out of curiosity and wonder," "to be challenged," and "because my husband can't—therefore he can vicariously share this with me." Her husband had slightly elevated blood pressure, which disqualified him.

Marsha managed her low screening dose of DMT well. The next day's high dose took her completely out of her body. She was startled to find herself in a beautiful domed structure, a virtual Taj Mahal.

I thought I had died, and that I might not ever come back. I don't know what happened. All of a sudden, BAM!, there I was. It was the most beautiful thing I've ever seen.

Marsha described in great detail what she saw, and how she was transformed, during her experience. It was an extraordinarily pleasurable morning. We listened to her report and didn't need to add much. She enjoyed it. There was little conflict and we shared in her happiness.

Marsha later participated in the cyproheptadine study. When it came time for her fourth double-blind session we were nearly certain, taking into account the effects of her previous sessions, that this final dose would be an unadulterated 0.4 mg/kg.

She began by saying, "I hope to meet some of my ancestors today, to help me deal with my current life stresses."

She talked about her marriage; her husband had been in therapy and his therapist was telling him to be more honest with her. As a result, he told her he didn't like that she was getting "fat," that it was a sexual turnoff. She wondered if I thought she was fat.

I sidestepped her question and suggested, "Maybe there's more going on that just how much you weigh."

She nodded, and we began preparing for the injection.

A few minutes before giving Marsha the DMT, her husband entered the room, ready to join us for the session. The atmosphere in the room was slightly sad, but also hopeful.

She began talking about 15 minutes after the injection.

I never would have imagined it would be like this. There was no transition. There was no universe with stars and a pinpoint of light like last time. You know what happened? I was on a merry-go-round!

There were all these dolls in 1890s outfits, life-sized, men and women. The women were in corsets. They had big breasts and big butts and teeny skinny waists. They were all whirling around me on tiptoes. The men had top hats, riding on two-seater bicycles. One merry-go-round after another after another. The women had red circles painted on their cheeks, and there was calliope music in the background. And there were some clowns, flitting in and out, not really the main characters, but busier, somehow more aware of me than the mannequins.

This sounded like a dream. It also was another encounter with clowns or jesters, something I had been hearing about for quite some time from other volunteers. However, they seemed less important than the merry-go-round and her feelings about it.

We had been talking about "therapeutic" issues before the injection. I decided to put on my therapist's cap and see what happened. When someone comes into a therapy session recounting a dream, I usually ask, and did this time, "What did it feel like for you?"

That's the wrong question, try another.

At that moment Marsha wasn't ready to "do work" with the dream, so I responded to the more superficial aspects of her experience, the carnival atmosphere.

"Was it fun?"

Yes.

Could we go deeper? "Was it *really* fun?"

Yes, but it was no Taj Mahal. I hoped to see my ancestors, a temple, or that I would see tall African people in old clothing.

"Instead you were at a carnival at the State Fair."

Big time! I was the only human there. They had these painted-on smiles, there was no change in their expression. I thought, "Hey, what's going on?"

She added,

There was a sexual energy of wanting more, of being stimulated, of wanting more. I've never felt that way on DMT. I guess the mannequins were so beautiful that it was a turn-on.

She lifted her eyeshades and looked at her husband, blurting out,

Let's fuck!

I laughed. "Sorry, you'll need to wait until you get home."

Her husband turned to me and said "Do people have sexual experiences during DMT?"

While a reasonable question, it did not quite fit in with the personal and emotional themes that were so active at that moment. I had to answer, but did so briefly and with the hope of regaining direction.

"There's sexual energy, but not usually sexual-intercourse types of feelings."

I knew I had to act fast if I were to be of any help in interpreting the dreamlike features of Marsha's session. What was the spirit molecule trying to tell us?

"Were the mannequins white? Were they Anglo?"

Yes, they all were. There were no colored people in any of the things I've ever seen from the gay '90s.

"It's interesting. DMT seems to have its own agenda. What do you make of this?"

I just can't figure it out. I'm exhausted and starved.

I ventured, "They sound like an exaggeration or a caricature of Anglo beauty. It's interesting within the context of what we were talking about—your concerns about your weight."

It's true, maybe I should have fun with my figure.

She looked at her husband and said,

I told Rick about your thinking I was fat, that that was part of your therapy.

He looked a little embarrassed.

When I was young I was quite thin. When my husband and I met I was 20 pounds less than I am now. I looked like a stick figure. That's not my culture at all. Rather, the desired form is heavy and full, big breasts and big waists and big rear. Skinny was terrible in my culture. They used a slang word that meant skinny but when they used it, I didn't know what it meant. It seemed like they were talking about ugly, ill, not well.

Marsha's husband excused himself to use the bathroom. Upon returning, he seemed to sense Marsha's need to talk about these things without him in the room, and he returned to work. She and I continued this discussion for a while longer, and then drifted onto other topics.

I usually was not as directive with volunteers as I was with Marsha that day. However, her DMT vision seemed so perfectly related to her current conflicts that I could not ignore the message the spirit molecule was giving us. Marsha's Anglo husband was comparing her with his image of the ideal woman, and she was lacking. Her figure was not "right." However, the "mannequin" Anglo women and men were lifeless, painted images, going round and round aimlessly. Marsha remembered the pride with which her family greeted the full figure of womanhood, and tried owning that herself. She felt her inherent sexuality was good enough. She wanted to have sex with her husband, to reconnect at that basic level. Surprised and nonplussed, it was difficult for him to address her emotional needs at that moment. It was a miniature version of their ongoing problems.

Another way in which DMT affects the mind and body in potentially useful ways is through creating a controlled and supported traumatic experience. *Trauma* derives from a Greek word meaning "wound." My dictionary defines trauma as "a severe emotional shock having a deep, often lasting effect upon the personality."

Traumatic experiences usually are out of our control. For example, we do not choose our abusive childhoods, exposure to natural or man-made disasters, or real threats to our life. Once we have experienced such events, the mind's natural tendency is to wall off the feelings of fear, helplessness, and anxiety that threatened to overwhelm us at the time.

Nevertheless, unprocessed trauma seeps out into our lives. We may find ourselves in situations that produce ghosts or shadows of those trauma-based feelings over and over again. It is as if we feel forced to repeat certain types of relationships that bring out feelings we couldn't master or control the first time, usually when we were powerless children. For example, an abusive spouse recreates the feelings brought on by an abusive parent. We may notice it's difficult to make deep emotional attachments because being close means being dangerously vulnerable.

If we are to move past the consequences of trauma, it is necessary to confront them head-on. Usually this requires a voluntary reexperiencing of the feelings caused by the trauma in a safe and supportive environment. The problem is how to access those feelings in the first place.

In many ways, a high dose of DMT is traumatic, bringing about a loss of control and annihilation of personal identity. "Shock" is a word we heard many times during the DMT studies. I even began using the term when I prepared people for their first 0.4 mg/kg session. Several volunteers recommended we print t-shirts with the words "I Survived 0.4" to hand out to those who successfully negotiated that morning's events.

I am certain that many of our volunteers were at some level attracted to the DMT project because it promised an overwhelming but structured voluntary traumatic experience. By experiencing absolute loss of control in a safe and supportive situation, it might be possible to more fully contact, and thereby own and let go of, certain painful emotions. Cassandra was one such volunteer whose incompletely expressed and felt emotions from past trauma hindered her current life.

Cassandra was twenty-two years old, the next-to-youngest volunteer, when she signed on for the DMT project. Her manner and appearance brought out conflicting feelings in most people she met, and I was no exception. She dressed and carried herself in a somewhat masculine way, and she was bisexual. Both men and women found her pleasing face and lithe, androgynous body type attractive. Her studiously casual attitude toward appearance and self-care made her seem somewhat waiflike, and it was easy to feel caring and maternal toward her—the older nurses on the research ward wanted to feed her and give her a bath. She also possessed sharp intelligence, laconic humor, and a direct manner. Cassandra was a complicated young woman, and it took some effort to see with whom you were really dealing.

Cassandra suffered in relationships. Her parents divorced before she was a year old, and her mother raised her neglectfully. This came to a head at the age of sixteen, when her mother left her alone with her stepfather for a week. He raped her repeatedly during that time, and this cemented her stark ambivalence toward men *and* women: distrusting and hating them on one hand, but needing their love and protection at the same time.

After this, she developed symptoms of a post-traumatic stress disorder, experiencing flashbacks of the rape during sexual relations in her first long-term relationship. When she was twenty, she decided that she never wanted to have children and had a tubal ligation.

Cassandra had been in and out of many short-term therapeutic and romantic relationships. At first she would idealize and romanticize the therapist or lover. Then she experienced disappointment and contempt in his or her inability to provide the empathy she needed so badly. She was friends with one of our male volunteers, and they became sexually involved after they completed the tolerance study. Soon after that she left the country, leaving no forwarding address.

I include Cassandra's story here although it could also belong in the entity contact or mystical experience chapters. Her sessions did include interactions with the "clowns" and led to a deep serene peace she had never previously known. However, the beings' primary effect was to make her feel loved and happy, and the mystical resolution to her conflicts came only after a painful psychological process. Cassandra's sessions were, like many of the ones I will present, hybrids of more than one type.

In addition, it felt as if I were doing psychotherapy with Cassandra, rather than spiritual counseling or interpreting "transdimensional" phenomena. So placement into the feeling-thinking, personal category of experiences relates to the type of response her session evoked in me as much as in her.

She had few stated expectations of her participation in our studies: "I want to see what DMT feels like." Also, she requested we not ask her a lot of questions, "so I could simply enjoy the effects."

We were not so offhanded in considering Cassandra's ability to manage high doses of DMT. We knew she could be volatile, and that it was important to be especially careful to avoid making her feel we were forcing anything on her. We didn't want to replay any rape themes in Room 531.

Cassandra's screening low dose of DMT was mild and pleasant. We met the next day for her non-blind, 0.4 mg/kg high dose.

As she began coming down, she said,

Something took my hand and yanked me. It seemed to say, "Let's go!" Then I started flying through an intense circus-like environment. I've never been that out-of-body before. First there was an itchy feeling where the drug went in. We went through a maze at an incredibly fast pace. I say "we" because it seemed like I was accompanied.

It was cool. There was a crazy circus sideshow—just extravagant. It's hard to describe. They looked like Jokers. They were almost performing for me. They were funny looking, bells on their hats, big noses. However, I had the feeling they could turn on me, a little less than completely friendly.

I want to do it again. I want to see if I can slow it down.

I called Cassandra the next day.

She said, "It's impossible to make sense of it. I'd rather do it again, to see what it's like. It's refreshing to get a change of perspective, to see how insignificant my everyday problems are. I felt peaceful this afternoon. There was a brief moment of wanting it to be over because it was so intense, but I remembered to breathe and settled back into it. It's so weird, impossible to prepare for, to know what to expect. I'd rather not introspect too much."

She agreed to participate in the tolerance study.

Cassandra was in a good mood when we met in Room 531 a month later.

She began, "I quit my job at the local restaurant where I've been working. I'm not sure what's next in my life now. I met a woman whom I really like; I think about her a lot."

I asked, "What are you thinking about the study today?"

"Coming down last month from the big dose, I really felt in my body for the first time in my life. I usually live in my head. I remember that feeling. It was therapeutic. I liked the feeling of being in my body."

"Can you carry it with you?"

She answered, "It's hard to do all at once. I've been out of touch with my body for so long, in a fight with it, I figure it will be a gradual process."

It turned out that this first double-blind tolerance day was active drug. We could tell at the 2-minute point, when Cassandra's heart rate and blood pressure jumped dramatically.

She didn't say much about her first dose that morning. She seemed to be getting her bearings, keeping her cards close to her chest. As she finished answering the first of the four rating scales, she said,

I thought a lot about my new friend. That was good, but this next one I want to be all my trip.

Once she was able to talk after her second dose:

It's funny. I let go more this time. This was no problem at all. It was all about feeling good. There was no revelation, no meaningful overtones. The

body is a real hindrance, isn't it? I definitely felt the presence of others. They were kind to me, nice and caring. They seemed small, as if they could enter my body and mind in that space. There was a total sense of losing my body, but the little presences know how to enter it somehow.

"How do you feel about the third dose?"

You should patent it. I guess it's too late for that. If I could only hold onto this feeling. If everybody did this every day the world would be a much better place. Life would be a lot better. The potential for good is so great. Feeling good within yourself. I guess meditation is supposed to get you to the same place.

"I'm not sure that's possible."

Me neither.

Ten minutes into her third dose, Cassandra started smiling. Just then, there also was a horrible coughing out in the hall.

I can still feel it. I hold all this stuff, the shit, in the left side of my abdomen. I got the message this time to let go of all that. I can still feel the relaxation. It's warm and tingly.

This seemed like an opening. If she retreated or attacked in response to my next few comments, I'd leave well enough alone. However, she seemed to be asking for some help.

"What do you hold on to?"

The pain.

"What pain?"

I guess all the pain.

She began crying.

I guess all the pain I ever felt.

"There's a lot there?"

Yeah.

She began crying more heavily.

"It's okay to feel it, and cry, and to let it go, too."

That's the good part, to let go of it.

At 15 minutes she sighed,

I feel like I have a new body. It's so much more aware.

"It *is* yours."

She laughed dryly, then began crying more deeply.

These aren't sad tears, they are tears of enlightenment.

"It doesn't matter."

I felt her bristle as she said,

Yes it does.

Reflecting back to her even more closely, I offered, "I guess they are a cleansing sort of tears."

Yes. I'll be a guru after this morning. You know how everyone's quest is to find the meaning or the purpose of life? Well, it's to feel this way. Life doesn't cut it normally.

"What do you mean?"

Everything about life. It's not very empowering. You aren't taught to focus on yourself. To realize the strength you have in yourself. Life throws you into the victim role. I know that's a trite expression, but I think it's true. Things do happen when you're out of control with your life. These DMT experiences are like the height of meditation, accessing inner power and inner strength. You know that question in your rating scale about "higher power or God"? Well, I'm uncomfortable with that idea because it implies outside, but I do contact something deeper and more inside. This session was more combined, in terms of the presences joining me and me being the focus of it more. The first trip was just me, and the second trip was more the presences; this was a combination.

"How do you feel about the fourth dose coming up?"

It'll be the best, it'll be even better. I am going deeper and deeper through these layers.

Immediately after giving Cassandra her last dose, people began talking loudly outside the door. At 6 minutes we heard a huge crash. Five minutes later she said,

I feel very loved.

"That's a nice feeling."

Yes, warm.

She looked sad and tapped the fingers of her right hand against the bed.

I'm feeling a lot.

There was a horrible sound outside the door, someone drilling in screws. I thought about how incredible it was that our volunteers could disregard all the chaos of a hospital ward and still have such profound experiences.

Cassandra lifted the eyeshades but kept her eyes closed. Then she opened her eyes half-mast, gazing straight ahead. She looked up at the ceiling and began crying again.

"What are you feeling?"

Everything will be okay. I don't need to worry about all my doubts. Things like "Where will I go? What will I do?" It's reassuring.

"An optimistic feeling?"

Yes, it's very refreshing. It feels like there are thousands and thousands of separate parts of me and this drug brings them all together. It feels very complete.

"You said you felt loved."

It was a feeling in my chest. It was warm. My whole chest felt inflated. It was a really good feeling. I was loved by the entities or whatever they are. It was very pleasant and comforting.

Cassandra and I spoke a few weeks later by phone.

She said, "There have been profound physical changes, very beneficial ones. It feels as if I got my stomach back. Now for the first time in years I'm able to breathe deep into my stomach. I'm more optimistic. That's worn off a little bit by now, but not extremely. I can remember the optimism in meditation. It's like having the deepest possible tissue massage. On the third trip I was really able to let go. I guess I was hurt in there when I was raped. That's where I hide things and protect myself, constantly clenching them. Years of keeping those feelings tightly kept in my abdomen. I feel a lot freer.

"DMT is far better than any therapy ever was for me. All therapy reminds me of is how bad things were and are. On DMT I saw and felt myself as a good person, as loved by the DMT elves."

I asked, "Elves?"

"There was a sense of many visitors. They were jovial, and they had a great time giving me the experience of being loved. With each dose there was more and more of a fulfilling safe and comfortable familiar feeling.

"It would be great to do DMT maybe once a year to put a perspective on things and see where I'm at and heal me. The freedom in my abdomen is still there. The clenching is back again a little bit, but on a more consistent basis I can remember that I was able to really clear it out."

I added, "It can be a useful reference point."

Freud coined the term *transference*, which refers to how people habitually react to others as if they were important figures from that person's earlier life. In therapy, *countertransference* feelings are those in the therapist similarly projected toward his or her client.

Cassandra's life was full of transference feelings for those with whom she became involved. Because there's never transference without countertransference, people reacted just as strongly to her. Sharing her comfort with me could be a trap or an opportunity. We needed to look at our relationship without the confusing dance of transference and countertransference.

The next month Cassandra returned for the second half of the tolerance study: four consecutive doses of placebo.

After we wrapped up the fourth dose of salt water, I said, "Thanks for your participation."

"Thank you. You've been easy to talk with."

I took this as an opening to do a little bit of work before saying goodbye. She was in a sober and steady condition, so I directly addressed the underlying theme.

"I wonder if you had some difficulty at first trusting a male physician who was going to incapacitate you with a drug."

She answered, "I went for it. I trusted you. I never really was worried about it. You changed my life."

Knowing Cassandra put people on pedestals before knocking them down, I countered very carefully, "I helped create the context for *you* to change your life."

"I guess. DMT strips you down to your soul. I know that there is nothing to worry about. DMT showed me how to see beyond it all. Everything will basically be all right. I remember an idea of Samuel Coleridge: If you have a wonderful dream and bring a rose back with you and then you wake up and the rose is in your hand, that meant the dream was real. When I came home and saw the bruises and the holes in my arm I really felt like that—that it really did happen, and that I really was where I was, and felt what I felt."

Cassandra's case shows us how critically important it is to respond appropriately to whatever issues DMT raises. I said the bare minimum to keep her process going, without trying to judge, take credit, or otherwise betray her trust. To do so would have derailed the important work she was doing, and most likely she'd experience it as another violation of her integrity.

With Cassandra, there was a blending of several different themes. However, the primary one seems to have been reencountering the psychological trauma of her rape through the symptom of her abdominal pain. DMT made it easier for her to make the emotional contact with what her physical pain represented and, indeed, where it began. The spirit molecule helped her by demonstrating that she could lose control, particularly around a powerful man, and be safe and loved at the same time. The issues of *who* loved her and told her she was good, and the nature of that love, take us into other categories, such as contact with beings and spirituality.

Both Marsha and Cassandra met up with clowns and presences who seemed to reside somewhere other than Room 531. Let's now examine these other worlds, and their inhabitants, to which the spirit molecule may lead us. They are neither personal nor transpersonal in nature. Rather, they are invisible, and for the volunteers and research team, quite startling and unexpected.

12

Unseen Worlds

In this chapter, we begin following the spirit molecule into more unexpected territory. This terrain is not so easy to recognize or understand because the experiences are less clearly related to the thoughts, feelings, and bodies of our volunteers. Rather, they suggest freestanding, independent levels of existence about which we are at most only dimly aware. These reports challenge our world view, and they raise the emotional intensity of debate: "Is it a dream? A hallucination? Or is it real?" "Where are these places? Inside or out?" These are the some of the questions we'll begin pondering as we review the following reports.

Volunteers have referred to these places already. Marsha journeyed to "the Taj Mahal," and Cassandra was yanked into "the crazy circus sideshow" full of clowns and other beings. In this chapter, I will focus on this issue of "where." Where *does* DMT take us by the hand and lead us to? This is a necessary part of mapping the spirit molecule's territory.

An interesting aspect to these reports is that they are mostly excerpts rather than records of entire sessions. Rarely did the DMT environment alone take center stage during someone's trip. Certainly the spaces in which volunteers found themselves were highly unusual. However, more important was the meaning or the feeling, the information, associated with where they were. Of course, once other "life-forms" began to appear in these spaces, it was difficult not to be completely swept up in their existence, and these reports rightly are the subject of separate chapters.

Despite their strange nature, these excerpts are introductory. They set the stage for the next layer of existence to which the spirit molecule leads. "Where" is the backdrop, the scenery. "Who" gets to the core of these matters. But first, let's get acquainted with the landscape.

At the most basic biological level was the perception of DNA and other biological components.

Karl was our first dose-response study volunteer: DMT-1. He began speaking within 2 minutes of getting his first non-blind low dose:

There were spirals of what looked like DNA, red and green.

Philip, about whose harrowing 0.6 mg/kg experience we've already read, also recognized the familiar double-helix pattern, this time on his double-blind 0.4 mg/kg dose:

The visuals were dropping back into tubes, like protozoa, like the inside of a cell, seeing the DNA twirling and spiraling. They looked gelatinlike, like tubes, inside which were cellular activities. It was like a microscopic view of them.

Cleo, whose enlightenment experience we will discuss in a later chapter, also met up with visions of DNA:

There was a spiral DNA-type thing made out of incredibly bright cubes. I "felt" the boxes at the same time that my consciousness shifted.

We will closely examine Sara's entity contact experience in a subsequent chapter. However, it's interesting to note her reference to DNA:

I felt the DMT release my soul's energy and push it through the DNA. It's what happened when I lost my body. There were spirals that reminded me of things I've seen at Chaco Canyon. Maybe that was DNA. Maybe the ancients knew that. The DNA is backed into the universe like space travel. One needs to travel without one's body. It's ridiculous to think about space travel in little ships.[1]

Some subjects experienced a less obviously biological representation of information than DNA.

Vladan, a forty-two-year-old Eastern European filmmaker, was one of our busiest research subjects; he volunteered for many of the pilot studies in which we worked out doses and combinations of medications to use with DMT. He also received more psilocybin in our preliminary dose-finding work than anyone else.

On a relatively low dose of DMT, 0.1 mg/kg, during the pindolol study, he encountered symbols that were rich with meaning:

There were visuals at the peak, soft and geometric. They were 3-D circles and cones with shading. They moved a lot. It was almost like looking at an alphabet, but it wasn't English. It was like a fantasy alphabet, a cross between runes and Russian or Arabic writing. It felt like there was some information in it, like it was data. It wasn't just random.[2]

Later, while participating in a pilot cyproheptadine session, Vladan received 0.2 mg/kg DMT and again saw alphabet-like figures.

Like seeing panels with a cut-out shape, rounded edges, hieroglyphics of some sort. They weren't painted on but more cut out, through which I saw the colors.

Another striking example of the visual transformation of language and numbers comes from Heather. At twenty-seven years of age, she was one of our most experienced volunteers. Heather had taken psychedelics close to two hundred times, had over a dozen experiences with smoked DMT, and was quite familiar with marijuana, stimulants, and MDMA. In addition, she had drunk the DMT-containing tea *ayahuasca* ten times.

Emerging from her first non-blind high dose of DMT, she began:

There was a woman speaking Spanish all the time throughout the trip. She had quite a unique accent. Maybe it wasn't Spanish, but it sounded like it. At one point she said, "Regular."[3] She threw a white blanket over the scene and then pulled it back repeatedly. It was really weird. There were numbers. It was like numerology and language. There were all these colors and then there were all these numbers, Roman numerals. The numbers became words. Where do words come from? The woman would cover them with her blanket—the words and the numbers.

It started out typically as DMT but then I went past it, beyond where I've been on DMT. There is that ringing sound as you're getting up there, and then I went to the language or number thing. It was totally inexplicable. Maybe it was trying to teach me something. The first number I saw was a 2 and I looked around and there were numbers all around. They were separate in their little boxes, and then the boxes would melt and the numbers would all merge together to make long numbers.

Eli was a thirty-eight-year-old architect and one of our most fearless research subjects. He previously had "regressed under LSD through childhood to a point where I was sitting above the room, watching myself." During a 0.4 mg/kg dose that he received during the cyproheptadine study, he noted,

What's interesting is that I began experiencing sets of hallucinations, and then I said to myself, "Ah, this is the Logos." There's the blue-yellow core of meaning and semantics, basically.[4]

I laughed at his use of the word "basically": "That's easy for you to say."

I know! It's like threads of words or DNA or something. They're all around there, they're everywhere. After the blue amoebic shapes, there were several pulsating places. I thought, "There are lots of these." It's a good feeling. Then it breaks into a ruffled reality. When I looked around, it seemed like the meaning or symbols were there. Some kind of core of reality where all meaning is stored. I burst into its main chamber.

Trying to keep up with Eli, I wondered, "It seems like some kind of membrane you break through, into a feeling of meaning and certainty."

It is! I don't know if it's because of my interest in computers or not, but it seems like it's the raw bits of reality. It's a lot more than only ones and zeros. It's a higher level, very potent bits.

Eli went on to describe the "room" into which he burst. With this report, the view DMT provides now starts enlarging.

I was in a white room, experiencing certain emotions and feelings that gave me an intense feeling of being a co-reality. Like a dream I had of bumping into some Hispanic kids with my car, into their car. They were really mad at me. I said to them "If you hate me, you hate yourself. Our cultures are merged, so there's no defending against that." Their culture, our culture, they were co-real, existing simultaneously. The white room consisted mostly of light and space. There were cubes stacked with icons on the surfaces, like a Logos of consciousness. It was light but there was a lot of other information coming in.

Other volunteers found themselves in rooms that seemed like "playrooms," or "nurseries," some sort of holding space, made especially for them, full of meaning and depth.

Gabe, a thirty-three-year-old physician, lived and worked in a remote rural community. He was one of the few volunteers who previously had smoked DMT. After receiving 0.4 mg/kg DMT in combination with cyproheptadine, he reported the following:

There were some scenes or forms like in a nursery. No babies, but there were cribs and different animals, vibrant. I went to a childhood scene, or feeling. It was like I was in a stroller, kid images. It was sort of scary. I can't describe it. I could draw it maybe. It was like being in a room, as a child, with a stroller. There were cartoonlike people in the room, but they weren't what I wanted to see.

Aaron was at the cutting edge of consciousness enhancement using legal technologies: electronics devices such as brain-wave-driving machines, supplements and vitamins, and Eastern spiritual disciplines. He was forty-six years old when he started working with us. Aaron was one of the few Jewish volunteers in our study, and I felt a certain kinship with him at that level. He was hopeful but skeptical, looking forward to the experience, but praying he would survive intact.

During his DMT-plus-pindolol session, he beheld two elements of unseen worlds: the informational language aspect, and the nursery/play-room theme.

There are no doors, there's nothing to go through. It's either over here—it's dark; or over there—there are images. You just can't do anything with them. It was Mayan hieroglyphics. It was interesting. The hieroglyphics turned into a room, like I was a child. There were toys there, like I was a kid. It was like that. It was cute.

On a slightly larger scale, the spirit molecule led another volunteer to an "apartment" of sorts. Tyrone was thirty-seven years old when he participated in the dose-response study. He was a former student of mine, a junior psychiatrist I had supervised for a year.

As he emerged from his double-blind 0.2 mg/kg dose of DMT, he reported:

It was a scene of apartments from the future!

He laughed at how unexpected it was.

Like living quarters, they were gorgeous. Pink, orange, those kinds of colors, yellow, real bright.

I asked, "How did you know they were of the future?"

The places to sit, do things, the counters, they were molded out of the walls. I've never seen anything like it. It was really modern looking. The almost organic nature of the apartment was beautiful. It wasn't just functional. There was life in the furniture, like it was molded out of something alive, an animal, a living being. I felt in awe of the apartments. An artistic appreciation, like looking at a beautiful painting and getting lost in it, lost in the happiness. At the end I went past, beyond the apartments. I entered into a space, a crack in the earth. It wasn't horizontal, it was vertical. A crack in space.

Aaron also participated in the EEG study. Several days after the session in which he received the 0.4 mg/kg DMT dose, he sent us handwritten notes that capture, better than mine, a description of where he went that day. Here we see some glimmerings of the inhabited nature of these strange spaces.

There was no turning back. After a moment or two I became aware of something happening to my left. I saw a psychedelic, Day-Glo–colored space that approximated a room whose walls and floor had no clear separations or edges. It was throbbing and pulsing electrically. Rising in front of "me" was a podium-like table. It seemed that some presence was dealing/serving something to me. I wanted to know where I was and "sensed" the reply that I had no business there. The presence was not hostile, just somewhat annoyed and brusque.

Phillip's double-blind 0.4 mg/kg dose was definitely easier to negotiate than his 0.6 mg/kg overdose, and he remembered it well. In this session, the venue expands to include even larger-scale observations.

The relentless scratchy, crackling visuals didn't last long. Then I was above a strange landscape, like Earth, but very unearthly. Mountains of some sort. It was very friendly and inviting. It was so real I had to open my eyes. When I did the scene was overlaid on top of the room. I closed my eyes, and that removed the interference with what I had been seeing. It was like a super-bright Day-Glo poster, but much more complex. I was hovering miles above it. I had the very distinct sense of doing this, not just the visual perception. There were some telescopes, or microwave dishes, or water-tower things with antennae on them. I wish I could take you by the hand and show you. A vast expanse of horizon. The sun was different, different colors and hues than our sun.

Let's close this chapter with Sean's description of a DMT world that seemed much like our own. However, that world had nothing to do with Room 531, and there were people other than Laura and me inhabiting it. I like this example because it combines the material from this chapter with the one that follows. In other words, it is "somewhere else" with "someone there" and "something happening," but so familiar as to deceive us about its "otherness."

We'll read about Sean's enlightenment experience in greater detail later. However, for our purposes, what's interesting to note is what he told us after his third 0.3 mg/kg DMT session during the tolerance study. Almost as an afterthought, before we began his fourth and final dose, he said,

Oh yeah, there were people and guides. I was with a Mexican family, on a porch of a house in the desert. There was a garden scene outside. There were kids and stuff. I was playing with the kids. I was part of the family. I had a sense of an old man standing behind me or around me someplace. I wanted to talk with him, but he let me know somehow that it was more important to visit with the young girl. It was pretty laid-back, benign. It seemed so natural and complete as it was happening. It wasn't a dream at all. I thought, "It seems like a pretty common day," and then I stopped and thought, "No, I'm tripping."

There were some black people, too, sort of pulling at me. There was a curious feeling of being extracted. It was a jarring feeling. I was being called away.

Trying to keep his train of thought going, I suggested, "It sounds like something out of Carlos Castaneda's books."[5]

It does, doesn't it? No, I hadn't thought of that.

Perhaps you think these perceptions are not so strange after all. We all dream of unusual places and things. However, our volunteers not only saw these things, but felt an unshakeable certainty that they actually were there. Opening their eyes at any time superimposed this reality with their now-manifest but previously invisible one.

Neither were they asleep. They were hyperaware and awake, able to tell themselves to do things in this new space. It's amazing how often I heard them say, "I looked around and saw . . ."

Listening to these experiences also began stretching my limits as a clinical psychiatrist and researcher. I made few comments regarding people's reports of these unseen realms. It was hard to keep up, and I didn't know what to say. It was at this point that I began having to fight a tendency to regard these stories as dreams, or figments of their DMT-amplified imaginations. On the other hand, I also began doubting my own model for what exactly happens on DMT. Were people *really* somewhere else? What exactly were they witnessing?

These are not trivial questions. As we saw in the previous chapter, sensitive, empathic, and encouraging responses are crucial in working with people under the influence of DMT. An offhanded, doubting, or skeptical remark could make someone feel badly and disregarded, which could rapidly lead to a negative or frightening outcome. We get an intimation of this in Sean's flat rejection of my suggestion that his Mexican family scene was based upon a memory of Carlos Castaneda books. He *was* with them; it wasn't something else.

In addition to the need for close tracking and empathic responses to volunteers' experiences, I also needed to help them understand what had happened to them. When it came to the invisible landscape, we all faced more difficult challenges in making sense of what was going on. As we'll see in the next two chapters, this became an even more pressing issue when contact with beings predominated people's sessions.

Contact
Through the Veil: 1

The material in this and the next chapter is the most unusual and difficult to understand. It is the weirdest and the easiest for me to skirt when
people ask "What did you find?"

When reviewing my bedside notes, I continually feel surprise in seeing how many of our volunteers "made contact" with "them," or other
beings. At least half did so in one form or another. Research subjects
used expressions like "entities," "beings," "aliens," "guides," and "helpers" to describe them. The "life-forms" looked like clowns, reptiles,
mantises, bees, spiders, cacti, and stick figures. It is still startling to see
my written records of comments like "There were these beings," "I was
being led," "They were on me fast." It's as if my mind refuses to accept
what's there in black and white.

It may be that I have such a hard time with these stories because they
challenge the prevailing world view, and my own. Our modern approach to
reality relies upon waking consciousness, and its extensions of tools and

instruments, as the only ways of knowing. If we can't see, hear, smell, taste, or touch things in our everyday state of mind, or using our technology-amplified senses, it's not real. Thus, these are "nonmaterial" beings.

In contrast, indigenous cultures are in regular contact with denizens of the invisible landscape and have no problems with straddling both worlds. Often they do this with the aid of psychedelic plants.

Many modern-day scientists possess an abiding faith in the spiritual. However, these same scientists are caught in a profound conflict between their personal and professional beliefs. What they say and what they feel may contradict each other profoundly. It is difficult to be "objective" about matters of the heart and spirit. Scientists may compartmentalize their faith and can't conceive of verifying or validating their spiritual intuition. In other cases they may water down the nature of those beliefs to maintain some consistency with their intellectual understanding. Perhaps they simply ignore the presence of angels and demons in essential scriptures, or regard them as symbolic or as hallucinatory manifestations of an over-active religious imagination.

Lack of open dialogue about these issues makes it much more difficult to even imagine enlarging our view of the reality of nonmaterial realms using scientific methods. What would happen to the study of spirit realms if we could access them reliably using molecules like DMT?

In addition to questions regarding the existence of nonmaterial or spiritual worlds, we also must consider expanding the notion of what we may perceive in them. Can our spiritual and religious structures encompass what truly resides within these different levels of existence? The stories we're about to hear go beyond reasonably "straightforward" encounters with the Divine or angels, nor are they especially neat, tidy, or in accordance with what we consider within the realm of "expectable" spiritual experiences.

I'm hopeful that these reports will accelerate interest in the nonmaterial realms, using whatever intellectual, intuitive, and technological tools we possess. Once there is enough interest in, and even demand for, information about them, such phenomena might become an acceptable topic for rational inquiry. Ironically, we may have to rely more upon science, especially the freewheeling fields of cosmology and theoretical physics, than on our more conservative religious traditions for satisfactory models and explanations of these "spirit-world" experiences.

I had expected to hear about some of these types of experiences once we began giving DMT. I was familiar with Terence McKenna's tales of the "self-transforming machine elves" he encountered after smoking high doses of the drug. Interviews conducted with twenty experienced DMT smokers before beginning the New Mexico research also yielded some tales of similar meetings. Since most of these people were from California, I admittedly chalked up these stories to some kind of West Coast eccentricity.

Therefore, I was neither intellectually nor emotionally prepared for the frequency with which contact with beings occurred in our studies, nor the often utterly bizarre nature of these experiences. Neither, it seemed, were many of the volunteers, even those who had smoked DMT previously. Also surprising were the common themes of what these beings were doing with so many of our volunteers: manipulating, communicating, showing, helping, questioning. It was definitely a two-way street.

As strange as the reports that follow are, our 1990s research was not the first in the scientific literature to describe DMT-induced "contact." There also are reports from the 1950s quoting volunteers to that effect. These older DMT cases are remarkable in their foreshadowing of the stories we were going to hear almost forty years later. What is even more striking is that I have been unable to locate any similar reports in research subjects taking other psychedelics. Only with DMT do people meet up with "them," with other beings in a nonmaterial world.

These older clinical excerpts derive from patients with schizophrenia, many of whom had been hospitalized for years, if not decades. They were not especially verbal, insightful, or personable. They received DMT in studies attempting to determine how similar the DMT state was to schizophrenia. Researchers also were interested in gauging whether naturally psychotic patients were more or less sensitive to DMT's effects.

A patient with schizophrenia in a study at Stephen Szára's former laboratory in Hungary reported the following after a high dose of intramuscular DMT:

I saw such strange dreams, but at the beginning only. . . . I saw strange creatures, dwarves or something, they were black and moved about.[1]

An American research team also gave DMT to patients with schizophrenia. Of the nine subjects, the only one who could say anything about her experience was an unfortunate woman who, after getting a robust dose of 1.25 mg/kg IM DMT, stated,

I was in a big place, and they were hurting me. They were not human. . . . They were horrible! I was living in a world of orange people.[2]

These little vignettes should keep us from becoming too complacent in believing that what our volunteers reported is purely a New Age, 1990s-in-Santa Fe phenomenon. The spirit molecule revealed unseen worlds, and their inhabitants, to Western science long before our research began.

Karl's early encounter with life-forms, like his visions of DNA described in the last chapter, offered a prelude to future, more elaborate stories from other volunteers. Karl was a forty-five-year-old blacksmith. He was married to Elena, whose enlightenment experience we'll read about later.

Eight minutes into his non-blind high-dose injection, he described this encounter:

That was real strange. There were a lot of elves. They were prankish, ornery, maybe four of them appeared at the side of a stretch of interstate highway I travel regularly. They commanded the scene, it was their terrain! They were about my height. They held up placards, showing me these incredibly beautiful, complex, swirling geometric scenes in them. One of them made it impossible for me to move. There was no issue of control; they were totally in control. They wanted me to look! I heard a giggling sound— the elves laughing or talking at high-speed volume, chattering, twittering.

In the last chapter, we heard about Aaron's experiences of unseen worlds. Let's return to his first non-blind high dose of DMT. He looked at me about 10 minutes after the injection and shrugged, laughing:

First there was a mandala-like series of visuals, fleurs-de-lis–type visions. Then an insectlike thing got right into my face, hovering over me as the drug was going in. This thing sucked me out of my head into outer space. It was clearly outer space, a black sky with millions of stars.

I was in a very large waiting room, or something. It was very long. I felt observed by the insect-thing and others like it. Then they lost interest. I was taken into space and looked at.

Aaron summarized his encounters with these beings after a subsequent double-blind high dose:

There is a sinister backdrop, an alien-type, insectoid, not-quite-pleasant side of this, isn't there? It's not a "We're-going-to get-you-motherfucker." It's more like being possessed. During the experience there is sense of someone, or something else, there taking control. It's like you have to defend yourself against them, whoever they are, but they certainly are there. I'm aware of them and they're aware of me. It's like they have an agenda. It's like walking into a different neighborhood. You're really not quite sure what the culture is. It's got such a distinct flavor, the reptilian being or beings that are present.

"How about the scary element?" I asked. "What's the worst they could do if they are unleashed with access to you?"

That's what it's about. It's the sense of the possibility that's so strange.

In a later chapter, we'll read about the physical problems Lucas encountered after his high-dose session. However, it's interesting to review part of a letter he wrote to us a few days after that experience:

There is nothing that can prepare you for this. There is a sound, a bzzzz. It started off and got louder and louder and faster and faster. I was coming on and coming on and then POW! There was a space station below me and to my right. There were at least two presences, one on either side of me, guiding me to a platform. I was also aware of many entities inside the space station—automatons, androidlike creatures that looked like a cross between crash dummies and the Empire troops from Star Wars, except that they were living beings, not robots. They seemed to have checkerboard patterns on parts of their bodies, especially their upper arms. They were doing

some kind of routine technological work and paid no attention to me. In a
state of overwhelmed confusion, I opened my eyes.

It was at this point in Room 531 that Lucas's heart rate and blood
pressure plummeted to nearly unrecordable levels.

We will read about Carlos's shamanic death-rebirth experience elicited
by his first non-blind high dose of DMT in chapter 15. During one of his
high-dose sessions, he also met beings who tried to help him with his
anxiety:

There's this whole different world with architecture and landscape. I
saw one or two beings there. The beings even have gender. The skin was not
flesh-colored. I communicated with them but there wasn't enough time. I
was so strung out, excited, agitated when I arrived there. They wanted to
try and reduce my anxiety so we could relate.

Gabe, whose transport into a nursery or playroom we read about in the
last chapter, felt an even greater sense of care and concern from "the
spirits" during his first high-dose DMT session:

There was an initial sense of panic. Then the most beautiful colors
coalesced into beings. There were lots of beings. They were talking to me
but they weren't making a sound. It was more as if they were blessing me,
the spirits of life were blessing me. They were saying that life was good. At
first it felt like I was going through a cave or a tunnel or into space, at a
fast rate, definitely. I felt like a ball hurtling down to wherever it was.

Many volunteers' encounters with life-forms in these nonmaterial worlds involved the powerful sense of an exchange of information. The type of information varied widely. Sometimes it concerned the "biology" of these beings.

Chris was thirty-five years old, married, and a computer salesman.
He was quite artistically talented, too, and performed in local theater
productions. He had taken psychedelics fifty to sixty times before starting
our research. He hoped his DMT sessions with us would "propel me into
a state of awareness I have been seeking during eight years of LSD use,
but have only had glimpses of previously."

His non-blind high dose was "the most reassuring experience of my life." The separation of his mind and body was effortless, and he decided that "if death is like this, there's nothing to worry about."

Chris returned for the tolerance study a few weeks later.

He lifted the eyeshades after the first dose and said,

There was a set of many hands. They were feeling my eyes and face. It was a little bit confusing. There were more individuals. They were recognizing and identifying me. It was more intimate. At first I thought it was the eyeshades on my face, but it definitely was not!

Filling out the rating scale, he added,

To get to that space I had to get through some sort of a non-benevolent space. It felt like there were talons and claws there trying to guard it in a way.

These were long mornings and he needed encouragement. I let my intuition guide me: "If need be, let them rip you to shreds, then you can get on with it."

Dismemberment is part of the shamanic initiation, isn't it? I felt a dragonlike presence. And, there were the same colors—red, golden yellows.

"The colors can be like a drape or a prelude or a curtain. Even though they're so pretty, you can get through them to the other side."

Coming out of his second dose he looked stunned, and he grasped for words that seemed inadequate.

It was wild. There were no colors. There was the usual sound: pleasant, a roar, a sort of an internal hum. Then there were three beings, three physical forms. There were rays coming out of their bodies and then back to their bodies. They were reptilian and humanoid, trying to make me understand, not with words, but with gestures. They wanted me to look into their bodies. I saw inside them and understood reproduction, what it's like before birth, the passage into the body. Once I established what they were communicating, they didn't just fade away. They stayed there for quite a while. Their presence was very solid.

I had been hearing about lots of encounters by then and could at least validate his experience: "You wouldn't expect it."

I try and program it and I go in with an idea of what to see, but I just can't. I thought I was developing tolerance, but then, Bang! There were these three guys or three things.

He looked awkward talking about his experience.

I empathized with his perplexity, saying, "It does sound odd."

It sure does. I wasn't sure as I was lifting my eyeshades if I wanted to talk to you about it.

Chris's third dose was relatively uneventful. He stayed aware of his body, his heart beating in his chest, his stomach growling from hunger.

His fourth dose built upon the themes of the previous three and concluded with many features of a mystical experience:

They were trying to show me as much as possible. They were communicating in words. They were like clowns or jokers or jesters or imps. There were just so many of them doing their funny little thing. I settled into it. I was incredibly still and I felt like I was in an incredibly peaceful place. Then there was a message telling me that I had been given a gift, that this space was mine and I could go there anytime. I should feel blessed to have form, to live. It went on forever. There were blue hands, fluttering things, then thousands of things flew out of these blue hands. I thought "What a show!" It was really healing.

It was part of me, not separate. It was a reassurance that this wouldn't go away, that it was mine, that a connection had been made. The whole thing was really crucial to my spiritual development. It's what I tried to do with LSD, a sort of self-initiation. With LSD, it worked in some ways and didn't in others.

Stranger yet are stories of procedures, more or less intrusive, performed by the life-forms of these nonmaterial worlds upon our volunteers during their DMT intoxication.

Jim, a thirty-seven-year-old schoolteacher, was a volunteer who didn't like to talk much about his experiences. During his tolerance study, we talked about going further through the bright colors, which he admitted were distracting him. He felt there might be "beings" behind the colors, and I encouraged him to see if there were. After emerging from his last dose, he said almost offhandedly, and with little emotion,

*I went with them as you suggested. There were clinical researchers prob-
ing into my mind. There were sort of long fiber-optic things that they were
putting into my pupils.*

This was years after we had stopped using the pupil measuring card,
so it had nothing to do with what was happening in Room 531. I asked Jim
what that was like for him.

It was pretty weird, but I figured it was just the drug.

Jeremiah, at fifty years of age, was one of our oldest volunteers. He had
recently retired from decades of service in the armed forces and was beginning a new phase of his professional life by obtaining training in clinical counseling. He was also starting his third family, and he underwent a
face-lift halfway through the dose-response study. He was a busy man.

During the first few minutes of his non-blind high dose of DMT,
Jeremiah burst out in several exclamations: *"Whoa!" "Wow!" "Incredible!"* He began beaming, a huge smile across his face. He seemed to be
having a great time.

*It was a nursery. A high-tech nursery with a single Gumby, three feet
tall, attending me.*[3] *I felt like an infant. Not a human infant, but an infant
relative to the intelligences represented by the Gumby. It was aware of me,
but not particularly concerned. Sort of a detached concern, like a parent
would feel looking into a playpen at his one-year-old lying there. As I went
into it, I heard a sound: hmmm. Then I heard two to three male voices
talking. I heard one of them say, "He's arrived."*

*I felt evolution occurring. These intelligences are looking over us. There
is hope beyond the mess we are making for ourselves.*

*I couldn't change the experience at all. I couldn't have anticipated it or
even imagined it. It was a total surprise! I tried to open to love but that was
silly. All I could do was observe it.*

I found this last comment especially interesting because it challenged
my assumption that what Jeremiah encountered was a product of his mind,
rather than a "true" perception. "Opening to love" is shorthand for an
effort to change the anxiety caused by an unexpected or unpleasant experience into love. If what Jeremiah had just encountered was only a product

of his own imagination, he may have been able to alter his reactions. The fact that his attempt felt "silly" reminded me of the futility of trying to "open to love" to a oncoming truck. "Opening to love" as he found himself instantly dropped into an alien nursery was such an ineffectual and inappropriate response that it seemed laughable.

Several months later Jeremiah received his double-blind 0.4 mg/kg DMT dose.

At 5 minutes he began,

That was much more intense than the first major dose. It's a different world. Amazing instruments. Machine-type things. There was one person operating some of this stuff. I was in a big room; he was in another part of it.

I feel a little shaky . . . a little hypersensitive . . . there are little tremors going through my body.

"Maybe closing your eyes might help. Here, let's put a blanket on you, too."

There was one big machine in the center, with round conduits, almost writhing—not like a snake, more in a technical manner. The conduits were not open at the end. They were solid blue-gray tubes, made of plastic? The machine felt as if it was rewiring me, reprogramming me. There was a human, as far as I could tell, standing at some type of console, taking readings or manipulating things. He was busy, at work, on the job. I observed some of the results on that machine, maybe from my brain. It was a little frightening, almost unbearably intense. It all began with a whining, whirring sound.

Jeremiah's last double-blind session was the less overwhelming but definitely psychedelic 0.2 mg/kg dose. At this session he was surrounded by the orthopedic traction cage, but he denied that it bothered him. Josette was filling in for Cindy that morning, as our nurse.

At 10 minutes, he began,

There were four distinct beings looking down on me, like I was on an operating-room table. I opened my eyes to see if it was you and Josette, but it wasn't. They had done something and were observing the results. They are vastly advanced scientifically and technologically. They were looking just over the traction bar in front of me. I guess they were saying, "Good-bye. Don't be a stranger."

Josette said that some of what Jeremiah described reminded her of some of her own "weird" dreams, and she went on to tell us about one of them.

Jeremiah replied,

That was a dream you described. This is real. It's totally unexpected, quite constant and objective. One could interpret your looking at my pupils as being observed, and the tubes in my body as the tubes I'm seeing. But that is a metaphor, and this is not at all a metaphor. It's an independent, constant reality.

Josette collected the last blood sample and left the room, closing the door behind her. Jeremiah and I relaxed quietly together.

DMT has shown me the reality that there is infinite variation on reality. There is the real possibility of adjacent dimensions. It may not be so simple as that there's alien planets with their own societies. This is too proximal. It's not like some kind of drug. It's more like an experience of a new technology than a drug.

You can choose to attend to this or not. It will continue to progress without you paying attention. You return not to where you left off, but to where things have gone since you left. It's not a hallucination, but an observation. When I'm there, I'm not intoxicated. I'm lucid and sober.

Dmitri's sessions continue to fill out themes of testing and experimentation upon volunteers once the spirit molecule brought them into nonmaterial realms.

Twenty-six years old when he started in the DMT research, Dmitri was of Greek extraction. He lived with Heather, whose experience of unseen worlds we read about in chapter 12. He was a writer and editor and was a seasoned and steady explorer of inner space. He had smoked DMT about sixty times and had taken LSD "hundreds of times," ketamine fifty to a hundred times, and MDMA about thirty times.

When I arrived in his room, Dmitri was casual about the day's schedule:

"I'm not too excited about this. I know it's just a low dose."

"Wait until tomorrow," I replied.

Ten minutes after I injected this low dose, Dmitri said,

It was pretty psychedelic, more so than I thought it would be.

The next day, Dr. V. and his assistant, Mr. W., joined us as guests. Dr. V. worked for the National Institute on Drug Abuse, the agency funding my research. He was developing a project that might treat drug abusers with the African hallucinogen ibogaine. He wanted to see the effects of a powerful psychedelic drug given in a research setting.

Mr. W. had been one of the most helpful people during my search through the regulatory labyrinth for human-grade DMT. I was happy to share with him the results of his assistance.

Dmitri's partner, Heather, was with us that day, too. Add Dmitri, Laura, and me, and there were six in all. It was a crowd in Room 531.

Almost immediately after the injection was complete, Dmitri began breathing deeply and rapidly. He repeatedly sighed and yawned as if to dispel physical tension. At about 9 minutes, he asked for some water, and thanked us when we gave him a few sips. After wetting his mouth, he began,

I feel like I'm in a mild state of shock. I feel really shaky.

"Here's a blanket."

Okay.

"Don't forget to breathe. There's a lot of energy being released."

I asked Laura to go out into the hall and turn off some beeping equipment outside. Dmitri wasn't quite sure what we were doing. He decided to ignore the fuss.

The first thing I noticed was a burning in the back of my neck. Then there was this loud intense hum. It was like the fan at first, but separate. It began engulfing me. I let go into it and then . . . WHAM!

I felt like I was in an alien laboratory, in a hospital bed like this, but it was over there. A sort of landing bay, or recovery area. There were beings. I was trying to get a handle on what was going on. I was being carted around. It didn't look alien, but their sense of purpose was. It was

*a three-dimensional space. I expected cartoonlike creatures, like a com-
mercial for LSD, but this was "Oh my gosh! Oh my gosh!" It was unlike
any other DMT experience I've had.*

*They had a space ready for me. They weren't as surprised as I was. It
was incredibly un-psychedelic. I was able to pay attention to detail. There
was one main creature, and he seemed to be behind it all, overseeing everything. The others were orderlies, or dis-orderlies.*

*They activated a sexual circuit, and I was flushed with an amazing
orgasmic energy. A goofy chart popped up like an X-ray in a cartoon, and
a yellow illumination indicated that the corresponding system, or series of
systems, were fine. They were checking my instruments, testing things. When
I was coming out, I couldn't help but think "aliens."*

*I am so disappointed I didn't talk to them. I was confused and in awe.
I knew that they were preparing me for something. Somehow we had a
mission. They had things to show me. But they were waiting for me to
acquaint myself with the environment and movement and language of this
space.*

The atmosphere in the room was surreal. It was bursting with people
and a very strange story. I hoped Dr. V. and Mr. W. were all right. I also
wondered if I might lose my funding the next week. Or see it doubled.

*It was not like any UFO abduction I've heard about. These beings were
friendly. I had a bond with one of them. It was about to say something to
me or me to it, but we couldn't quite connect. It was almost a sexual bond,
but not sex like intercourse, but a total body communication. I was filled
with feelings of love for them. Their work definitely had something to do
with my presence. Exactly what remains a mystery.*

Let's close this chapter with one of the most striking interventions performed on a volunteer by these otherworld beings. In Ben's experience,
they not only tested and probed him, but also implanted something into
his body.

Ben was twenty-nine years of age and had recently relocated from
Seattle. He was a drifter, having held thirty jobs in just ten years. He was
an old friend of Chris, about whose entity-contact encounter we just read.

During one of his longest stints of employment, Ben had served as a military policeman for two years.

Ben was an intense fellow—short-cropped, nearly shaven head, a muscular build, and a very direct manner. He actively sought novelty and change, so it's not surprising that in his written statement about why he wanted to participate in the New Mexico research, he replied: "I am an explorer, and I expect this will be an interesting experience."

As with Dmitri, Ben's non-blind, low-dose DMT session was relatively powerful. His high sensitivity to DMT warned us that the next day probably would be one of the biggest psychedelic experiences of his life. I told him to be ready.

While a little nervous the next day, Ben was eager for his non-blind high dose to begin. I spent a little more time than usual getting him ready, advising him to try and take some big deep breaths as the DMT went in.

"You may take in a breath and have that be the last thing you remember; you may not even notice the out-breath. That means you're there."

Ben tried to breathe deeply as the drug was going in. Then his breathing settled down as he obviously fell under the influence of the drug. His heart beat visibly in his chest. At about 3 minutes, his neck showed some hives, something that had also happened to several other volunteers who had truly astonishing stories to tell us later.

At 8 minutes, several total body spasms occurred, and he cleared his throat.

It was time to try and ground him. "We're going to put a blanket on you. Try to breathe into that tension if you can."

He slowed his breathing and starting calming down, a big smile on his face. He stayed silent for 36 minutes, longer than most of our volunteers, before I felt the urge to rouse him.

It started with a sound. It was high-pitched like a tightly taut wire.

There were four or five of them. They were on me fast. As crazy as this sounds, they looked like saguaro cactus, very Peruvian in color. They were flexible, fluid, geometrical cacti. Not solid. They weren't benevolent but they weren't non-benevolent. They probed, they really probed. They seemed to know time was limited. They wanted to know what I, this being who had shown up, was doing. I didn't answer. They knew. Once they decided I was okay, they went about their business.

His eyes were open, glazed, staring at the ceiling. He seemed unable to grasp what he had just undergone.

"I know. It sounds incredible to you. To us, too, but it happens."

Haltingly, as if he weren't really sure he wanted to tell us:

I felt like something was inserted into my left forearm, right here, about three inches below this chain-link tattoo on my wrist. It was long. There were no reassurances with the probe. Simply business.

Laura asked "Was there any fear?"

Maybe at the onset, at just having my ego brushed aside. When they were on me, there was a little bit more confusion than fear. Kind of like, "Hey! What's this?!" And then there they were. There was no time for me to say, "Who the hell are you guys? Let's see some ID!"

There are surprising and remarkable consistencies among volunteers' reports of contact with nonmaterial beings. Sound and vibration build until the scene almost explosively shifts to an "alien" realm. Volunteers find themselves on a bed or in a landing bay, research environment, or high-technology room. The highly intelligent beings of this "other" world are interested in the subject, seemingly ready for his or her arrival and wasting no time in "getting to work." There might be one particular being clearly in charge, directing the others. Volunteers frequently comment about the emotional quality of the relationships: loving, caring, or professionally detached.

Their "business" appeared to be testing, examining, probing, and even modifying the volunteer's mind and body. Sometimes testing came first, and after results were satisfactory, further interactions took place. They also communicated with the volunteers, attempting to convey information by gestures, telepathy, or visual imagery. The purpose of contact was uncertain, but several subjects felt a benevolent attempt on the beings' part to improve us individually or as a race.

I was baffled and nonplussed by the sheer volume and bizarre nature of these reports. My crude and minimal responses to volunteers' tales in this chapter clearly reflect my quandary. At first I tried to avoid the pitfalls attendant to developing any explanatory model, either for my benefit or for that of the subjects. After a while, however, we all needed to make sense of these types of sessions.

As a clinical research psychiatrist, I entertained the idea that the regularity and consistency of these reports, and the strength of the sense of reality behind them, supported a biological explanation. We were activating certain hard-wired sites in the brain that elicit a display of visions and feelings in the mind. How else could so many people report similar experiences: insect-like, reptilian creatures?

I believed that these experiences were hallucinations, albeit rather complicated ones—simply products of brain chemistry brought on by a "hallucinogenic" drug, like a waking dream. Several volunteers' eyeballs did rotate in their sockets during high-dose DMT sessions, reminding me of rapid-eye-movement sleep, when dreaming occurs. Maybe DMT was inducing a wakeful dream state.

However, research subjects tenaciously resisted biological explanations because such explanations reduced the enormity, consistency, and undeniability of their encounters. How could anyone believe there were chunks of brain tissue that, when activated, flashed encounters with beings, experimentation, and reprogramming? Neither did suggesting that it was a waking dream satisfy volunteers' need for a model that made sense and fit with their experience. Many even prefaced their reports by saying, "This was not a dream," or, "I couldn't have made it up if I wanted to."

At a slightly more abstract level, I tried a psychological explanation. That is, these experiences were symbolic of something else: wishes, fears, or unresolved conflicts. However, these "symbolic" explanations weren't any more successful. Even gently persistent interpretations fell flat. How could these experiences reflect unconscious psychological issues like aggressive or dependent wishes?

In some volunteers the need to make sense of the strangest sessions was almost academic: "It was just the drug."

For others, however, this need took on a pressing urgency. How could they have possibly undergone the experience they just did? Was it their imagination? How could their imagination generate a scenario that felt more real than waking consciousness? If it were "real," how does one now live his or her life, knowing that existing right now are multiple invisible realms inhabited by intelligent life-forms? Who are those beings? What is the nature of their relationship to the volunteers now that they had made "contact"?

At a certain point I decided to suspend my reductionistic, materialistic, "I know what this is" approach. Not that doing so helped me feel any more comfortable with what I was hearing. But at least I no longer would risk making things worse by explaining away people's experiences as something else. Interpreting, explaining, or otherwise reducing their reports usually caused volunteers to shut down, and I knew I would be missing valuable and important pieces of the entire story if I couldn't encourage them to talk.

So, as a thought experiment, I decided to act as if the worlds that the volunteers visited and the inhabitants with whom they interacted were real, as real as Room 531, the hospital bed, the research nurse, and myself. There now was freedom to respond more empathically, and to see where it led. It also made it possible to start considering other ways of understanding research subjects' eerily consistent reports.

Nevertheless, there was a nagging discomfort in taking this approach in responding to reports of contact. I began wondering if I were starting a descent into some sort of communal psychosis.

So did the volunteers. Upon hearing of similar encounters by their comrades at our post-study socials, several subjects decided to form a DMT support group that met every month or two. Their reason? "I can't talk with anyone about these things." "No one would understand. It's just too strange." "I want to remind myself that I'm not losing my mind."

Contact
Through the Veil: 2

This chapter will describe two of the most complex cases of contact with beings we saw in our New Mexico research. While qualitatively similar to the reports we read in the previous chapter, they stand out by virtue of their detail and intensely personal meaning to the volunteers, Rex and Sara. Their stories exemplify how far DMT, the spirit molecule, can take us into worlds and vistas that we cannot begin to imagine. These particular sessions are the full blooming of this absolutely unexpected and profound series of experiences.

They also left me feeling confused and concerned about where the spirit molecule was leading us. It was at this point that I began to wonder if I was getting in over my head with this research. The experiences were such that my models of the mind, the brain, and reality started seeming too limited to absorb and hold the nature of what volunteers like Rex and Sara were undergoing. They also caused me to start wondering how adequately we were able to support, understand, and help our volunteers integrate these otherworldly experiences. Were we opening up Pandora's box? How were volunteers going to live their lives from that point on, after having experienced such an inexplicable but certain reality? What could we tell them that would ease their confusion?

Sara was DMT-34 and Rex was DMT-42. By the time they volunteered for the studies, more than two and a half years after the DMT project began, we had gained a familiarity, albeit an uneasy one, with tales of encounters with intelligent life-forms. If their sessions had taken place earlier in the research, we might not have been as supportive of their telling, nor learned the level of detail we did.

Rex's and Sara's sessions may have been so extraordinary because they quickly suspended their disbelief and shock when the spirit molecule threw open the doors to the unseen worlds and introduced them to the inhabitants of those places. They both had been through a lot in their lives and were remarkably able to keep their wits about them in stressful and frightening circumstances. They entered those types of situations trying to learn everything they could from them, disregarding nothing, accepting as much as they possibly could.

Rex was forty years old when he volunteered for our studies. While in the armed services, he had taken some PCP, or angel dust, thinking it was THC, the active ingredient in marijuana. The resulting psychosis landed him in a psychiatric hospital for a week. He had gone to college for several years, but financial hardship and homelessness ended his studies. He suffered an episode of depression after a divorce in his twenties. Despite these setbacks, his current emotional health was good, and we had few concerns about his ability to manage our studies.

Rex was a rugged-looking fellow, but he was much more mild-mannered than he appeared. His dark eyes, hair, and mustache were accentuated by his pale skin. He was the only volunteer who referred to me more often as "Dr. Strassman" than as "Rick." While a journeyman carpenter by trade, he had also won some local awards for his creative writing. He was loosely allied with the Wicca religion, a nature-based practice and community.

These were Rex's reasons for volunteering: "I want to explore the potentials of the mind, the nature of actual and perceived reality and our relationship to reality, and to God. I hope to gain at least greater self-knowledge."

Rex's response to his first dose of DMT, the non-blind low dose, was surprisingly strong, and I knew he would be a having some powerful experiences the next day. At 5 minutes after the low-dose injection, he said,

There was a humming sound. I couldn't tell if it was the air conditioner. Then I felt like I was suddenly in the presence of an alien or of aliens, vaguely humanoid. There were serpentine colors surrounding them, producing an outline of their shape. Based on my reading, I expected leprechauns, not anything like this.

The bed was spinning, rocking, it was uncomfortable, alarming. There was some constriction in my chest. That feeling then turned into the alien presence. I tried to make contact and relax into it. It seemed a lot more in control than I was. It was interested in my fear and in me.

I remember that feeling from when I was a kid. When I was scared I would relax and say to myself, "The worst thing that can happen is I'll go to God" when I was afraid.

I knew that the next day he would have a potentially cataclysmic encounter with the beings he had just encountered. It seemed only fair to warn him, to prepare him, as best I could, based upon other's experiences. Nevertheless, it felt strange to hear myself say,

"They do seem interested in you, in people, especially in their feelings."

He tried to sound casual,

Cool.

"Be ready to be dismembered tomorrow. I know that's a grim suggestion, but it sounds like you may be in for a fairly rough ride."

I awoke nervous that next morning. How would Rex do? We both were alarmed by his reaction to a dose one-eighth of what he'd receive today.

We got right down to business. He told me, "I guess I'm most afraid of the vertigo, of getting sick."

His comment reminded me of a Tibetan meditation practice I had learned many summers before. The method was simply to ask yourself over and over again, "Is this what I am?" With whatever answer you gave— "my body," "my job," "my relationships"—it was important to ask again, "Is *this* what I am?" My body, mind, identity, opinions, feelings, all began falling away. This meditation upset me so much that I ran outside and vomited.

I wondered if something similar weren't occurring with Rex:

"Sometimes nausea and vertigo can relate to something that you're not wanting to acknowledge, something deep but obvious. Is there anything important these days that you're trying not to think about?"

"I broke up with my girlfriend about six weeks ago and I called her this morning. I'm not sure if it was a good idea to break up with her."

Women. Relationships. Trust.

"How about your marriage? What was that like?"

"She was diagnosed a paranoid schizophrenic. She was horrible. She did terrible things to me."

Time for a leap. I suggested, "So, there's a commitment fear in a way. Commitment means getting exploited by somebody who is totally crazy."

"Yes." And he made the connection: "Also, I was afraid of the physical reaction to the drug, that I was going to get sick and die from the allergic feeling that I had to it. I wondered if I was allergic to it, with that pressure in my chest and head."

Steering back to his emotions, not his body's symbolic dealing with them, I pressed Rex, saying, "The commitment issue is important. A commitment to yourself and then the commitment to not having a self once that happens. I guess ultimately a commitment to a faith that you will be looked after, and not be abused when you're in need."

We went on in this vein for a while. Within half an hour, Rex seemed much calmer, although I was feeling sick to my stomach and dizzy. That seemed a signal that he had expelled his fear, and it had landed in me. I told him we could probably start now. I walked briskly up and down the hall a few times, splashed my face with cold water in the bathroom, and felt relatively normal.

Rex lay very quietly for the first few minutes after the injection. I see in my notes the following comment after remarking upon how still he was: "Thank God."

At 7 minutes, hives began forming on his neck. Laura pointed to the vial of antihistamine we had handy in case the hives became too severe or the allergic reaction spread to his lungs and he began to wheeze. He *did* have an overactive allergic system. As if sensing our concern, he reached out his left hand and Laura took it.

At 10 minutes, Rex removed his eyeshades. He started,

When I was first going under there were these insect creatures all around me. They were clearly trying to break through. I was fighting letting go of who I am or was. The more I fought, the more demonic they became, probing into my psyche and being. I finally started letting go of parts of myself, as I could no longer keep so much of me together. As I did, I still clung to the idea that all was God, and that God was love, and I was giving myself up to God and God's love because I was certain I was dying. As I accepted my death and dissolution into God's love, the insectoids began to feed on my heart, devouring the feelings of love and surrender.

It's not like LSD. Things really closed in around me, in comparison to the spaciousness that I feel with LSD. There was no feeling of space. Everything was in close. I've never seen anything like that. They were interested in emotion. As I was holding on to my last thought, that God equals love, they said, "Even here? Even here?" I said, "Yes, of course." They were still there but I was making love to them at the same time. They feasted as they made love to me. I don't know if they were male or female or something else, but it was extremely alien, though not necessarily unpleasant. The thought came to me with certainty that they were manipulating my DNA, changing its structure.

And then it started fading. They didn't want me to go.

Remembering many previous stories, I said, "Yes, they are interested in us and our feelings. And, no, they don't want us to go."

The sheer intensity was almost unbearable. The forms became increasingly sinister the more I fought. I'm going to need therapy after this—sex with insects!

Still grasping at a psychological explanation for these strange experiences, I tried this: "That's them. Your fears, your limits."

Rex wouldn't bite:

Mmmm. Maybe, I don't know. It was nonverbal communication. "Even here? Even here?" was not spoken in words. It was an empathic communication, a telepathic communication.

At about 28 minutes, he didn't yet quite seem "back."

"How do you feel now?"

Right now? My body doesn't feel quite my own. There is still something of the other dimension flowing through it. I feel permeated by something else.

"How about emotionally?"

Emotionally, emotionally . . . I'm slightly euphoric.

"Glad to be alive?"

He laughed, looking at me in a more focused manner:

Yes! Glad to be alive!

"You may have passed out as they were feeding on you. I wouldn't be surprised. That would probably make most people faint."

That's right. That's true. Depending on the person, it could throw them over the edge. Is it self? Is it other? I just don't know. I just don't know where these things come from.

As was often the case, answering the rating scale helped Rex fill out some of the gaps in his description. He echoed what many volunteers stated when they thought about the reality of their encounters with these otherworld beings:

This question about "being high"—I don't know. I had my capacities. I was able to observe quite clearly. I didn't feel stoned or intoxicated; it was just happening.

Rex came in for several pilot-study days for the pindolol project. First he would get a dose of DMT. After all effects were gone, we would give him an oral dose of pindolol and then administer the same dose of DMT 90 minutes later. At that point, the pindolol would be exerting its maximum effect on serotonin receptors.

The 0.05 and 0.1 mg/kg DMT doses without and then with pindolol were relatively uneventful. We used the time to process his high-dose encounter with the feasting alien insects.

I now have the feeling that there's something more that I can't access in my daily life. I guess it's the feeling of having made alien contact. I guess I have an expectation of that contact in everyday life. I hope for it. I know it's there.

I had to ask, "What is the nature of alien sex? Would you say it is like intercourse, or is it more the feeling, or what?"

It's positive and warm. Maybe it's like an after-sexual effect, feeling alive and alert.

Rex then came in for two 0.2 mg/kg doses, one with and one without pindolol. He seemed moderately affected by the first 0.2 dose:

I realize the intense pulsating-buzzing sound and vibration are an attempt by the DMT entities to communicate with me. The beings were there and they were doing something to me, experimenting on me. I saw a sinister face, but then one of them somehow tried to begin reassuring me. Then the space opened up around me. There were creatures and machinery. It looked like it was in a field of black space. There were brilliant psychedelic colors outlining the creatures and the machinery. The field went on forever. They were sharing this with me, letting me see all this. There was a female. I felt like I was dying, then she appeared and reassured me. She accompanied me during the viewing of the machinery and the creatures. When I was with her I had a deep feeling of relaxation and tranquility.

I was happy he finally was finding some support within his trips: "At last, a friend!"

Yes. She had an elongated head. I guess the guardians were keeping me from seeing her.

Trying again to interpret his experiences psychologically, I said, "The guardians are your own stuff. They're just the things that prevent you from seeing what's there."

And again, just like last time, Rex gently rebuked me:

I know, but they do seem like something else. They seem like guardians, gatekeepers.

He continued,

They were pouring communication into me but it was just so intense. I couldn't bear it. There were rays of psychedelic yellow light coming out of the face of the reassuring entity. She was trying to communicate with me. She seemed very concerned for me, and the effects I was experiencing due to her attempts at communicating.

There was something outlined in green, right in front of me and above me here. It was rotating and doing things. She was showing me, it seemed like, how to use this thing. It resembled a computer terminal. I believe she wanted me to try to communicate with her through that device. But I couldn't figure it out.

We returned in about 90 minutes, knowing this session, 0.2 mg/kg DMT with pindolol, might be the most intense DMT experience Rex would ever undergo. I warned him, "Considering how intense your first 0.2 session was, this may be pretty wild. Are you ready?"

"I guess!"

Rex's blood pressure was quite high at the 2-minute point, 180/130, and I gestured for Laura to check it again at 3 minutes. It remained high, and his heart rate was slowing, a normal physiological defense mechanism to protect the brain and other organs from too high a pressure. However, he looked well.

At 5 minutes his diastolic blood pressure (the bottom number) remained over 105. I thought to myself, "This is too high a blood pressure response." At 12 minutes, he took off his eyeshades, looking shocked:

I have a sensation that is really strange. It's kind of like lying in a hot bath.

"Are you warm?"

Mmm, a little. Mostly I'm drowsy. Things about the room look funny. It came on real strong. I thought it would last and last and never go away. It was the same place, neon lights defined everything. I was in a huge infinite hive. There were insectlike intelligences everywhere. They were in a hyper-technological space.

He lifted his arms above his head, looked at his right hand, and laughed.

At one point I felt wet stuff hitting me all over my body. They were dripping stuff on me. Everything in there was friendly. I don't think I lost consciousness but I can't bring it all back.

He stared at the ceiling, perplexed.

I'm sorry, doctor. I can't remember.

"It's okay. You came back. That's all that matters."

Struggling:

There was one that was with me by my side. There was the same pulsating vibration. They wanted me to join them, to stay with them. I was tempted.

"Maybe that's where you went, that you can't recall."

I was looking down a corridor that was stretching out forever. That may be where I lost it. The buzzing and kaleidoscopic shifting was intense and went on for a long time. Then it let up and I was in that hive. There was another one helping me, different from the one I saw earlier this morning.

It was very intelligent. It wasn't at all humanoid. It wasn't a bee but it seemed like one. It was showing me around the hive. It was extremely friendly, and I felt a warm sensual energy radiating throughout the hive. I decided it must be a wonderful thing to live in a loving and sensual environment such as that. It said to me that this was where our future lay. I don't know why it said that or what it meant or if that's a good thing or not. I recall telling myself as I was coming down, "I want to remember. I want to remember," but I can't.

Where had Rex gone? Who were the insectlike beings with such a keen interest in and complex relationships with him—devouring and consuming, but also loving and nurturing? My attempts at suggesting a personal psychological meaning fell on deaf ears, something that routinely occurred in our volunteers whenever I tried to help them interpret their experiences in that manner.

Rex was at peace with his experiences, and he incorporated them into his understanding of the increasingly complex and symbol-rich dreams that began developing. He also started reading more seriously about psychedelic plants and shamanism.

Before one of his last pindolol days, he asked me to look at a festering mole on his leg. I urged him to immediately consult with a dermatologist, who diagnosed malignant melanoma. Rex could not be in any more studies until his cancer was worked up and treated. Thankfully, the melanoma had not spread, and he was treated successfully with simple removal of the tumor. By that time, though, I had left New Mexico.

Sara entered the DMT project when she was forty-two years old. She was living with her second husband, Kevin, their young child, and two older children from her first marriage. Sara worked as a freelance writer and was attending graduate school. She was a solidly built woman with red hair and twinkling blue eyes. Her manner was direct, and her mischievous grin often emerged during conversations about any and all topics.

Sara probably had suffered from the most serious depression of any of our volunteers, having overdosed on prescription tranquilizers in her mid-twenties. She had to be involuntarily hospitalized for two weeks after her suicide attempt and subsequently took antidepressants for several years. Nevertheless, her mood had been excellent without any medication for over a decade, and she was one of our most content and insightful research subjects.

Sara told us that an "angel" had visited her once when she had had a high fever as a child, and she now had "spirit guides" with whom she communicated for advice and support. She considered herself "more sensitive than most people to healing and psychic energies." Sara practiced the Wicca religion, as did Rex, and they knew each other through the greater Wiccan community.

Sara volunteered for this study for "personal understanding and expansion of consciousness. I hope I will come to a deeper understanding of myself and my relationship to the universe and unseen worlds." Her fears hinged on "being lost in an abyss, and of not being brave enough to face the challenge."

Sara's low-dose experience was typical of that of the other volunteers—pleasant, relaxing, with a sense of more to come. Her high-dose session the next day, however, was deep and profound. Let's turn to her notes, which she sent me within a week of that morning's events:

"Rick said, 'All right; we're going to start now in about 15 seconds.' His hand was cool on mine, a comforting last connection to reality. I tried to count the heartbeats, something intellectual to hold on to. I got to three beats."

There was a sound, like a hum that turned into a whoosh, and then I was blasted out of my body at such speed, with such force, as if it were the speed of light. The colors were aggressive, terrifying; I felt as if they would consume me, as if I were on a warp-speed conveyer belt heading straight into the cosmic psychedelic buzzsaw. I was terrified. I felt abandoned. I'm completely and totally lost. I have never been so alone. How can you describe what it feels like to be the only entity in the universe?

There are sounds: high-pitched singing, like angel voices. But they aren't comforting. They are very impersonal and don't care about me. They are simply part of the background noise of blasting through the void of the universe. It felt like going backward from life in a physical body to life as simply an energy form with no body. The essence of who I am was alone in the void, back in the staging area for life where souls wait to incarnate. I was in a place where there are no physical life-forms, only colors and sounds. The singing angels were there only to observe me, not to comfort me. But even though they didn't comfort me, I did bring back an incredible sense of Love.

A male presence tries to communicate with me, but I don't understand. I use my mind to ask, "What?" The reply is garbled. It (he) is trying to tell me I will see something. But what? I try to ask, "Will I know it when I see it?" The presence tells me I will see something. Is it by the horizon's light I see in the vast darkness? There is a great roaring sound. It interferes with the voice because I know it is a jet "out there." I'm coming back. The Voice is gone.

It starts with my face seeming to harden up, become firm rather than nebulous. I feel the blood pressure cuff inflate. The rest of my body comes together, and I know I'm completely back. I lift up the eyeshades. I feel a deep and poignant love for Laura and Rick, whom I see first. I turn my head to see Kevin. What a beautiful relief.

Sara also came back for the tolerance study. Let's again refer to her notes from that remarkable day. They require almost no additions from the ones I took at bedside.

Dose #1:

The first trip was lots of spinning colors. I was scared, but I kept telling myself, "Relax, surrender, embrace." Then I saw what I can only describe as a Las Vegas–casino type of scene, all flashing and whirling lights. I was rather disappointed. Here I'm expecting this profound spiritual experience and I get Las Vegas! But then, before I had much time to be disappointed, I "flew" on and saw clowns performing. They were like toys, or animated clowns. I had the overwhelming urge to laugh. I was kind of self-conscious about it at first, but I couldn't contain myself and I laughed out loud watching those clowns.

Rick told me the clowns are a common experience. In fact, he said, "Oh, you saw the clowns?" as if they were old friends or something. Then he said, "Yes, they're hilarious." I felt more confident and not as scared.

Dose #2:

This time the aggressive spinning colors were almost familiar. Suddenly, a pulsating "entity" appeared in the patterns. It sounds weird to describe it as "Tinkerbell-like." It was trying to coax me to go with it. At first I was reluctant, because I didn't know about finding my way back. By the time I made up my mind that I did want to go with it, I could tell the drug was starting to wear off, and I wasn't "high" enough to follow it. I told it, "I can't go with you now. See, they want me back." It didn't seem to be offended and, in fact, "followed" me back until I sensed it had reached its boundary. I felt like it was saying good-bye. Reentry was slow, and I was reluctant to take off the eyeshades.

Everyone's eyes were so sparkling when I took off my eyeshades!

I knew Sara was on the verge of some breakthrough, but that her strong reaction to the colorful hallucinations were somehow holding her back.

"Can you stop short of contact with the colors? You can't help seeing them, but you can stop yourself from responding to them."

She asked, "Is it best to hope and intend for something, like to see that little pulsating shining creature again?"

"The best is to have no intention. If you intend something and it doesn't happen, you'll bump against it. You'll react against it. Just feel your body lying in bed and try and empty your mind."

She nodded, and we all paused to look out the window, remarking on the beauty of the thunderheads building in the spring sky.

Sara looked exhausted.

Dose #3:

I realized what Rick said was true, that the most intense part of each trip was spent tangled up in these colors. This time, I quickly blasted through to the "other side." I was in a void of darkness. Suddenly, beings appeared. They were cloaked, like silhouettes. They were glad to see me. They indicated that they had had contact with me as an individual before. They seemed pleased that we had discovered this technology. I felt like a spiritual seeker who had gotten too far off course and, instead of encountering the spirit world, overshot my destination and ended up on another planet.

They wanted to learn more about our physical bodies. They told me humans exist on many levels. I needed to reconnect with my body in time for the blood pressure check and blood sampling. It was as if they, rather than Laura, were collecting the information, and they appreciated my doing it for them. Somehow we had something in common. They told me to "embrace peace."

I could feel myself begin to slip away from them as the drug wore off. As I started to come down, I saw these things from their world that I really can't describe. I thought of how the South Pacific natives could see only Captain Cook's small boats, and not his big ships, until they actually climbed on board and touched them.

The reentry was very difficult. I felt sort of lost, but I sensed a tractor beam of Kevin's love and followed it in.

My notes state that Sara got up to use the bathroom. Upon returning she said, "I'm tired, but I'm ready for the fourth dose."

"This is the last dose. You can really go for it."

Kevin added, "Make sure you return."

At 5 minutes, her blood pressure and heart rate went up higher than they had all morning, even compared to her 2-minute reading, when people's responses are usually greatest. She obviously was exerting herself, but at what, we would find out only later. At 10 minutes, my records indicate that she murmured,

We have things we can offer you too. Spirituality. . . . Okay, hurry up. Right there, right there. I did it for you. There, you can go out.

Sara's notes from dose #4:

I went directly into deep space. They knew I was coming back and they were ready for me. They told me there were many things they could share with us when we learn how to make more extended contact. Again, they wanted something from me, not just physical information. They were interested in emotions and feelings. I told them, "We have something we can give you: spirituality." I guess what I really meant was Love. I tried to figure out how to do this. I felt a tremendous energy, brilliant pink light with white edges, building on my left side. I knew it was spiritual energy and Love. They were on my right, so I reached out my hands across the universe and prepared to be a bridge. I let this energy pass through me to them. I said something like, "See, there I did it for you. You have it." They were grateful. I was coming down off the DMT, losing altitude. I would have to go back.

I was a little disappointed that experience was spent "giving" when what I wanted was spiritual enlightenment. Should I have asked for something to take back first? I guess I don't feel comfortable in my role as an earthly spiritual emissary. But I did my best. I always knew we weren't alone in the universe. I thought that the only way to encounter them is with bright lights and flying saucers in outer space. It never occurred to me to actually encounter them in our own inner space. I thought the only things we could encounter were things in our own personal sphere of archetypes and mythology. I expected spirit guides and angels, not alien life-forms.

My own notes add this little exchange toward the end of her session:

I saw some equipment or something, sticks with teardrops coming out of them. It looked like machinery.

"It may have been machinery."

Sara's notes describe her state of mind after these sessions:

"It's difficult to sort through all this. Was it real? It certainly seemed real, but so do dreams when they are happening. But there was something about this that was different from a dream, even the lucid dreams I sometimes have.

"Were there really other life-forms out there? Did I really send them the power of Love and spirituality? Even more disturbing, did they somehow mark me? Are they watching me somehow? It makes me feel a little crazy and very confused. Even worse, I feel very isolated in my experience. How can anyone except someone who has been there understand? Maybe this stuff did make me go nuts. I know it sure changed my life. Now, what am I going to do with it? How do I keep something this big inside?"

I was not at all familiar with the alien abduction literature before beginning the DMT study. Neither were many of our volunteers. I knew almost nothing about it, and had little desire to learn more. It seemed much more "fringe" than even the study of psychedelic drugs! However, once we began hearing so many tales of entity encounters, I knew I could no longer plead ignorance of the larger phenomenon. Despite my better judgment, I now feel compelled to weigh in with my opinion regarding the experience of contact with "alien life-forms."

Let's review the popularly reported "alien abduction" experience. We will see the striking resemblance between these naturally occurring contacts and those reported in our DMT study. This remarkable overlap may ease our acceptance of my proposition that the alien abduction experience is made possible by excessive brain levels of DMT. This may occur spontaneously through any of the previously described conditions that activate pineal DMT formation. It also might take place when DMT levels rise from taking in the drug from the outside, as in our studies.

Our current culture is fascinated with the alien abduction experience. Psychiatrist John Mack has published many reports from "abductees," people whom he now calls "experiencers," in his books *Abduction* and *Passport to the Cosmos*.[1]

As the event begins, Mack says, "consciousness is disturbed by a bright light, humming sounds, strange bodily vibrations or paralysis . . . or the appearance of one or more humanoid or even human-appearing strange beings in their environment." Mack emphasizes the sense of high-frequency vibrations many abductees report, which may cause them to feel as if they are coming apart at the molecular level.

Some find themselves in familiar environments, like "a park with swings," and figures "emerge" out of the background. Abductees also often find themselves on some type of examining or treatment table. Experiencers are absolutely under the aliens' control. Despite the obviously unexpected and bizarre nature of what they are undergoing, there is no doubt in their minds that it really is happening. Thus, they describe their experiences as "more real than real."

Varying degrees of anxiety occur in this preliminary stage, especially if it feels as if one's consciousness is separating from the body. For many, the experience of fear is by itself somehow transformative. "Letting go" into the terror seems to change the nature of the experience from negative to positive. The individual may "float" or otherwise make their way "into a curved enclosure that appears to contain computer-like and other technical equipment." Once the person arrives, "[s]trange beings are seen busily moving around doing tasks the experiencers do not really understand." Abductees commonly report seeing energy-filled tunnels and cylinders of light in these environments.

The "typical" alien looks like the ones portrayed commonly in the media: large head, skinny body, big eyes, small or no mouth, gray skin. However, Mack also reports frequent descriptions of reptiles, mantises, and spiders.

Some abductees feel there is some kind of neuropsychological reprogramming, or an enormously rapid transfer of information between the beings and experiencer. Aliens may communicate using a language of universal visual symbols rather than sounds or words.

Many abductees report a complicated scenario revolving around the aliens using their reproductive machinery to breed "human-alien hybrids." However, Mack reports that the hybrid project "is by no means all that happens. . . . They may be gazed at closely . . . and otherwise examined, probed, and monitored. Sometimes the experiencers feel that their health is being followed, especially through ano-rectal and colonic examinations, and they even report healings. . . . On other occasions, the experiencers report probes being inserted into their brains through the nose, ears, and eyes, and they may feel that their psyche has been transformed. . . . Implants are inserted under the skin . . . and they may feel certain that these represent some sort of tracking or monitoring devices."

Abductees report "that the beings appear to be greatly interested in our physicality and emotionality, seeming, as is said of angels, to envy our embodiment . . . they need something that only human love can provide." This may even take the form of alien-human sexual encounters. These experiences "can range from cold and bodiless to ecstatic, beyond what is known to them in earthly love."

As Mack describes, the "experience of connection between one or more of the alien beings and the abductees with whom they relate is a powerful and consistent aspect of the experience. . . . Commonly the initial memories . . . are of cold, indifferent contacts in which the aliens (especially the gray reptilian or praying-mantis-like beings) render the person altogether helpless." It is common for abductees to feel as if there is one alien in particular with whom they have a special relationship. It's as if this alien is "in charge."

The relationship may later evolve into a greater sense of familiarity, meaningful connection, and even love between the abductee and the alien. Several of Mack's subjects report that they are "greeted" by the aliens when they emerge into their reality; the aliens say telepathically, "Welcome back!" Some report a life-long series of encounters beginning in childhood.

Experiencers often report that the aliens are urgently notifying them that Earth is in danger. Their abduction relates to this, inasmuch as they either provide reproductive material for the hybrid project or decide to spread the message of environmental degradation to a wider audience.

As Mack's work with his subjects has progressed, he notes another common, perhaps even basic, element of the abduction experience. This is the transformational and spiritual nature of the encounter: "[t]he collapse of space/time perception, a sense of entering other dimensions of reality or universes . . . a feeling of connection with all of creation." Abductees' sense of belonging in that realm may be so acute as to create a yearning for it—a desire "not to come back." Many abductees no longer feared death, knowing that their consciousness would survive the body's death. One even considered the idea of killing himself so that he could return to the blissful state he encountered during his abductions.

The resemblance of Mack's account of the alien abductions of "experiencers" to the contacts described by our own volunteers is undeniable. How can anyone doubt, after reading our accounts in these last two chapters, that DMT elicits "typical" alien encounters? If presented with a record of several of our research subjects' accounts, with all references to DMT removed, could anyone distinguish our reports from those of a group of abductees?

Shocking and unsettling as they were, contact with life-forms from another dimension was never on the list of volunteers' reasons for participating in our research. Neither was it something I expected with any frequency. Rather, it was the transpersonal, mystical, and spiritual states to which they aspired. It is to these that we now will shift our attention.

15

Death and Dying

Since Raymond Moody published *Life After Life* in 1975, and Kenneth Ring *Life at Death* in 1980, the expression "near-death experience" has been a part of our vocabulary.[1] These highly unusual altered states of consciousness occur when the body faces life-threatening circumstances, such as when a rock climber free-falls off a cliff. They also may occur when the body actually has begun to die, such as after a massive heart attack or when drowning.

The broad outline of a near-death experience (NDE) includes the sensation of rapid travel through a tunnel, sometimes accompanied by voices, songs, or music. There is the presence of "others"—living or dead relatives, friends, and family members. These beings also may take the form of spirits, angels, or other "helpers." The realization may come that one really is dead.

Many experience feelings of great peace and calm, although others report terrifying images and emotions. Some experience a "life review," the organized and rapid recollection of personal memories ending at this present moment. Some feel "commanded" to return to life because it is not yet time for them to die.

The NDE may climax with a merging into an indescribably loving and powerful white light that emanates from the divine, holy, and sacred. This leads to a mystical or spiritual experience in which time and space lose all meaning. Those who undergo an NDE feel embraced by something much greater than themselves, or anything they previously could have imagined: the "source of all existence." There's a certainty that consciousness exists after death. Those who reach the mystical level of the NDE emerge with a greater appreciation for life, less fear of death, and a reorientation of their priorities to less material and more spiritual pursuits.

The sense of reality of what near-death experiencers see and feel is undeniably certain, and it's common to hear expressions like "it was more real than real." It is difficult for those "coming back" from an NDE to describe it; they often say it is "beyond language."

Since one of the theories motivating my DMT research was the belief that the spirit molecule is released by the pineal gland when we die, or nearly die, I listened carefully for these types of experiences. If outside-administered DMT replicated features of the NDE, it would strengthen my hypothesis that endogenous DMT mediates naturally occurring NDEs.

However, in only two research subjects, Willow and Carlos, did themes of death and dying clearly dominate the sessions. Therefore, based upon what we actually saw during our research, I now think this original expectation was naïve.

The problem with anticipating frequent NDEs in our volunteers concerns set and setting. Clearly, many of our research subjects experienced a radical and complete separation of consciousness from their bodies. For most of us, this would make us feel as if we had died. However, many of our recruits had already undergone this type of dissociation in their previous psychedelic experiences. They knew what it was when it happened at the Research Center. They realized they weren't dying or near death, and therefore they could watch the unfolding of effects with far greater balance and poise. They did not panic, but instead kept alert and focused on observing and remembering what was going on. Within a few minutes, the DMT started wearing off, and they reentered their bodies.

Certainly, if their out-of-body state lasted much longer than a few minutes, and if we actually were making efforts to resuscitate them, a more "classic" NDE might have developed. However, our volunteers were undergoing experiences probably only inexperienced and unprepared individuals would have interpreted as death or near-death.

Let's first proceed to several volunteers' sessions that make passing reference to death themes. In them, they almost casually referred to the "death-like" nature of the high-dose DMT experience. Then we'll look more carefully at Willow's and Carlos's sessions, in which death and near-death themes took center stage.

Elena's high-dose DMT sessions partook of many elements of a spiritual enlightenment experience. We will hear about them in the next chapter. For now, however, I will share a comment she included in a letter she sent to me a year after finishing her DMT study:

More than once, the DMT sessions gave me the gift of truly subjectively knowing the phenomenon described in "Introductions to the Dead" in The Tibetan Book of the Dead. *Even greater is the gift of knowing that I have had practice dying and returning.*

Elena's comments were not the only time we heard reference to *The Tibetan Book of the Dead.* In this centuries-old text, Tibetan Buddhist practitioners have "charted" out the various *bardo* states that one enters along the path from dying to rebirth into one's next life-form. *Bardo* is sometimes defined as "intermediary state," that is, between life, death, and rebirth. Many descriptions of the *bardos* echo unerringly reports gathered from those who have had an NDE.[2]

Sean, whose spiritual enlightenment experience we also examine closely in the next chapter, made this remark on one of the days he helped us develop the dosage schedule for the tolerance study:

It's so far out, so weird, so out of control, you have to learn something.

I think I've learned what it's like to die, to be completely helpless in the throes of something. That's been helpful.

Eli, whom we met in chapter 12, wrote to us after his first high dose of DMT:

Stunned, I felt myself holding back. I relaxed and the environment began to change noticeably. I knew I was going through the first bardo of death, that I had been here many times before, and it was okay. "This is just like the last time," I thought. Enough continuity with my waking consciousness gave me this thought next: "But this is my first time crossing over." I concluded I had broken out of time and space and either was experiencing my "normal" pattern of dying or was connected to a time in the future when, once again, I will know "this is the time I was in, back then, now."

Some months later, in another study, Eli said,

I no longer fear death. It's like you're there one minute and then you're somewhere else, and that's just how it is. So I think it had that effect. These experiments are helping me in my reading of the Tibetan Book of Living and Dying.[3] *I know what it's like to be totally free.*

Joseph, a thirty-nine-year-old Italian–Native American businessman, also noted how deathlike the DMT experience was:

I think the high dose is like a death trauma. It knocks you out of your body. I could have tolerated death or some major physical leaping-out-of-this-plane type of experience under DMT. This would be a good drug for people in a hospice program or the terminally ill to have some acquaintance with.

Unlike these other research subjects, death and near-death themes dominated in Willow's and Carlos's high-dose journeys with the spirit molecule. Let's now turn to their stories.

Willow was thirty-nine years old when she joined the DMT project. She was married and lived in a semirural part of the county. She was a medical social worker who treated drug-abusing professionals. She saw the irony in her own participation in our study and appreciated our overriding concern with confidentiality and anonymity.

Willow used psychedelic drugs two or three times a year and had taken them around thirty times in total. She volunteered for the DMT project due to her "curiosity, and the opportunity to experience deeper or higher states of consciousness, to gain insights about my own functioning."

Willow's low non-blind dose produced stronger-than-average effects.

I've never had so many visuals.

I warned her about tomorrow's session, saying, "It's kind of like falling off a cliff."

I like to think of myself as daring, jumping off a cliff.

The next morning we got right down to business, spending very little time catching up or chatting. It was not even 8 A.M. by the time I finished administering the DMT to Willow. Her body made a small jerk.

Even though a jet flew overhead at 3 minutes, the room and ward had taken on the deep solid silence that every so often blessed our high-dose DMT sessions. Willow laid nearly perfectly still for the next 25 minutes. Then I started getting restless and gently asked her how she was doing.

Good. It's a very enchanting place. I almost don't want to leave it. Transitions are completions. How I am. Who I am.

First I saw a tunnel or channel of light off to the right. I had to turn to go into it. Then the whole process repeated on the left. It was intentional that way. It was as if it had a source, further away. It got bigger farther away, like a funnel. It was bright and pulsating. There was a sound like music, like a score, but unfamiliar to me, supporting the emotional tone of the events and drawing me in. I was very small. It was very large. There were large beings in the tunnel, on the right side, next to me. I had a sense of great speed. Everything was unimportant relative to this. Things were flashing, flashing by, as if from a different perspective. It was so much more real than life.

The left and right tunnels joined in front of me. There were gremlins, small, faces mostly. They had wings and tails and stuff. I paid them little attention. The larger beings were there to sustain and support me. That was their realm. A sort of good and evil thing: the gremlins versus the tall beings. The tall beings were loving, smiling and serene.

Something rushed through me, out of me. I remember thinking at some point, "Here comes the separation." I felt my body only when I swallowed or breathed, and that really wasn't a physical feeling as much as a way of setting ripples through the experience. I felt strongly, "This is dying and this is okay."

I had heard of the bright light tunnel, but I didn't expect it to be the way it was here today. I thought it would be primarily in front of me, but this took turns on both sides and then joined in front. Nor was it as bright as I thought it might be.

I'm amazed DMT is in the body. It's there for a reason. It's there for dying today. I had a sense of dying, letting go and separating, after the beings in the tunnel helped me along.

"How do you feel about returning, being back in your body?"

It's okay for now.

She sounded wistful.

The other side is very, very different. There are no words, body, or sounds there to limit things. I first saw deep space, white with stars. Then there was this multidimensional experience starting. It was alive. *It was the aliveness that I heard. My body was trying to say, "Remember the body" as I was going into that place. It wasn't a desperate cry, but an attempt to keep it real, make the experience real from the point of view of the senses. The body wanted me back.*

I thought I could see light down below, the world's light. It was like a little flap was lifted, like a simultaneous alternate reality.

A few months later, Willow reexperienced another high dose of DMT in the menstrual phase study. As she stirred, she began speaking:

It's like a cosmic joke. If we all knew what was waiting for us, we'd all kill ourselves. That's why we stay in this form for so long, to figure that out. That's also why it's so hard to remember the immediacy of it.

I've been reading books about the near-death experience: Saved by the Light *and* Embraced by the Light. *They really do a good job describing the DMT state. I'm reading them in such a familiar manner.*[4]

Everyone should try a high dose of DMT once. I don't know if the beings today were saying "Try death once" or "Try life once." That place is so full and so complete that the idea of this *place is to try and be as complete as possible. Yet when I came back into my body it was so heavy and so confining. Also, time here seems so strange. Eternity is an attribute of the place. It would have to be.*

While it's never a good idea to call anyone's experiences on DMT "classic," I think it's not too far afield to use that term in describing Willow's near-death experiences. Her consciousness separated from her body, she moved rapidly through a tunnel, or tunnels, toward a warm, loving, all-knowing white light. Beings helped her on the way, and some even threatened to drag her down. Beautiful music accompanied her on the early stages of the journey. Time and space lost all meaning. She was tempted not to return, but realized she needed to share the incredible information she received with this world. There were spiritual and mystical overtones to her joining with and basking in the white light.

Willow's dawning awareness of a "light down below, the world's light" also reminds us of one of the last *bardos* in *The Tibetan Book of the Dead*. This is the stage in which the soul starts looking for a new body in which to incarnate, sees the lights of the world, and starts its descent.

Her comment about everyone committing suicide if they knew how great the "afterlife" is points out another similarity between Willow's experiences and those of "naturally occurring" NDEs: That is, those who have had an NDE do not rush off to suicide. Rather, they reside in the knowledge that there is "life after death," and that transition loses its sting. Thus, they are able to live life more fully, because the fear of death that drives so many to distraction is now so much less.

I was interested to hear that she found reading popular books describing the near-death experience to be like reviewing her own DMT sessions. I needed little more validation to believe we were on the right track in relating high levels of DMT to the NDE.

Carlos was a challenge. Exuberant, outspoken, and playfully confrontational, he was forty-four years old when he joined the DMT research. He hailed from Hispanic and northern Mexican-Indian families, had been married for nearly twenty years, and had two grown children. Carlos was a full-time software programmer and had attended the University of New Mexico for several years. He also was a practitioner of urban shamanism. In this capacity, he led a group in which chanting, visualization, and his teachings provided his students with a wide range of alternative states of consciousness. He had his feet in several worlds at once.

Carlos was well-versed in many mind-altering substances. He had taken psychedelics "over one hundred times" and described their effects as "complete strangeness." He recently also had used the seeds of *Datura stramonium*, or jimsonweed, a highly toxic and dangerous plant that induces delirium and, at times, terrifying breaks with reality. There is not much difference between psychedelic and lethal doses of these seeds.

Carlos was not expecting much from "white man's medicine." This set up a curious dichotomy within me. On the one hand, I wanted to "show him who's got the better drugs." Not the most noble reaction, but true! On the other hand, I was concerned that his scoffing at DMT was not wise, and that he might be unpleasantly surprised by the intensity of its effects. Perhaps his cavalier attitude hid deeper fears.

The morning of his non-blind low dose, we found Carlos sitting in the rocking chair I used. He had arrived almost two hours early. He was leaving nothing to chance and was not-so-subtly challenging my "seat of authority."

"This will be a trip around the block to the local convenience store, rather than a trip to someplace else," he opened.

Before we began, he wanted to bless the DMT to "the four directions" and for the good of the community. This was traditional shamanic preparation of a mind-altering substance. His benedictions were simple but profound. They successfully established a feeling of deeper reverence for the work than was usually the case.

His low-dose experience that morning seemed relatively mild. That is, until he began shaking at 15 minutes after the injection. First were only fine tremors, but these quickly progressed to rather pronounced whole-body shakes.

I hate this part. My own body, my energy starts to shake. It's like after any spiritual trip. It's like an aftershock. Every time I do any kind of psychoactive drug I shake for awhile. Do other people do that?

An unexpected vulnerability.

I answered carefully, seeing an opening to a more honest and deeper relationship. "Sometimes, especially after the high dose. Not usually after the low dose. I wonder if it's fear."

He actually seemed quite uncomfortable, shaking, looking somewhat frightened.

Don't worry, this is nothing. It doesn't matter if it's a big dose or little dose of anything. I shake because of the post-traumatic effects.

His shivering started going away while he filled out the questionnaire. He felt fine after completing it, ate a light snack, and left for the day.

Later, Laura and I talked about Carlos's reaction to this little dose of DMT. While he described its effects as "miniscule," his body had a rather different reaction to it. We thought it best to bend the rules a little and give him 0.2 mg/kg before jumping to 0.4.

When I told him, Carlos offered no resistance to the plan: "You guys know best."

This foresight seemed warranted. As I entered the room the next week, Carlos was shaking badly in response to the ward nurse having failed three times to start his IV line.

In the offhanded manner we were beginning to recognize, he said, "This started in the 1970s when I went into a church once."

I started leaning toward being more concerned for his welfare than that our white man's DMT "wouldn't be enough."

I warned him, "This will push you. It will give you an idea what twice this amount might be like. It is a psychedelic dose."

"Okay, I'm looking forward to it. I'd like to have some more of a psychedelic effect."

The injection went smoothly. At 12 minutes, he laughed loudly and exclaimed:

Oh, boy! There is no spiritual value . . . none! Ask me some questions.

"Well, what happened?"

I was wondering, "What is this?" Then it came to me. This is the drug. This is what it does. There was too much to process. It's like trying to listen to music that is just loud. I didn't know what was going on. I wondered if I'd died. I've taken so many psychedelics and nothing like this has ever happened. My nervous system was squashed. My spirit was smashed.

"What do you mean by 'spirit'? It sounds to me like you are talking about your self-image, your identity."

Well, we could argue about terms.

"When I think of spirit, it's the unborn and the undying. That which is before and after and doesn't depend on the body."

I'm used to the "I" that is the body, and I can leave that, so it's not dependent on the body.

Our conversation seemed to increase his enthusiasm.

I saw who I am at a fundamental level. You know sonically or visually there is a certain spectrum that one can tune into that is one's individual self? That was just totally bare and it was there.

"Remember . . . this is only half of the big dose."

That's a frightening thought.

It was my turn: "Now you're getting it!"

Did he really want to take twice this amount of DMT? I would rather he quit now than all of us regret it later.

"How *do* you feel about double this dose?"

What is the value? How can this experience help me or humankind or my community? If I had brought back a wonderful truth, that would be great.

I laughed and said, "Well, you've been talking twenty minutes non-stop about 'nothing.'"

However, as he finished up the rating scale, he said,

I guess I will complete this study. I'll take the 0.4 and then I'll do the pindolol study. But I don't think I will do anymore. I think that the shamans in South America use other plants to fill out and make the DMT more reason-able. Pure DMT seems empty or hollow.

The morning of Carlos's 0.4 mg/kg dose, he was sweating and shaking when I entered the room.

Carlos said, "It's a body fear primarily. It's stress. This is no chance to build up to it. It's just there so fast. With *Datura*, I have the fear of death but you can build up to it gradually. On that 0.2 dose last week, I thought you gave me the wrong drug, that I was poisoned, that I had died. The duress is terrible. I take substances to leave my body, not to put it under duress."

I tried to provide some consolation: "This dose will be more, but not qualitatively different."

He began chanting as I started giving him the drug. His chanting abruptly stopped halfway through the flush. He let out a big sigh at 2 minutes. He resumed chanting, more softly this time, at $3^1/_2$ minutes.

At 12 minutes he said,

Please remove my eyeshades.

Laura did so.

It was really quite special. I wasn't human for about three and a half minutes. This dose creates a level of stress that's unparalleled in the annals of Carlos's history.

He cleared his throat and said,

I met myself as the Creator.

"Creator of . . . ?"

The Creator of all. I've had that realization before, but not at this level.

"One of our volunteers likes to say 'You can still be an atheist until 0.4.'"

This is true.

Carlos took a deep breath and began telling us what had happened. It was difficult to keep up with his rate of sharing his incredible story.

There was the sound of the entire universe, more like a hum. It was pervasive, overwhelming. I thought, "Holy moly, how did I get into this?" Things weren't right and were getting more wrong all the time. Then my ability to perceive as a human being winked out. There were no more emo-tions, because emotions work only up to a certain point.

I saw a man lying in a hospital room. He was naked with a person on either side of him, one female and one male. At first they didn't look like anybody I knew. They were perfect generic human beings. I recognized, in context, that they were me, you, and Laura. The way of knowing was totally different from this reality. I didn't know I was in a study of any kind.

There was something wrong with him. He was there to get better. The hospital was a healing center. What was wrong with him was death. The naked person was dead. What killed the person was the stress from the DMT. None of my guardians or protectors made an appearance. They were out of the loop.

He was healed, more than healed. He was reborn. He got cured from death, healed from death. And then he became the creator of a whole universe.

I gradually became more and more solid and moved toward my everyday presence. I watched the universe's creation down from fundamental mental energy to a vibratory rate to material things. I realized I was re-creating the hospital and the room. As the world jelled more and more, I wanted to see it and asked to have the eyeshades taken off. I became fascinated with my fingers, like a newborn.

I've taught classes on how the universe is a construct of your own mind. And here it was happening. My attitude was different when I knew you were my creations. I felt as close to you as to my own son and daughter.

I would have to say my experience was a classical death/rebirth experience. I had done it before, but never in the same way as with DMT. It was spectacular in imagery, texture, and atmosphere and had incredible lighting and effects. Boil it down and it's very, very classic.

The 0.2 was harrowing—this was way beyond. I knew the boundary beyond life existed. I never thought I'd be there, though, at such an early age. It's one of those things that old men talk about, like "once I got there." It's just the wrong place and time. I expect these sorts of things in the mountains with my friends in a more ceremonial setting.

While I was impressed with the features of his session, I also wondered about other reasons for it. "Creating" Laura, me, and the hospital environment reversed the balance of power in the room. He no longer needed to fear us or the DMT. Nevertheless, there was no point in making such an interpretation. Carlos certainly would have seen little merit in it. Instead I simply dealt with the feelings that came through as he spoke.

"You were surprised."

A true surprise.

Carlos did not have the type of near-death experience about which we hear so often in today's popular clinical literature. Willow's case exemplifies this more contemporary version of the NDE. However, Carlos's high-dose DMT session did partake of many features that practitioners of shamanism report as part of the initiation into the more advanced realms of their practice; that is, the death-rebirth experience.[5]

Carlos experienced himself as dead rather than dying. He saw his lifeless body lying on the bed, although not quite the way he left it, as he was wearing all his clothes before the spirit molecule entered his brain. As he was reborn, so was his universe reconstituted. Here again we see a mystical culmination of the near-death experience. He experienced creation in a way similar to Sara's first high-dose experience in the last chapter, and to Elena's in the next: vast energy slowing to vibrations, finally resulting in matter. Carlos, feeling like a newborn, marveled at his fingers the way an infant is fascinated with his newly discovered body.

There is a progression from the personal to the transpersonal series of experiences DMT elicits. It's possible to work through one's own psychological and psychosomatic problems with the spirit molecule's light and power. The near-death encounter spells what seems to be the end of those concerns by simulating or foretelling what it's like once our individual bodies fall away.

Near-death experiences seem to have the greatest impact on those who take the next step within that mysterious experience—the leap to a mystical level of awareness. It was these realms, into which DMT might lead, that the volunteers and I believed held the greatest promise of significant personal transformation. It is into these fields of DMT's sight that we now enter.

Mystical States

One of the most compelling factors fueling my decision to make a career of psychedelic research was the similarity between high-dose psychedelic experiences and mystical experiences. Years later, it was these types of sessions I hoped to see, study, and understand in our New Mexico DMT volunteers.

The debate regarding the spiritual relevance of psychedelic experiences has raged on for as long as people have used these chemicals for their profound psychological effects. For example, books such as *The Varieties of Psychedelic Experience* make the obvious connection to William James's early-twentieth-century book *The Varieties of Religious Experience*. Recently, *Entheogens and the Future of Religion* continues a long and controversial tradition of recommending that any deep spiritual practice include psychedelic sacraments.[1]

In my early visits to the Zen Buddhist community at which I studied, I raised this question with many of the young American monks. Nearly everyone I asked at this training center answered that psychedelic drugs, especially

LSD, first opened the doors to a new reality for them. It was the pursuit of stabilizing, strengthening, and broadening their initial psychedelic flash that led them to the discipline of a communal, meditation-based ascetic life.

Naturally, I wondered if psychedelic drugs could speed up and simplify attainment of sublime states of mind free of the "side effects" of institutional practice, such as ritualistic behavior and withdrawal from the everyday world.

The answer that did emerge from our New Mexico research was complicated. Yes, psychedelics could induce states similar to mystical experiences; but no, they didn't have the same impact. Even more revealing than these relatively straightforward answers was my Buddhist community's reaction to even asking and discussing these questions. However, I am getting ahead of myself.

In order to establish the close similarities between spiritual experience and what is possible with the spirit molecule, I will first review briefly the features of a mystical experience.

The three pillars of self, time, and space all undergo profound transfiguration in a mystical experience.

There no longer is any separation between the self and what is not the self. Personal identity and all of existence become one and the same. In fact, there is no "personal" identity because we understand at the most basic level the underlying unity and interdependence of all existence.

Past, present, and future merge together into a timeless moment, the now of eternity. Time stops, inasmuch as it no longer "passes." There is existence, but it is not dependent upon time. Now and then, before and after, all combine into this exact point. On the relative level, short periods of time encompass enormous amounts of experience.

As our self and time lose their boundaries, space becomes vast. Like time, space is no longer here or there but everywhere, limitless, without edges. Here and there are the same. It is all here.

In this infinitely vast time and space with no limited self, we hold up to examination all contradictions and paradoxes and see they no longer conflict. We can hold, absorb, and accept everything our mind conjures up:

good and evil, suffering and happiness, small and large. We now are certain that consciousness continues after the body dies, and that it existed long before this particular physical form. We see the entire universe in a blade of grass and know what our face was like before our parents met.

Extraordinarily powerful feelings surge through our consciousness. We are ecstatic, and the intensity of this joy is such that our body cannot contain it—it seems to need a temporarily disembodied state. While the bliss is pervasive, there's also an underlying peace and equanimity that's not affected by even this incredibly profound happiness.

There is a searing sense of the sacred and the holy. We contact an unchanging, unborn, undying, and uncreated reality. It is a personal encounter with the "Big Bang," God, Cosmic Consciousness, the source of all being. Whatever we call it, we know we have met the fundamental bedrock and fountainhead of existence, one that emanates love, wisdom, and power on an unimaginable scale.

We call it "enlightenment" because we encounter the white light of creation's majesty. We may meet guides, angels, or other disembodied spirits, but we pass them all as we merge with the light. Our eyes now, finally, are truly open, and we see things clearly in a "new light."

The import and momentousness of the experience stands alone in our history. It may serve to focus the rest of our life toward the completion, filling out, and working through of the insights obtained.

Some of these types of experiences occurred in our volunteers within the context of another more compelling category of encounter, such as mind-body healing, being contact, or near-death experiences. For example, Willow's near-death experiences partook of a deep spiritual nature. And Cassandra's DMT-tolerance sessions involved more than simply working through personal trauma; she also experienced the presence of deeply loving and healing beings. In this chapter, we'll hear about spiritual experiences that predominated the volunteers' sessions.

These DMT sessions were some of the most satisfying of the research. Since Elena's and Sean's came relatively early in the studies, they supported the validity and importance of studying the spirit molecule's more sublime properties. By the time Cleo's spiritual experience took place, I had already begun the process of leaving the university. Therefore, I cast a somewhat less idealistic eye on her sessions. Nevertheless, if everyone's encounters with DMT had been as rewarding as hers, there would have been less reason to stop the research when I did.

Supervising these sessions was relatively easy, at least at first. I knew the territory based upon training, study, and experience. The difficulties emerged in the interpretation of these effects, and my sense of their importance. Were they "real" enlightenment experiences? How would I know? And with whom could I consult about them?

While Cleo's spiritual experience took place later than Elena's and Sean's, it was somewhat less complex than theirs. So I'd like to start with hers. It gives us a good introduction to where the other two subjects' encounters will lead us.

Cleo was forty years old when she started our study. She was legally blind due to a genetic eye disorder. Nevertheless, she had persevered, having earned an academic degree and massage therapy certification. She now was enrolled in a master's program in counseling. Red-haired, petite, and with a fiery spirit, Cleo was born into a Jewish family but later began practicing nature-oriented rituals within the Wiccan faith. Once, while on LSD, Cleo saw a "past-life experience" in which she was burned at the stake for being a witch.

Her father had molested her sexually when she was a child, memories of which emerged for the first time during a recent psilocybin mushroom trip. Curiously, Cleo had suffered from a phobia to snow as a child, hyperventilating and vomiting whenever she was out in it. She no longer was troubled by this irrational fear, having worked it through on psilocybin several years before. I usually don't use the word "indomitable," but Cleo is as close to exemplifying that attitude as few people I know.

Her reasons for volunteering reflected her pioneering, altruistic spirit: "I am curious. I think I am ready for the next step. I believe in this type of research—from an academic stance—and believe there may be a valid clinical/therapeutic use for hallucinogens."

When I met Cleo in Room 531 the afternoon of her screening low dose, she was drawing tarot cards from her deck. The ones she picked were of butterflies and voyagers—optimistic themes.

At 15 minutes after the injection, she commented,

There was the lightest feeling of a beckoning for me to follow something. It was like a light on the horizon, like two roads merging with the horizon. There were some eyes looking at me, friendly. They wanted to see who was there, and seemed to say that I would follow them later.

The next morning Cleo asked about the advice I had given her the day before regarding how to prepare for her large dose: "What did you mean when you suggested I 'go through' the colors?"

I replied, "It seems like people can get entranced by the colors. If they can go through the curtain that the colors seem to represent, there often is more information and feeling than just the colors themselves."

At 19 minutes after her high-dose DMT injection, it started snowing outside. I recalled Cleo's old phobia to snowflakes. Laura rose from her seat and turned up the thermostat.

Rick, I can see why you became a psychiatrist.

"Why?"

To give this to people.

I told her she was right.

I had the expectation that I would be going "out," but I went in, into every cell in my body. It was amazing. It wasn't just my body . . . themselves . . . themselves . . . it's all connected. Oh, that's what I did. Okay.

She laughed at her inarticulateness.

By 30 minutes, she spoke more clearly:

I felt the DMT go in and it burned in my vein. It was hard to breathe into it. Then the patterns began. I said to myself, "Let me go through you."

At that point it opened, and I was very much somewhere else. I believe it was at that point that I went out, into the universe—being, dancing with, a star system.

I asked myself, "Why am I doing this to myself?" And then there was, "This is what you've always been searching for. This is what all of you has always been searching for."

There was a movement of color. The colors were words. I heard what the colors were saying to me. I was trying to look out, but they were saying, "Go in." I was looking for God outside. They said, "God is in every cell of your body." And I was feeling it, totally open to it, and I kept opening to it more, and I just took it in. The colors kept telling me things, but they were telling me things so I not only heard what I was seeing, but also felt it in my cells. I say "felt," but it was like no other "felt," more like a knowing that was happening in my cells. That God is in everything and that we are all connected, and that God dances in every cell of life, and that every cell of life dances in God.

In a letter she sent several days later, Cleo wrote,

I am changed. I will never be the same. To simply say this almost seems to lessen the experience. I don't think that anyone hearing or reading this can truly grasp what I felt, can really understand it deeply and completely. The euphoria goes on into eternity. And I am part of that eternity.

Cleo was ready and well-prepared for her DMT sessions. Thus, when the spirit molecule called in Room 531, she leapt up to answer. In her session we see many of the hallmarks of a mystical experience: the suspension of normal boundaries of time and space, the ecstatic nature of the encounter, and how poorly words function in describing it. She experienced the certainty of her own divine nature and that all her questions were answered in these brief but intensely felt moments.

Elena was one of our earliest volunteers and was thirty-nine years old when she began. She was short, wiry, dark, and intense, and her manner was playfully blunt. She lived with Karl (DMT-1) and her daughter in a little village outside of Taos.

Elena had taken psychedelics about twenty times in her life. More recent were her almost one hundred MDMA experiences, which she believed contributed to her decision to slow down her professional life's trajectory. She sold her counseling business and house and began an intense process of inner work. She hoped her participation in the DMT study might "lead to a clearer understanding of my spiritual truths."

Elena and Karl were a fun couple. I had known them socially for years. They offered steady and consistent support during the grueling time I describe in chapter 6. Thus it's no surprise they became DMT-1 and DMT-2.

Elena's non-blind low-dose session was uneventful. However, she was extraordinarily apprehensive the next day as I readied the syringe full of eight times the previous amount of DMT. Her heart rate soared from 65 to 114 and her blood pressure from 96/66 to 124/70 just while watching me prepare the drug! Her widely dilated pupils reflected and contributed to a powerful and unpleasant tension in the room. I tried dispelling the anxious atmosphere by putting the syringes down and quieting myself as best I could. No effect. The energy bordered on out of control. Karl and Cindy felt it, too, and looked restless.

"Well, how about it?" I offered hopefully.

Elena gave a game smile. "I'll be okay. I'm just scared of what the unknown will bring. Let's get started."

Within 45 seconds of finishing the injection, Elena began groaning, sighing, and sucking her breaths in and blowing them out. The strength of her movements made it impossible to get her 2-minute blood pressure and heart rate. Her hands were cold and damp, and the color drained from her face. Her pulse climbed even higher, to 134, by the time I got her 5-minute recording, but her blood pressure held steady. Her head rocked back and forth slowly, and she nodded occasionally. She licked her lips, yawned, sighed, and seemed unable to get comfortable. By 4 minutes, she finally began settling down.

The color returned to her face at 13 minutes, and she lay there quietly. Ten minutes later she began spurting out laugher, which grew to an uproarious level. She began to talk excitedly at 30 minutes. While I took notes, the report she wrote the next day does a better job of capturing what she experienced than does my shorthand.

Before you spoke the words, "Okay, we're done," there arose in me an energy so forceful that no words could describe it. It drove my heart. The swirl of color reminded me of the visual experience the day before, but multiplied a millionfold. I could only hold on, remembering not to fall off into the distracting light show. Then everything stopped! The darkness opened to light, and on the other side of space all was utterly still. Then the words "just because it is possible" emerged out of nothingness and filled me.

The great power sought to fill all possibilities. It was "amoral," but it was love, and it just was. There was no benevolent god, only this primordial power. All of my ideas and beliefs seemed absurdly ridiculous. I never wanted to forget this. I was aware I could open my eyes and relate to those around me. But first I had to wait for all this to solidify, to allow the fullness of the experience to congeal, so I could bring it back to the others.

I wondered, "Why come back?" I was reluctant to open my eyes. When I did, the room seemed very bright, but otherwise quite as I had left it.

Several months later, in the dose-response study, Elena had a chance to revisit this state with a double-blind high dose. This time she was much less anxious before we started.

At 20 minutes she began:

It came on fast and big, and an incredible pressure arose in my head, pushing me back. It blasted me into the realm in which pure living energy begins to take form. As it began to slow down, I saw the process of separated awareness. This slowing down creates form and consciousness. Before the slowing down, it's not there. It's not unconscious, but not conscious. It's real, of its own substance, not fragmented. It's amazing how slowly things move here on Earth!

Going out and slowing down into the periphery, to the fringes of it, into form. There is the endless outflow of creation, effortless, and then this vast process takes it back in. My little piece of energy goes in and out, too, not more or less than any other piece. You can't die. You can't go away. You can neither add nor subtract. There is a continual outflow that is immortality. The "I am" notion goes around and around. I have the certainty of that.

There were loads of paradoxes. I was not disoriented but there was no orientation. I didn't know where or who I was, but there was nothing to know who or where it was. I didn't have to wonder what to do next. There are no empty spaces, they were all filled up.

While Elena described the essence of her encounter as "amoral," her joy and wonder suggest she found it anything but cold or lifeless. Rather, "it was love," and she was so happy there she considered not "coming back." She understood the cycle of birth and rebirth with the resulting personal certainty of immortality. Like Carlos in the last chapter, she also saw what modern cosmologists propose is the source of the universe. First there is nothing, then the Big Bang, out of which slowed-down and cooled particles become the elements of matter. From matter comes our own separate bodies and minds.

Sean's story is remarkable for its combination of features. His sessions partake of unseen worlds and entity contact as well as mystical states. However, his enlightenment experience is the climax for which the other types of effects paved the way.

Thirty-eight years old at the time we began working together, Sean received more DMT than any other volunteer. He participated in every double-blind placebo-controlled experiment as well as the pilot studies in which we determined the best doses of DMT to use in combination with pindolol and cyproheptadine. He also came in for the DMT EEG study and several psilocybin sessions in our preliminary work with that compound.

Sandy-haired, fair-skinned, of medium height and build, he was mild-mannered and low-key in the extreme. Only after spending some time with him did you appreciate Sean's solid character, keen and searching intellect, and wry sense of humor.

He was a lawyer at a major Albuquerque firm. However, he worked only part-time so as to allow himself the freedom to pursue his other love: growing a wide range of native trees.

He previously had taken LSD around thirty-five times, and psilocybin mushrooms and mescaline once or twice each. His reasons for participating in the DMT studies were modest, in line with his general approach to life: "To experience another hallucinogen. I don't know what to expect at all—but I'm *not* afraid of new experiences or myself or what I may do."

Sean's non-blind low dose of DMT went well, but the high dose the next day was an aberration. The IV line had worked itself loose, and I inadvertently injected the drug under his skin rather than into his vein. We suspected this but were not certain until he was well into the full double-blind dose-response study. He got much higher on several of these doses than on what we thought was his first "large" dose.

The effects of this initial non-blind 0.4 mg/kg dose were quite slow to develop and not much more than those from his low dose the day before. The injection did feel odd as I gave it, but it did not fully dawn on me that it missed his vein. I didn't think to repeat it. Maybe he was one of the people I anticipated might have little reaction to the drug.

During one of the double-blind study days, Sean received what turned out to be 0.2 mg/kg. Because of his reaction to this unknown dose, I started thinking that indeed there must have been a problem with that first high dose. He thought so, too.

I'll bet this is the high dose, and that I didn't get the high dose last time. I've never been so high. The grain in the door just opened up!

Sean participated early enough in the studies that we hadn't begun using the eyeshades regularly, and at first he liked keeping his eyes open. This gave me the opportunity to help him think more deeply about the DMT visuals, and their sometimes distracting nature.

"I wonder if you could focus on that space within the grains of the wood, rather than the grain itself. You might go further once you're more familiar with what happens on DMT. The visions and display are not all that's there."

I was just at the edge of losing it. I had no sense of what you two were doing, just that you were around. I was glad I knew you both; I would have been self-conscious if you were strangers.

His comments about being comfortable with us also speak to the crucial, but rarely discussed, variable of the relationship existing among those who give and take psychedelic drugs. Comfort with the sitters allows for letting go; anxiety or mistrust creates the opposite.

A few weeks later he received placebo, which gave him time to reflect upon his previous session.

I believe the last trip was a near-death experience. Everything is more alive now. I'm not bored, even when I should be! It was the awe and fear of God. I thought about barely anything else for the first day or two afterward. The desire to talk about it to anyone and everyone faded after three or four days.

It's curious that Sean had such a deep experience without any of us knowing about it at the time. It reminded me to remain alert to how different people were in their comfort or ability to discuss the contents of their sessions, especially right after they occurred.

Sean volunteered for the tolerance pilot work, in which we worked out the appropriate dose of DMT as well as how much time should pass between each injection. One morning he received four 0.2 mg/kg injections at hourly intervals. As he came down from his third dose, he said,

I couldn't watch it all, it was so busy. Something asked me, "What do you want? How much do you want?"

Sean mentioned this rather casually. It was his first time he had spoken of hearing "the other."

I answered that I wanted to see fewer things, but more of it. That reduced the intensity of the busy, crackling, colorful Chinese-like panels. It became more manageable and focused. I'm feeling freer about going out there. I'm not lost. I'm asking questions and getting answers.

Sean then came in for four 0.3 mg/kg doses at one-hour intervals. He had an extraordinarily moving day. While my bedside notes capture much of his sessions, the letter Sean later sent to me does an even better job:

The first session was a lot of fun. I felt myself lifting off the bed three or four feet. The visions rapidly developed into an almost sparkling electric blue-green light pattern. I asked, "Are you here again?" No answer, so I watched a low-lying city on a flat plane on the far horizon mutate through a variety of colors and hues, with many ill-defined "things" floating in the "air" above the city.

Then I noticed a middle-aged female, with a pointed nose and light greenish skin, sitting off to my right, watching this changing city with me. She had her right hand on a dial that seemed to control the panorama we were watching. She turned slightly toward me and asked, "What else would you like?" I answered telepathically, "Well, what else have you got? I have no idea what you can do."

Then she stood up, walked up to my right forehead, touched it and warmed it up, and then used a sharp object to open up a panel in my right temple, releasing a tremendous amount of pressure. This made me feel much better than I'd felt before, even though I realized I'd felt fine in the first place.

Sean's second dose was difficult because a loud vacuum cleaner passed by the room and a garbage truck screeched terribly outside the window. Temporarily confused and anxious, he regrouped but could do little else with the session.

Dose 3:

For the first time ever, I went into a blank state before the DMT injection. I had no thought, no hopes, no fears, no expectations.

The trip started with an electric tingling in my body, and quickly the visual hallucinations arrived. Then I noticed five or six figures walking rapidly alongside me. They felt like helpers, fellow travelers. A humanoid male figure turned toward me, threw his right arm up toward the patchwork of bright colors, and asked, "How about this?" *The kaleidoscopic patterns immediately became brighter and moved more rapidly. A second and then a third asked and did the same thing. At that point, I decided to go further, deeper.*

I immediately saw a bright yellow-white light directly in front of me. I chose to open to it. I was consumed by it and became part of it. There were no distinctions—no figures or lines, shadows or outlines. There was no body or anything inside or outside. I was devoid of self, of thought, of time, of space, of a sense of separateness or ego, or of anything but the white light. There are no symbols in my language that can begin to describe that sense of pure being, oneness, and ecstasy. There was a great sense of stillness and ecstasy.

I have no idea how long I was in this confluence of pure energy, or whatever/however I might describe it. Finally I felt myself tumbling gently and sliding backward away from this Light, sliding down a ramp. I could see myself doing this, a naked, thin, luminescent childlike being that glowed with a warm, yellow light. My head was enlarged, and my body was that of a four-year-old child. Waves of the Light touched me as my body receded from it. I was almost dizzy with happiness as the slide down the ramp finally ended.

Of course, we had no idea what Sean was experiencing. My notes at 9 minutes after this third injection simply indicate that Sean stated,

I think I'm down.

After filling out the rating scale, he said,

It's interesting. I chose to enter a bright light.

I offered general support and encouragement: "I'm glad you chose to go into it rather than waiting and observing."

It wasn't too conscious a choice.

"Faith can be leaping off the cliff optimistically."

It wasn't that scary.

He paused and smiled,

I can't believe I'm doing this. That you're doing this.

Let's return to his letter for notes on his fourth and final dose that day:

There were wire people everywhere riding bicycles, like programmed people, like video-game people having fun. I watched them. They were blue-green, running all around me. Like being in a parking tower. I forget what happened at the end. They did it for a long time! I kept wondering if anything else would happen. Slowly the trip ended, but I can't remember how.

The morning was almost over. Sean's face was pale as he removed his eyeshades. He bent his knees up toward his chest.

Laura said, "You look tired."

No, I'm not tired, I just feel fuzzy.

He looked around the room and at us and sighed,

What a day!

Clearly there are striking similarities between naturally occurring spiritual experiences and those induced in certain individuals by DMT. Cleo's, Elena's, and Sean's high-dose sessions were ecstatic, insightful, revolutionary, and profound. All three volunteers were steady and solid people with knowledge of religious concepts. The words they used to describe their sessions are remarkably like those we read from the great mystics of the ages.

DMT reproduces many of the features of an enlightenment experience, including timelessness; ineffability; coexistence of opposites; contact and merging with a supremely powerful, wise, and loving presence, sometimes experienced as a white light; the certainty that consciousness continues after death of the body; and a first-hand knowledge of the basic "facts" of creation and consciousness.

While gratified and in awe of these sessions, larger questions began to loom as I heard more of them. Because DMT can elicit mystical experiences, are the experiences necessarily beneficial? Or, put another way, do they have a spiritual effect in those who've undergone them? If they did, I'd feel justified in labeling these encounters truly spiritual. In addition, the occasional negative effects of DMT might be easier to accept in the presence of real transformational experiences in others.

These thoughts lead to two separate clinical issues: adverse effects from, and long-term benefit wrought by, encounters with the spirit molecule. In order to begin looking at the overall balance sheet, let's turn to the dark side of DMT.

Pain and Fear

In preparation for writing these chapters on the DMT sessions, I reviewed every page of my bedside notes. It took a month to look over all of them, cutting and pasting people's reports into various groupings of experience. One of these categories was "adverse effects," in which I placed difficult or troublesome responses to DMT. Parts of twenty-five people's sessions landed in this "bin." These adverse effects ranged from being subtle, minor, and extremely brief to those that were terrifying, dangerous, and lingering.

Twenty-five out of sixty volunteers seemed like a lot. At the time, I never sensed that nearly half of our volunteers were having problems. Was I minimizing difficulties in my desire to forge ahead in the research under any and all conditions?

This number was even more surprising because I hoped to reduce the incidence of frightening reactions to DMT by studying only normal volunteers with previous psychedelic drug experience. This seemed a safer path than enrolling those who had no idea what to expect, or who were already psychologically troubled.

Looking more closely at these sessions, it became clear that the vast majority of these problems were, if not especially minor, very brief. This reassured me to some extent. One of the primary reasons I chose DMT as the drug with which to resume clinical psychedelic research was that its effects were so short. I anticipated that no matter how bad things became, at least they wouldn't last too long.

The research setting was ripe for the development of negative responses to the drug, and this may have contributed to the high frequency we saw. The clinical environment was quite unpleasant, even though it reassured some research subjects about our ability to respond to medical emergencies.

In addition to the actual physical environment of the Research Center, the research attitude also created a tension that does not normally exist in typical psychedelic settings. The blood drawing, questionnaire administration, and various other experimental manipulations impacted our relationship with the volunteers. We wanted something from them other than just their own psychedelic experience, and that expectation was impossible to ignore.

I expected nearly everyone to feel some anxiety as the DMT effects began. I knew many people would find themselves struggling to keep their bearings, especially with the higher doses. My respect for the deeply disruptive properties of DMT made it easier for volunteers to feel understood in their natural apprehension before getting big doses of the spirit molecule.

We did our best in attending to such details as smells, gestures, speech, emotional state, and the behavior of everyone in the room. This attention to detail went a long way in protecting our subjects from unnecessarily anxiety-provoking or otherwise disruptive influences. We realized that supportive, caring, and understanding attitudes and responses were the best insurance against serious adverse effects, and the best initial treatment should they emerge.[1]

The issue of adverse effects becomes extraordinarily important when we assess the risk-to-benefit ratio in working with psychedelics. Do benefits outweigh risks? Are the negative consequences of psychedelics' use worth accepting in light of their positive effects? This chapter addresses the dark side of DMT, while the next looks at how helpful the volunteers' experiences were in the long run.

The older research literature hinted at what types of negative reactions we might see with DMT.

One of Stephen Szára's subjects for a 1950s DMT EEG study was a female physician. As effects of the intramuscular DMT peaked, she exclaimed,

It is frightening because I cannot terminate it [by opening my eyes]. . . . How unpleasant! Oh, how bad. It would be better to fall down in a faint. Will it endure still for one hour? Give me something so that I shall die quickly, it would be better to die. How were you capable to do such?[2]

Szára later summarized the five "paranoid or delusional" reactions in his thirty original volunteers:

"These subjects reported 1 to 2 days later that they were convinced that someone wanted to kill or poison them during the experiment. DMT was the poison, and the person conducting the experiment was the murderer. One subject became very violent during the experiment and had to be restrained forcibly."[3]

Szára's descriptions are unusually forthcoming for a psychiatric researcher. It usually is rather difficult to get a clear sense of what exactly happens during psychedelic drug sessions in the research environment. This is especially common when adverse reactions occur in studies when the research team has a vested interest in demonstrating the drug's beneficial effects.[4]

Our New Mexico volunteers' negative reactions to DMT were not qualitatively different from those of volunteers in the other types of sessions about which we've read. They included characteristics of all the previous categories: personal psychological issues, unseen worlds and contact with nonmaterial beings, and near-death and spiritual experiences. What made the effects adverse was not the experience itself, but the volunteers' reaction to it. The subjects' responses to the anxiety-provoking elements subsequently determined whether they'd continue the fearful descent or pull out of it into a more positive resolution.

Ida was one of the few volunteers who dropped out of our research after the non-blind low dose.

Thirty-nine years old when she volunteered for the DMT studies, Ida met my former wife at a woman's spirituality workshop in Albuquerque. She had three children and had been unhappily married for nearly most of her adult life. She had a dry sense of humor that seemed to hide a great deal of anger and resentment. It was difficult to relax around her because it wasn't easy to tell if she was laughing with you or at you.

She was interested in the DMT research because of her fascination with shamanism. She had taken LSD and psilocybin mushrooms about twenty times in her life, but not once since beginning to raise her family nearly two decades previously.

Walking into Room 531 the afternoon of Ida's non-blind low dose, I was surprised to see her sitting on her bed reading a *New Yorker* magazine. This was the first and only time a volunteer ever prepared themselves for their first DMT session in this way. She looked nervous.

She continued riffling through pages as I gave her my orientation. There was an uneasy tension in the room, and I found myself stuttering my way through my usual speech, which alerted me sooner than did my conscious mind to Ida's intense anxiety.

At 4 minutes after the injection her eyes opened briefly. She looked at me, then quickly looked away. A minute later, she began,

I didn't like it. I didn't like the feeling. My head got real hot. I was out of my body. It was hard to breathe.

"It's pretty quick, isn't it?"

For you maybe.

"I mean the onset. Did it seem to last a long time?"

I was waiting for it to get over with immediately after I started feeling it. I felt the effects while the flush was going in. I couldn't have moved if you'd asked me to. I looked down at my feet and didn't recognize them as my own. It was scary, and I didn't feel safe.

There was no way I could give Ida eight times this dose tomorrow.

"Some people just don't like the drug, you know."

I hated it.

"Let's call it a day, and chalk it up to experience. No need to press our luck."

Okay.

The kitchen brought her an awful lunch. Mystery-meat tacos. A fitting end to a difficult session.

I called Ida that night. She felt fine, but confirmed her desire never to take DMT again.

For some volunteers, their high-dose experiences were powerfully unsettling, and several research subjects dropped out after these sessions. Ken was one of these.

Twenty-three years old, Ken had been in Albuquerque only a few months before embarking on our research project. Sporting long, permed hair and a flashy motorcycle, he was one of our more flamboyant volunteers. He moved to New Mexico to obtain training at one of the alternative health colleges, having dropped out of another university because of "feeling like a sheep."

He had taken MDMA quite often and admitted to having problems limiting his use. He enjoyed the "fun, celebration, love, bonding, depth, and spirituality" it provided. Curiously, he neglected to answer the drug-use questionnaire on the typical psychedelic drugs. I didn't notice that until after he had dropped out of the studies. If I had, it may have alerted me to some misgivings about his experiences on these more powerful drugs.

There was something just a little unsettling about Ken. He seemed ever so slightly "too cool" and "New Age," and Laura and I both wondered about his shadow side. Where were his edges, his anger, and his boundaries? What really made him tick? He seemed to be flitting through life rather than really taking it in. In retrospect, naturally, this seems to have been the basis for his subsequent difficulties, but there was little way we could have truly predicted his negative response to DMT.

Ken's low 0.05 mg/kg DMT dose went without difficulty.

It's a little calming and energizing, like MDMA. There were a few colors. It was pleasant. I wonder how the big dose will be tomorrow.

I wasn't sure how he'd hold up the next day, either. In my mind, MDMA is a mild drug. People who prefer it to the typical psychedelics tend not to do well when stressed, either by life or by taking more potent mind-bending drugs. MDMA is what I like to call a "love and light" drug, one that accentuates the positive and minimizes the negative. If only life were so simple.

Ken wore baggy, tie-dyed thin cotton pants the next day and a wild psychedelic T-shirt. The nurses at the front desk commented on how cute he was.

His breath seemed to catch in his throat as the flush cleared whatever remained of the high dose of DMT from his IV line. Based upon Philip's and other volunteers' reactions to high doses of DMT, this small choking sound almost always was a sign of a powerful effect. Ken's head rocked back and forth, and his feet, involuntarily it seemed, flopped up and down on the bed, as if to discharge the excessive tension he felt.

He settled down at about the 5-minute point, but grimaced and shook his head. Within a couple more minutes he took off his eyeshades and stared straight ahead. His pupils remained large, so Laura and I sat quietly, waiting for him to come down further. At 14 minutes, looking shaken but keeping some composure, he started,

There were two crocodiles. On my chest. Crushing me, raping me anally. I didn't know if I would survive. At first I thought I was dreaming, having a nightmare. Then I realized it was really happening.

I was glad he didn't have the rectal probe in place, this being a screening day.

Tears formed in his eyes, but stayed there.

"It sounds awful."

It was awful. It's the most scared I've ever been in my life. I wanted to ask to hold your hands, but I was pinned so firmly I couldn't move, and I couldn't speak. Jesus!

His experience was over, so there was little advice we could give about letting go, or trying to get past his reptilian assailants. He had been stuck, and the most we could do was try and help him accept, and maybe even learn something from, his session.

"What do you make of it?"

I haven't the slightest idea. It was as if I were being punished.

He looked directly at me and asked:

Will future doses be this big? I don't think I could do this much again.

Ken lay on the bed quietly, absorbing what had just happened to him. He didn't want to talk much, but answered the rating scale without too much difficulty. He was calmer and more composed after eating breakfast.

I reentered Room 531 after completing my notes in his chart. He looked refreshed and was waiting for me before leaving the hospital.

"How are you feeling now?"

I don't think this is the drug for me. I prefer the mellowness of MDMA. This is too hard and intense.

"That's fine. There are other big experiences in store for you in this study. It's a good idea to stop now."

I continued to wonder about the content of his horrific encounter: "Do you have any idea why crocodiles came up for you?"

Not really. I like reptiles; I used to own a pet iguana.

He laughed,

Maybe it's some sort of Egyptian past-life experience.

We stayed in touch with Ken, although he soon left Albuquerque and moved to California. His reaction had been so traumatic that I was concerned he might have some permanent psychological damage. We wondered if perhaps he had been sexually molested as a child. He did not recall any such episodes, so this remains speculation.

In a way, Ken's session scared him straight. His reptile rape had become a bad memory, one that he rarely thought about, but whose effects continued to ripple outward. He stopped taking any psychoactives, including MDMA, and cut back significantly on his marijuana use. He found work at an herb store and was living with his girlfriend. It could have been a lot worse for him.

It's easy, with hindsight, to relate Ken's negative entity-contact experience on a high dose of DMT to his habit of fending off any dark, shadowy aspects of himself. His psychological defenses were just too weak to function under the spirit molecule's powerful influence.

While earth-shattering high-dose DMT sessions could turn and stay dark and menacing, some volunteers did a remarkable job of turning them around. For example, Andrea was terrified when the spirit molecule pulled her toward a near-death experience. However, she used her initial fear as a catalyst for some important personal work.

Andrea was thirty-three years old and lived north of Santa Fe with her husband and two children. They were software developers and were quite familiar with mind-altering drugs. She had taken psychedelics over one hundred times and had used a lot of cocaine and methamphetamine several years previously.

As a child Andrea began experiencing what we call "sleep paralysis" and "hypnagogic hallucinations." Upon drifting asleep, she would be unable to move and would see brief, frightening visual scenes. Her mother, a strict Catholic, told her it was Satan coming to torture her and that she should pray to Jesus for protection. These frightening experiences continued even now, although rarely.

This inability to comfortably drop into the sleep state worried her when she thought of taking DMT at the Research Center. Perhaps she wouldn't be able to completely relax into the rush of effects. She thought she might have a near-death experience on DMT and wondered about her ability to give up awareness of her body.

Despite her concerns, Andrea enjoyed her low dose. She summed up her feelings with her first words:

That was fun!

The next day she began by saying, "I woke up this morning with a momentary fear. Then I thought that since things had been so easy yesterday, things would be fine this morning."

For some reason I placed the "emergency kit"—Valium for panic and nitroglycerin pills for severe high blood pressure—on the blood pressure machine. I couldn't remember when I had ever done that before a high-dose session.

Andrea coughed before I had half-finished the DMT injection.

She sighed deeply a time or two while the flush was going in.

She then bellowed,

NO! NO! NO!

For the next minute, she cried,

No! No! No!

Andrea's legs kicked and flailed. Her husband rested his hand on her leg, gently patting and massaging her. I placed my hand on her other foot.

At 2 minutes she was sighing, no longer screaming, and seemed to be settling down a little.

I said, "You're doing fine. Just breathe."

She replied softly,

Okay.

I noticed tears forming under her eyeshades at about 4 minutes.

"You can cry."

She began sobbing, continued for about five minutes, and then started relaxing a little.

Did I scream?

"A couple of times."

I thought so. It was hard to let go.

"There's a lot of feelings in there."

She laughed quietly,

I volunteered for this, right?

"Yes, I have your informed consent at home."

I never really left my body. I fought it all the way. I thought I was going to die. I didn't want to die. I was afraid. I realized that I had a body for a reason and that I have work to do in this body.

Andrea now turned her fear into a challenge, rather than a defeat.

When I was coming down, I wasn't sure if I ever wanted to do this again, but now I think I do. I don't think it will be as scary next time. It was death. I saw myself in that void, the void. It was just black, just too much. I've never had anything like that happen before. On LSD and mushrooms you can build up to things and you are still in your body and you can move in and out of it. With this you have no choice. I was just totally unprepared and startled and scared.

When I returned to the front desk to work on Andrea's chart, several of the ward nurses asked if everything was all right. They were alarmed by the screams coming out of Room 531.

"She got off to a rough start, but she's fine now."

Andrea looked pretty good at the 30-minute point, and she filled out her rating scale. Within an hour she was eating breakfast. How amazing the speed with which DMT hurls us through the abyss and then returns us!

When we spoke by phone a day later, she said, "Things I want to do with my life before I die are more clearly defined now. I'm not ready to go yet. We had originally moved to New Mexico so I could go to college, particularly in bodywork. I got discouraged and never followed through. My life is finite, though, and if I am to go to school, this is the time to do it."

Andrea returned for the tolerance project the next month.

Before getting started, I steered her toward her fear.

"Are you afraid of being unconscious? If so, it's all right to black out. You can just pass out. Go for it. You can lose your mind, you will get it back, it'll be all right. Four doses of DMT *will* wear you down today. Hopefully, you'll just give up without too much pain and fear."

"I'm just worried about where I will go. Will I be all right?"

She let out a brief muffled cry as the first 0.3 mg/kg dose went in. However, anticipating this, her husband, Laura, and I quickly responded by placing our hands on her arms and legs. She calmed quickly, and throughout the morning she worked on developing the theme that had emerged on her first high dose: a fear of death related to the fear of how to live her life fully.

As was the case with so many of our tolerance study volunteers, Andrea broke through into an ecstatic resolution of her anxiety and confusion during her fourth session.

Eighteen minutes into this session, she said,

That was a real gift, this last one. I was in such angst and pain for the first doses, especially the third one, and I thought, "Oh God, am I going to do this again in this last dose?" and I thought, "Yes, I'll do it again." I just never gave up. And then it was easy.

There was literally a flood of beings saying, "Okay, remember when you were young and idealistic and wanted to learn how to do bodywork?"

There's no reason I can't do that now.

When we spoke by phone later that week, she said, "I am really grate-ful for the experience. I really wanted to blow things out.[5] It's changed my perspective. It's helped me refocus on my interest in healing work. There is so much I want to do.

"There is no feeling of 'It's all fine.' There was no white light during my session. I still have a lot to work on. Part of my joy at the end was a feeling of accomplishment."

Andrea could have continued fighting against painful and frighten-ing feelings, making a bad situation worse. We knew she might have difficulty letting go after she told us about her mother's comparing her sleep-related symptoms to demonic attacks. Nevertheless, with her husband's and our support, she continued on through her fear and found the sadness and confusion that lay behind it. Facing her anxiety and fears, giving up resistance, she emerged with a clearer sense of who she was, what she desired, and plans for carrying out her goals.

Some of the most immediately hair-raising DMT sessions involved real life-and-death issues related to blood pressure that rose or fell to danger-ous levels. Lucas's blood pressure dropped to almost shocklike levels, while Kevin's rose to frighteningly high ones.

At fifty-six, Lucas was one of our older volunteers. A writer and en-trepreneur, he lived in a remote village in northern New Mexico, where his greenhouse contained all manner of exotic mind-altering plants. He was articulate, intelligent, and fearless.

Luca's outpatient clinic screening electrocardiogram (ECG) tracing was not 100 percent normal. His heart rate was rather slow, in the high 50s, and he had what is known as a "sinus arrhythmia." This means that when breathing in and out, his heart rate slowed down and sped up more than was the case with most people. I called the cardiologist who inter-preted his ECG, and he told me that if Lucas had no signs or symptoms of heart disease, there was little to worry about. It was a "normal variant."

Lucas's low dose gave us some idea that he might have a big session the next day. Like Rex, who passed out upon entrance to the futuristic beehive (see chapter 14), Lucas also reported a swaying, rocking, slightly dizzy feeling:

It feels like the bed is gently rocking. Like a hammock swaying back and forth.

Part of Lucas's non-blind high-dose session the next day, in which he approached a space station landing bay where he was accompanied by numerous humanoid automatons, is described in chapter 12. Let's now review the more frightening aspects of that morning.

Immediately after finishing the injection, Lucas became pale and sighed restlessly. He bent his legs at his knees up and down several times, then looked at Cindy.

Jesus Christ! I had no idea what it would do to me!

He retched once. I looked around. There was no "emesis basin" into which he could vomit. Cindy pointed at a gown that was crumpled into a pile behind me. That was all we had, and I offered it to him. He put the gown into his hands and looked at it uncomprehendingly.

Hunnh??

"Try that," I offered.

He retched once into the gown but did not throw anything up.

Jesus Christ!

While retching into the gown, he began sliding off the bed headfirst toward Cindy's feet. I got up, walked over to Cindy's side of the bed, and helped pull him back onto it. He was holding the gown up against his face.

At 5 minutes his blood pressure dropped from 108/71 to 81/55, and his pulse from 92 to 45. He was pale; in fact, he was turning green. Holding his head and trembling, Lucas was going into shock.

Two minutes later his pulse was 47 and his blood pressure was 87/49.

We tried to adjust the bed—to raise his feet and lower his head—to increase blood flow to his brain. In the confusion, it was impossible to operate the controls. Should I call the cardiac emergency team? Get ready some drugs to raise his blood pressure? DMT causes such robust rises in blood pressure that I worried that if his circulation did recover on its own, and we gave him a big dose of adrenaline to treat his shock, we might overshoot and cause a stroke from too high a blood pressure.

I said, "You're doing fine. Take some deep breaths, focus on your breathing."

He looked baffled and ill.

His vital signs recovered on their own over the next 2 minutes. At 12 minutes, his blood pressure was 102/78, and his pulse was 73.

At 15 minutes he began describing his approach to the space station. More relevant to his terror, he described what he saw upon opening his eyes:

I looked at Cindy and she had incredible clown makeup on. It was not funny. It was malevolent. I was afraid to look at her face. I don't really know you, Cindy, but you seem real nice. It was the drug. I had just a flash of you, Rick—like a stainless-steel face, with intimations of protuberances and knobs. Cindy was bad enough. I couldn't look at you directly. It would have ruined your bedside manner forever.

He started to relax and moved on to excitedly describe his outer space voyage. It was difficult for me to pay attention, thinking about how close to disaster we all had been.

His truck broke down on the way home. His wife picked him up, and she spent the drive back to their house describing horrific memories of childhood incest that were emerging in her therapy. Two messages awaited them upon their arrival: a friend had shot his head off in a suicide, another friend was dying rapidly of cancer.

When we spoke the next day, he wondered, "What's real? What's not? It felt like a boulder was dropped into the pond, not a pebble, and the wake was being felt everywhere. The man who killed himself did so at just about the time I took the DMT. It makes me believe in synchronicity of some sort or another."

I had little choice but to tell him, "I've been thinking it would be safest to hold off on any more studies. While I think you're a great person to have in the research, I would hate to damage you physically."

Lucas weakly protested, but he understood. Nevertheless, the day's events had seriously rattled him. He asked me to come by to visit him. Later that week I drove to his house and spent the day with him, the first and only house call for the DMT studies. We went over his session, what had happened, and how he felt about it. By the end of the afternoon he had somewhat regained his bearings. He felt pretty well within a few days and resumed his normal routine. He attended nearly every one of the post-study socials over the next several years and came to look back appreciatively at his DMT experience.

Kevin was thirty-nine years old and married to Sara, whose story we read in chapter 14. He was a rather serious individual, and in his career as a mathematician found a certain predictability that suited him. He had taken psychedelics nearly two hundred times and found them "useful for emotional and spiritual growth."

Kevin was a big and burly man, one of those people whose body seems to provide a certain protective role in fending off the outside world. He had a dry wit and a sparkle in his eye, but there seemed to be a certain fearfulness that he spent lots of energy keeping at bay. One of the ways he expended that energy was in being hyperlogical and extremely talkative.

Kevin also barely squeezed through the cardiac screening gates to our study. His blood pressure was just below our cut-off point, and his ECG showed some "nonspecific" abnormalities, meaning they did not indicate any particular type of heart disease. Showing tremendous determination to get into the tolerance study, he began exercising regularly, dropped almost fifteen pounds, and stopped drinking coffee. He paid for an independent cardiologist examination and an exercise treadmill test, both of which gave him a clean bill of health.

His low-dose session was thankfully uneventful, but I worried about his attitude.

At 2 minutes after his low dose, he said,

So when does it start, or is that all there is?

Oh, I feel some physical effects. My heart's speeding up, and the blood pressure cuff feels odd.

He seemed too cavalier. I wanted to shake him up, get him ready for a big trip tomorrow. I felt this even more so when he said Sara and he were going to have a big meat-and-cheese pizza and beer with some friends that night!

I warned, "I would go into it tomorrow as if you were going to die. Be prepared for that. Approach it with fear but faith. That's the way that I get prepared for people's sessions when I come into the room.

"I suggest a lighter meal, too. You really want to be nice to yourself tonight and tomorrow."

That next morning he looked nervous lying in his bed. Sara sat near the foot of the bed, ready to offer assistance.

He said, "I'm worried about my blood pressure."

"So are we, but it should be all right. We've had some pretty high blood pressures and they resolved quickly."

His breathing sped up after the infusion was done, but he remained still. His top blood pressure number, the systolic, shot up to 208 at the 2-minute recording. An alarm I didn't know existed on the blood pressure machine began ringing piercingly. Laura couldn't locate the switch, so she turned off the entire machine. I passed her a note: "Turn it back on at 4 minutes."

Let's turn to the notes that Kevin sent us a few days later for his account of what happened:

I feel a tingling in my body. A strange lifting sensation. I see colors coming at me in the darkness. Then I see a light, a matrix of cells that looks like skin under a microscope, with white light behind them. All of a sudden off to the upper right I see a figure. She looks like an African War Goddess. She is black, carries a spear, a shield, and appears to have a mask on. I have surprised her. She takes a defensive and aggressive posture. She says, "YOU DARE TO COME HERE?!" I mentally reply, "I guess so."

The scene before me erupts in a way that I can only relate to what it looks like in the TV show Star Trek *when the spaceship shifts into a faster-than-the-speed-of-light acceleration. I feel a tremendous rush in my chest. My heart is hammering. I feel waves coursing through my body. I think, "This is it. Rick and Laura have killed me." Then my subconscious or someone said to me, "You're dying, don't die." Far away I hear what sounds like an alarm. I think something's gone very wrong. I think of Sara and my little son. I fight. I'm not going to die. I feel as if I've dived off a 10-meter platform, hit the water, and am at the bottom of the pool. I swim for the surface.*

The effects are wearing off. I am hypersensitive to people in the room. I can hear their breathing and their movements. I feel their tension.

My notes indicate that at about 3 minutes Kevin said,

I'm still here.

"Good."

His 5-minute systolic reading was only two points lower, 206, and the alarm went off again. Sara looked worried. Laura turned to me questioningly. What to do? The situation began hovering near chaos.

Is that an alarm?

"It's okay, your blood pressure's dropping a little."

That was incredible!

My bedside notes indicate that as Kevin began speaking, he rubbed the back of his head.

His blood pressure continued slowly dropping.

He said,

I have a little headache at the base of my neck.

His headache mostly likely resulted from the arteries leading to his brain stretching, but thankfully not tearing, under the assault from his high blood pressure.

Kevin then added,

It would be interesting to see if the black woman warrior were there again during the next sessions. Maybe she wouldn't be taken by surprise next time.

I thought, "Next sessions?"

Kevin's blood pressure was normal by 30 minutes. He was tired, but felt good. I knew I had escaped a collision with something very dangerous.

I spoke with Kevin later in the day from my office. He sounded upbeat and pressed to continue in the research.

"I have had many psychedelic experiences in my life," he said, "but nothing could compare with or prepare me for what happened today. I feel I have come back a changed person. I realized that there are many more realms than the one we exist in. Even though it was terrifying, I am looking forward to participating more. I want to let go next time and see where I go and what I experience. I want to know more about the spaces that I went to."

Laura and I conferred about bringing him in for four 0.3 mg/kg doses for the tolerance study. While this was slightly less than the 0.4 mg/kg high dose, we kept asking ourselves, "What if he suffers a stroke?" The answer was, of course, "We can't take that risk."

Kevin was disappointed, but we tried to make the most out of what he had undergone.

I said, "You have lots to mull over. You experienced a high dose of DMT, something few people ever do. I probably shouldn't have bent the rules in the first place with your abnormal cardiogram."

On the drive home through the mountains at the end of that day, I wondered how the road signs I passed on the highway would have looked if Kevin were dead. Exhausted, I ate dinner listlessly and went directly to bed.

Effective screening and preparation was key to keeping serious adverse effects as infrequent as we did. While the rate of negative effects may have been even lower with better screening, it's difficult to see how we could have improved upon our methods. Looking back on it now, one thing I should have done was to trust more deeply my intuition about certain volunteers' psychological suitability or cardiovascular health.

Perhaps our doses of DMT were too high. This was a razor's edge. Too small a dose would have fallen short of the psychedelic threshold, but too high a dose, as we saw in Philip's case (as described in the prologue), was dangerous. In retrospect, 0.3 mg/kg may have been better as our top dose. No one experienced this as "sub-psychedelic." We chose 0.4 mg/kg based upon clinical judgement and our research aims. Nevertheless, this high dose of DMT may have compromised the safety and well-being of the minority of volunteers who lost their way, struggled to find it, and were traumatized in their journey.

When all is said and done, the fact remains that the spirit molecule does not always lead us to love and light. It can open our eyes to terrifying realities, too, and mark us with those experiences for as long as do any beatific ones. DMT is a potentially dangerous drug. For that reason, we must think long and hard about using it in ourselves and on one another.

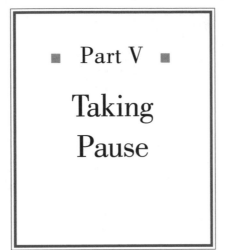

■ Part V ■

Taking Pause

18

If So, So What?

Our volunteers unquestionably had some of the most intense, unusual, and unexpected experiences of their lives during the DMT research. The spirit molecule dragged, pushed, pulled, and thrust research subjects into themselves, out of their bodies, and through various planes of reality. We've read about all manner of sessions, many of which seemed to help people better understand their relationship with themselves and the outside world. We've also read about the toll some experiences took on our recruits.

Was it worth it? Were those who participated in our research any better off for their involvement? Did they undergo any positive changes in their lives? Did anything really good stick to their ribs? In other words, "If so, so what?"

The answer to these questions, I will tell you now, is "It depends." It depends upon what we call "benefit." Are subtle changes in attitude, perspective, and creativity adequate reasons to take the risks about which we've read? Or do we require more visible grounds for believing something truly beneficial happened? What would that proof look like? If not much really resulted, why not? Did the fault lie in the drug, the set, or the setting?

Before beginning the study, I expected people would have profound psychedelic encounters. However, we all know how fleeting most of these insights, understandings, and realizations can be. My hope was that with a safer, more consistent and reliable clinical environment, our volunteers would be able to get even deeper and further into the psychedelic experience than ever before. Perhaps under these circumstances there might be more long-lasting effects.

What would be testimony to a fuller commitment to putting into effect the ideas, perceptions, and feelings to which the spirit molecule provided access? A change in career. Entering psychotherapy. Beginning a regular meditation practice, within or outside of an organized spiritual discipline. Concerted efforts to modify lifestyle, such as increasing exercise, improving diet, or discontinuing potentially harmful drugs or alcohol. Donating time or money to charitable or community organizations. In other words, did more enlightened behavior result from their enlightened experiences?

As volunteers came in for their last session in any particular experiment, I asked how they felt about their participation. "What did you get out of your involvement in the study?" was how I began such conversations.

This was a relatively short-term assessment of any benefit, as experiments generally lasted three to six months. In this context, most did think they had grown in some ways, especially in response to their high-dose encounters with the spirit molecule. These were informal, casual impressions obtained in Room 531, where managing sessions and gathering data competed for our attention.

We also gathered some longer-term follow-up data from the first group of volunteers. Laura contacted as many of the original dose-response research subjects as she could and arranged for more formal personal or telephone interviews with them. By the time I left New Mexico, we had completed only eleven formal follow-up interviews. Longer-term follow-up for the nearly fifty additional volunteers is obviously of great importance, and I hope to have the opportunity to complete this in the future.

We read about Sean's mystical experience during the tolerance study. On a day during the cyproheptadine study when he received placebo, we had time to talk about things other than his immediate response to DMT.

He thought for a minute after I asked him about the overall effects of his research participation, then said, "It seems like you create your own world in a way. It's amazing what the mind can do."

"Are you referring to your big experience during the tolerance project?"

"Yes," he said. "I call it a mystical experience. I took my mother to church the other day. It was a ceremony having to do with Easter: Paul on the road to Damascus. He was blind for three days after he encountered Christ. I think that's what happened to me. But I don't know how it's really affected my life. I guess part of it was asking for permission each of the three times. Maybe a lot of that has been involved in my life changing. I can do more with my life now. I give myself permission to get involved in new experiences and then do so."

Mike was a thirty-year-old graduate student whose sessions were enjoyable but always a little anxiety-provoking. He wasn't sure if he remembered his entire first 0.4 mg/kg session, and he didn't like losing his bearings. He received placebo on the last day of the dose-response study, and I asked about what he had gotten out of his time with us.

He replied, "I think about that sometimes. When I read now, I'm increasingly interested in fringe areas of my field. When I took LSD when I was younger, it opened my mind to other possibilities I wasn't otherwise aware of. DMT may have had some of that effect, too. Before the study, I was grinding away. Now I'm looking at other things. I can't think of anything else that would have nudged me in that direction."

However, he was less enthusiastic two years later:

"It was an experience of being poked and stuck and having my brain assaulted with chemicals—not a life-changing experience. Thoughts of the high dose might wander through my mind every month or two. I've not changed as a result, though. It only reminded me of taking drugs in my twenties, when I was more carefree and had lots of time on my hands."

We read about Willow's near-death experiences in chapter 15. After a low dose of DMT one day, she reflected upon her life since involving herself in the study:

"DMT's teaching me about transition, change, and death. When my husband's father died recently, it was clear to me that much has happened with my views about death. I knew he had transitioned rather than disappeared.

"DMT is about death and dying. I had a near-death experience on it. It's not a blank death, it's full. I liked it really. I no longer fear death. Not that I need to wait to die to be unafraid and know what dying is like. Rather, I'm more accepting and serene about living."

Tyrone was the dose-response volunteer who found himself in the "organic apartment of the future." During a placebo day, we had a chance to look back upon his participation.

"Maybe I get drunk less," he admitted. "I still have one to two beers at night to get a little buzz, but drinking five at a time, on a Saturday or Friday night, I'm doing that less. Things are more or less as usual. My girlfriend wants to get married. I've never been married. It's a big decision. I'm thinking more of settling down permanently. Maybe it's a function of the study, maybe it's a function of where I am now with my life. It may have helped a little, but not really."

At follow-up two years later, he remarked, "There were some insightful thoughts at the time, but I didn't necessarily follow through on them. They were pleasurable to think about, though. However, I haven't really thought about it much since the first three or four months.

"I think overall I'm getting healthier, but I don't see this as related to DMT. I went through a big move and career change after the study, although this was in the works all along. There haven't really been any changes I can attribute to the DMT experiences themselves."

Stan, about whose therapeutic experience we read in chapter 11, described some possible effects of his DMT exposure on his subsequent sensitivity to psychedelic mushrooms. We had this conversation toward the end of his double-blind low dose in the dose-response study.

Stan said, "I've taken mushrooms two times since I've been in the study, and I've never been so high on psychedelics before. I had the experience of going into and never coming out of the white light. Previously, I never felt the choice was mine to stay or come back. I saw how the white light is all there is, and that this world is just shadows and plays of light."

"How about any positive emotional changes?"

"The psychic channels may have been opened," he replied, "but the trips were mostly without content or insights. Maybe I'm a little more empathic, in tune, receptive. If that's the case, it's very subtle. And it's not because of the DMT. Maybe if I looked at the last couple of months there have been some changes, but the DMT experiences themselves have not caused them directly."

We followed up with Stan after he finished the tolerance study. He remained rather reticent about the impact of his DMT sessions:

"Maybe my self-concept has been affected. Taking a ride like that can cause you to feel a little better about yourself. However, it can go both ways. There weren't any insights, however, neither spiritual or psychological. It did have a cleansing effect, though, and it laid the foundation for some other things."

I've described some of Aaron's experiences in chapter 12, "Unseen Worlds," and chapter 13, "Contact Through the Veil: 1." He received placebo one day during the pindolol study and had a chance to reflect on DMT's effects on his life:

"The long-term effects are very interesting. It leaves me in a different state. It's not altered, per se, but more open to synchronicity, magic, and unexpected opportunities."

In the longer-term follow-up Aaron said, "DMT shook some things loose, as it was so shattering. I now find I have more control over my reality by letting go; it's a paradox. I've found that the DMT experience intensified verbal, visual, and musical abilities. Overall, DMT showed me another level or process I needed to see. Nothing I thought or felt made any difference in terms of controlling the sessions. I learned the beneficial aspects of losing control."

Sara, who made such complex contact with nonmaterial beings in the tolerance study, also participated in the pindolol study. On the last of those four sessions, we had a chance to look back upon her involvement in the research.

"Things have broadened out. I have an awareness of worlds on the other side of this reality. I have the feeling of remembering those entities. My experience of them was so real it doesn't fade with time like other things do. They want us to come back and teach us and play with us. I want to go back and learn. I wish you didn't control who gets DMT!"

Before Rex underwent his overwhelming 0.2 plus pindolol session described in chapter 14, "Contact Through the Veil 2," he received a lower dose of DMT with pindolol. As that session wrapped up, I asked him how he had been feeling about his participation.

"I've had more creative urges," he answered, "and I've been writing more. As chaotic as they are, the DMT sessions have helped me be more centered. Having gone through it gives me more of a sense of strength in myself.

"I have written some poems of the Other. Many were written before, but some after getting started in the study. DMT made me face aspects of my unconscious that I didn't know were there, like my fear of dying."

We read about Ken's terrifying encounter with sexually violent crocodiles. A few months after that, I called him to see how things were. He sounded surprisingly philosophical:

"It's really changed my feelings about death. I'm not nearly as afraid to die as I was before. It has also really changed my view of life—about how things are basically not as they seem. There is a certain falling away of expectations.

"I'm also less afraid of my own insanity. There's this Jewish guilt to fit in and be normal but I feel less inclined to be that way now. I'm not as interested in people or social lubrication situations that don't have a lot of meaning to me. Friendships that aren't that important are fading away."

We haven't met Frederick before; his experiences with DMT were not especially noteworthy above and beyond the "average" 0.4 mg/kg encounter. One morning, however, after receiving a low dose of the spirit molecule, he had this to say about how the effects of DMT spread out over time:

"I'm more relaxed now in general after that 0.4 dose. It seems to have cleared out some energy blocks. The momentum from two years of pushing really hard at my job is hard to get rid of. When I was coming down from the big dose, I saw how the energy was blocked by fears and holding on to things. Nothing specific, but more alertness and awareness of my state. I'm not in such a hurry to get things done now. I am more relaxed in general. I am less goal-oriented. If things don't get done now, they will sooner or later."

Gabe, the physician whose nursery and being contact experiences we read about earlier, described some positive repercussions from his meetings with the spirit molecule. This conversation took place during the morning he received four saline injections in the tolerance study.

He said, "I've been feeling a peacefulness from having been in the study. It's a whole different realm than other high-dose psychedelics. I can access deep stuff in the psyche. It's right there, it's like a movie screen. It's in your face. With LSD it's not as much a movie as with DMT. For two or three weeks after the tolerance study, I was much more there for the people I work with. I was super-there."

Philip's 0.6 mg/kg DMT overdose occurred in the initial stages of the study, when we were testing to find the right dosages for "high" and "low" DMT sessions. He went on to develop over the next several months mild panic symptoms whenever he found himself in unfamiliar or uncertain circumstances. It was as if he had become overly sensitive to any inkling of losing control. Nevertheless, he worked these through himself and successfully negotiated his way through the dose-response project.

At his follow-up interview with Laura he stated,

"I now have a much more tangible sense of cosmic and divine consciousness with an altered sense of selfhood in relationship. A more real sense of connectedness to all around me. I am more integrated. My own divinity is less of an abstraction. Thinking and feeling overlap more now."

While he also believed this had changed his capacity for engaging in psychotherapy with his clients, he didn't believe it was outwardly obvious. Philip had reduced his use of psychedelics since his participation in the DMT work. He now took them every two or three months, instead of several times a month, and used them more carefully, in a supportive group context. He wasn't sure how much of this was the result of other changes in his life—moving and getting divorced—and how much was from his DMT experiences.

Don was a thirty-six-year-old waiter and writer. His transpersonal high-dose DMT sessions destabilized his world view so much that he stopped writing for the first time in years. As opposed to Elena, when Don met face-to-face the vast and impenetrable nature of the source of all existence, he despaired. Elena was steeped in Eastern mysticism, while Don was raised in, and continued believing in, the Catholic faith. Elena saw the love behind the "impersonal" void. Don, on the other hand, felt shocked, stunned, and betrayed by the absence of a personal God or Savior behind it all. DMT had knocked away his spiritual and philosophical underpinnings, and he found himself at a loss for something to replace them.

When I called to request his participation in additional studies, he declined, but updated me. He was feeling quite well.

He told me, "I'm doing better than I was before the study. I have more enthusiasm for life, as it was a death experience for me. I've gotten back into writing and found a patron to support me part-time. There's a little bit of my DMT sessions in my writings, but not too much."

We read a brief excerpt from one of Ray's high-dose DMT EEG sessions in chapter 15, "Death and Dying." When we spoke with him some years later, he had this to say about long-term effects of his high-dose sessions:

"I've adopted a few new words into my mental vocabulary to describe the psychedelic experience. I see people more as organisms. I think the DMT experiences validated certain spiritual ideas, particularly a belief in the value of the subjective, beyond or in addition to the validity and value of the scientific."

He also sent us a photograph of his young son, whose middle name was Strassman.

Lucas, whose real-life near-death experience nearly ended in circulatory collapse, nevertheless felt he got something positive out of the session.

"I don't see the world in quite the same way since DMT," he said. "I'm more open-minded and laid-back. The experience reconfirmed my path and what I'm involved in. As far as my beliefs and spiritual perspectives, everything was reinforced."

Elena, about whose mystical experience we read in chapter 16, sent me a letter one year after she finished the dose-response study:

"Most of my experiences fade with time. Not so with DMT. The images and ordeals from my sessions have grown more clear and refined. I recall being able to face the eternal fire of creation and not be burned, to bear the weight of the entire universe and not be crushed. This brings some perspective to my mundane life and I am able to relax and embrace it more easily. Outside me, not much is different. Inside, I rest in the comfort of knowing my soul is eternal and my consciousness endless."

Let's summarize this small number of follow-up conversations and interviews. Volunteers reported a stronger sense of self, less fear of death, and greater appreciation of life. Some found they were better able to relax, and they pushed themselves a little less. Several volunteers drank less alcohol or noted they were more sensitive to psychedelic drugs. Others believed with greater certainty that there are different levels of reality. We also have heard about powerfully felt validation and confirmation of previously held beliefs. In these cases, views and perspectives became broader and deeper, but not essentially different.

Thankfully, there also were no long-term negative effects in Philip, Lucas, and Ken. While we did not formally interview Kevin after his high blood pressure episode, we saw each other socially a few times afterward, and he seemed to have suffered no ill effects.

The few examples of visible change in volunteers' "outside" lives all were underway in some form or another before they met the spirit molecule. Several divorces occurred in our subjects, but none were directly brought on by the effects of DMT sessions. Perhaps Marsha's high-dose DMT encounter with white porcelain carousel figures, described in chapter 11, convinced her that she belonged "with [her] culture" on the East Coast. She divorced her husband and left New Mexico. However, she had been married and divorced twice before and clearly knew how difficult was her current marriage.

No one left an established career for a more heartfelt vocation. Peter, one of our recruits, had images while on DMT of a community in Arizona to which he had been considering relocating. He made the move after completing the dose-response study. He was wealthily retired, however, so the move was easy and natural for him.

Sean, too, made good decisions about his career, cutting down on his backbreaking hours as an attorney so he could "tend his garden" and plant more trees on his remote rural acreage. In addition, he weathered his then-girlfriend's departure with grace and began a new, more satisfying relationship during his DMT participation. In Sean's case, many of these events also were in motion by the time he began working with us.

Andrea, whose screams of "No! No! No!" rang through the Research Center, seemed like one of the most likely people to make major shifts in her life. Her high-dose DMT sessions showed her the preciousness and limits of the body and helped her remember some youthful idealism regarding her career. However, by the time I left New Mexico two years later she had gone no further than obtaining some catalogs from local natural therapeutics schools.

Even in Elena's case, I was not convinced that she really had benefited from her experiences in a practical way. We remained friends and I continued to be involved in her and Karl's life, and there did not seem to be evidence of basic changes in her everyday pattern of interactions and reactions to her world. Hers was one of the earliest cases causing me some reluctance in accepting at face value the transformative power of even the most profound and incredibly spiritual experiences.

It was especially disappointing that no one began psychotherapy or a spiritual discipline to work further on the insights they felt on DMT. The few people for whom therapy was an issue returned to therapy, or restarted antidepressants, because of relapses into depression at some point after their high-dose DMT sessions. That is, they sought help for possible adverse effects rather than capitalizing on psychological or spiritual breakthroughs from their sessions.

Why wasn't there more obvious benefit to our volunteers?

Within sessions, we were not focusing on helping people with problems. These were not treatment studies. Volunteers were relatively well-adjusted. Neither did we intend to treat our research subjects. We planned to, and mostly did, sit by and support them rather than steer or guide them in any particular direction. When we did apply psychotherapeutic principles or techniques, it was out of clinical necessity or prudence. We scrupulously avoided working on a psychological level with the vast majority of our volunteers. In fact, one of my most pressing questions was whether a neutral environment would lead to positive responses in those having powerful DMT experiences.

Another answer became clearer only as the study progressed. This was the deep and undeniable realization that DMT was not inherently therapeutic. Instead, we again had to face the crucial importance of set and setting. What the volunteers brought to their sessions, and the fuller context of their lives, was as important, if not more so, than the drug itself in determining how they dealt with their experiences. Without a suitable framework—spiritual, psychotherapeutic, or otherwise—in which to process their journeys with DMT, their sessions became just another series of intense psychedelic encounters.

As the years passed, I began feeling a peculiar anxiety about listening to volunteers' accounts of their first high-dose DMT sessions. It was as if I didn't want to hear them. These psychotherapeutic, near-death, and mystical sessions repeatedly reminded me of their ineffectiveness in effecting any real change. I wanted to say, "That's very interesting, but now what? To what purpose?" By extension, these sessions' lack of lasting impact began eroding the basic foundations of my motivation for performing this type of research. Additionally, the reports of contact with invisible worlds and their inhabitants, while utterly amazing, left me grasping at conceptual straws as to their reality and meaning. My attitude to high-dose sessions started turning from hope for breakthroughs to relief at volunteers emerging unharmed and intact.

The need to shift the focus of the psychedelic research in Albuquerque was clear. Risks were real, and long-term benefits vague. I began looking for a way to improve the benefit-to-risk ratio. This required a more concerted effort to develop a therapy study, one that would involve working with patients instead of normal volunteers. It also called for using a longer-acting drug that would allow time to perform psychological work during the acute intoxication.

In the next two chapters, I will describe how the cessation of my work began with research involving the longer-acting drug psilocybin and with plans to treat patients. Events from both within and outside of the research environment combined to exert tremendous personal and professional pressure. At a certain point I felt I had less to lose, and more to gain, by discontinuing the psychedelic research.

19

Winding Down

A wide range of difficulties began affecting our psychedelic drug studies. Their cumulative effect led to my leaving New Mexico and stopping the research. I will begin describing those events in this chapter.

Some difficulties were built into the study from its very inception, and it was only a matter of time before they began causing problems. The biomedical model was the most obvious of these concerns.

Others resulted from a series of unfortunate events. Such was the case of the university's Human Research Ethics Committee not allowing us to take the psilocybin project out of the hospital into a more pleasant environment.

Many of the stumbling blocks were ones I dimly saw but chose to minimize, hoping they might "take care of themselves": There should have been little surprise that a critical mass of collaborators at the University of New Mexico failed to materialize as promised. I suspected, but needed to see for myself, that there would be few sustained beneficial effects on our volunteers from isolated high-dose DMT sessions. I kept on the research team an especially troubled and troubling graduate student. I chose to disregard reports I had heard about contact with beings on DMT and was unprepared for dealing with their frequency in our work. I ought to have predicted what would be my Buddhist community's response to publicly linking psychedelics with Buddhist practice.

Certain developments truly were completely unexpected, but in retrospect they appear related to the strain of performing the research, and its effects on those around me. My former wife's sudden development of cancer falls into this category.

The repercussions of working with spirit molecules are so complex, so widespread and far-reaching, that no one who was not there from the very beginning could really understand what this research was like. However, the purpose of this book is to tell the entire story. Part of every story is its end. For those who are now working, or wish to work, with psychedelic drugs, it's important to convey these details, in a spirit of "informed consent." You'd better know what you're getting yourself into.

There were several threads running through these projects, and early on they all lined up rather neatly. I wanted to give a lot of DMT, see what various doses did, and then give more. The first two projects, the dose-response and the tolerance studies, felt like the appetizer and the main course. Single high doses of the spirit molecule were incredibly psychedelic, and repeated dosing made it possible to assimilate and work more effectively with the access it provided to profound altered states. However, the model that allowed me to begin also negatively constrained subsequent research projects with DMT.

The biomedical model's explicit task is to dissect, dig deeper, and explain-by-describing the biological phenomenon under examination. Since this model holds sway in psychiatric research, I learned it thoroughly and presented the DMT studies in those terms.

In the dose-response and tolerance studies, the biological measurements were less personally compelling than were the psychological effects of DMT. We drew blood and measured vital signs and temperature, and with these data we could mathematically demonstrate that something *really* was going on. The rating-scale data also nicely straddled the clinical and objective realities; that is, the questionnaire provided objective validation of subjective effects. Nevertheless, the most fascinating and rewarding data were obtained by listening to and watching our volunteers in Room 531.

However, once we began the required mechanism-of-action research, the biomedical model was going to exert greater restrictions upon the types of studies we would be allowed to perform. In chapter 8, "Getting DMT," I described these follow-up DMT studies, which examined the effects of pindolol, cyproheptadine, and naltrexone. We combined these receptor-blocking drugs with DMT and compared responses to this combination with those of DMT alone. We thus could infer the role of the relevant receptor in mediating specific effects of the spirit molecule.

These types of studies no longer placed the subjective effects of DMT at the forefront of our inquiry. The mechanisms were now more important than the experience. The explicit setting had shifted in a titanic manner. These protocols now approached our subjects less as individuals undergoing a psychedelic experience and more as biological systems with which we could define drug mechanisms more precisely.

It wasn't easy to be as enthusiastic about these studies as the earlier ones. In fact, volunteers did as much to encourage me to perform them as I did to request their participation. Adding to this discomfort was my sense that I had learned something deep and basic about the workings of the spirit molecule. In the last chapter, I describe this conclusion—that is, that lasting or substantial benefit from high-dose DMT sessions in our setting was difficult to see. Combined with the gradually growing incidence of adverse effects, I saw the risk-to-benefit ratio turning less favorable. I needed to change the model to one in which people might benefit from participating in the studies.

The two frameworks that might contain projects where people "got better" were the psychotherapeutic and the spiritual. A spirituality-based project was unlikely in a clinical research environment. So I began work on a psychotherapeutic project, a psilocybin-assisted psychotherapy study with the terminally ill.

It was at this point I felt most acutely the lack of a larger psychedelic research community at the university. While the Research Center and Department of Psychiatry were consistently and unquestionably supportive of my studies, there were no local psychiatric colleagues familiar with psychedelic drug research.

A large part of why I began our work with a strictly biomedical model related to promises by other psychedelic research scientists, especially psychotherapeutically oriented ones, to join forces with me once the New Mexico research started. I was willing to take the set and setting risks inherent in the biomedical model in anticipation of colleagues later helping me shift to more treatment-based activities.

There's a widespread and far-flung network of scientists and clinicians interested in psychedelic drugs throughout the United States, many of whom have close affiliations with the academic and the private sectors. I met nearly all of them at various meetings before the DMT research began. This psychedelic research network seemed more altruistic and cooperative than the larger biomedical research community. Perhaps scientists who believed in psychedelics' power could join forces, rather than compete.

At these meetings was a unanimous complaint that "the government won't let us study these drugs." If only somewhere someone could begin, that place would become the center of a psychedelic research renaissance. As it became apparent that I would receive permission to give DMT and would obtain some funding for the study, it seemed that the University of New Mexico would become just that center of psychedelic research.

I was willing to accept the short-term drawbacks associated with the animal-biology-based model as the price for initiating studies. However, I hoped that after establishing safe use of psychedelics under medical supervision, more therapeutic studies would begin with my colleagues' assistance. It would be a smooth transition from our dose-response and tolerance work to psychedelic therapy projects.

Topping off this ambitious clinical research framework was the development of new psychedelic drugs with unique properties. With the full range of clinical facilities available, it would be easy to assess the effects of new medications in normal volunteers and in specific patient populations.

It sounded good. The University of New Mexico is the premier university in the state and has dozens of undergraduate and graduate departments, professional schools, and a highly ranked medical school. I believed that once research began in Albuquerque, the half dozen or so carefully positioned colleagues throughout the country would quickly join me. They said they would.

After the Food and Drug Administration approved the DMT study and we began work in late 1990, I asked my colleagues to come on board. The opportunity for which we all had been waiting had arrived.

Here is how they answered:

"My wife thinks Albuquerque's too small. There aren't enough malls. My daughter doesn't want to leave her friends."

"We have to wait until our son graduates from high school in seven years."

"The University of New Mexico is second-rate. I'd never take my research there."

"We've already moved enough. I can't commit to another move unless I know it's the last one I'll ever make."

"I have to wait until I get my Ph.D. I don't know when that will be."

"I don't want to work that hard. I like my part-time job at a mental health clinic. I get to take a lot of vacations and go on meditation retreats."

In retrospect, I had succumbed to my own wishful thinking. It was easier to talk about the transformative value of the psychedelic experience than it was to put into practice some of its contents. My colleagues may have had inspiring experiences, but they were not committed to goals that required work and sacrifice.

There were, of course, other less explicit reasons for everyone's sudden change of heart about the importance of joining forces to generate a critical mass of psychedelic researchers. One of these undoubtedly was the normal and reasonable, although difficult to admit, anxiety about really doing this sort of work. Anyone who knows anything about administering psychedelics gets nervous just thinking about it.

Another issue concerned political motives. That is, who was going to lead the way in psychedelic research? Rather than combining our efforts, some colleagues saw the breakthrough occurring in Albuquerque as an opportunity to establish their own research foundations, putting themselves at the head of such organizations.

While the lack of support by psychedelic colleagues was an emotional loss, I could deal with that. More problematic was being left holding the ball. I now was committed to a course of research out of which I had planned to transition as soon as I could with the aid of those collaborators.

As the dose-response study neared completion, I needed to decide how to design subsequent grant applications and study designs. It seemed reckless to begin proposing full-fledged psychotherapy protocols. I had no training in that field of research and knew that any such proposals would fail to attract funding. There was momentum to continue biomedically based studies. We had the data and Research Center support, and it was my area of expertise. These mechanism-of-action follow-up studies would not be controversial, and there would be support for funding them.

I could delay this process by performing dose-response and perhaps tolerance studies with other drugs, such as psilocybin and LSD. However, the brain-science projects would increasingly take precedence. Any psychotherapeutic studies would be minor, informal, and peripheral to the main thrust of my work. I designed several mechanism-of-action experiments and received approval and a generous grant to perform them. At the same time, I also received approval and funding to perform a dose-response study with psilocybin.

Psilocybin, the active ingredient in magic mushrooms, is closely chemically related to DMT. It's orally active and much longer-acting. It also is significantly more popular than DMT, so learning about its effects has greater relevance to public health issues of drug abuse.

Psilocybin's six- to eight-hour duration was attractive in many ways. We'd be able to study its effects in a more leisurely manner than with DMT. Volunteers could participate in experiments while intoxicated with psilocybin in ways that were impossible in the case of DMT's debilitating and brief peak effects.

However, the setting of the Research Center was an obstacle to designing and thinking about psilocybin protocols. Many of our DMT volunteers would have leaped at the opportunity to participate in a psilocybin project if it were not for the prospect of spending an entire day in an altered state of consciousness in the hospital.

The short duration of DMT's effects usually allowed us to find a window of tranquility at the Research Center. Even so, there were many times when the sounds of jet planes, laughing and debating medical personnel, crashing carts, groaning and screaming patients, the overhead duct fan, and roaring compactors had a major negative impact on people's DMT sessions. The smells of burning food, medication, and powerful disinfectants were especially grim. And the rare but regular occurrence of hospital service personnel walking into Room 531 was a constant source of anxiety. They all would combine to make a full-day psilocybin session an exercise in tension.

The university owned several small houses within a city block of the hospital. There was a relatively steady turnover of clinical, administrative, and teaching personnel in them. Several had little courtyards and gardens, and they seemed perfect for taking the psilocybin research "off-site."

I approached the Research Center nursing and administrative staff, the University Hospital legal counsel and risk-management office, and the Department of Psychiatry about moving the psilocybin research out of the hospital. They all considered my request reasonable, prudent, and within the realm of possibility

However, the Human Research Ethics Committee, many of whose current members were not familiar with our research, was not comfortable with the safety issues off-site studies might raise. They wanted to make sure that security guards were close at hand to manage any volunteers who might act dangerously, and they wanted us to keep studies in the more contained hospital setting. As is so often the case, their fears led to exactly the outcome they hoped to avoid.

Several brave DMT volunteers agreed to come in for some psilocybin pi-lot work in which we would determine what were "low," "medium," and "high" doses of the drug. A few people dropped out after low-dose expe-riences, finding the hospital room and setting too restrictive. There were no significant problems with these research subjects other than that they felt cramped and bored. Then we had a serious incident.

One of these volunteers was Francine, a physical therapist I had met while working in the hospital as a consulting psychiatrist. She was thirty-five years old when she volunteered for the DMT-pindolol study. She had taken a lot of psychedelics in college, but stopped using them upon enter-ing graduate school, after which she got married and raised a large, successful family.

I was concerned by her tales of driving long distances, swimming in lakes, and undertaking other tasks requiring focus and attention while under the influence of psychedelics. Perhaps she was trying to fend off the effects of the drugs with her hyperactivity. She was physically rather robust, but it didn't seem as if her physique was the only thing contribut-ing to the sense she exuded of being tightly wound, bunched up, and restricted. Nevertheless, careful questioning on my part failed to turn up any sign that she could not manage situations that came up while she was under the influence.

Francine tolerated the low screening dose of DMT without difficulty, but she kept the head of the bed maximally elevated, at an almost ninety-degree angle. She looked terribly uncomfortable, but denied feeling any awkwardness. She talked throughout the entire session, from the time I began giving the drug until all effects were gone. I gave her fair warning about the next day's high dose of DMT.

I doubt it will be that big. After all, I've taken a lot of LSD with little effect in the past.

We asked her to put on the eyeshades and lie down before we began with the following morning's high dose. If she were less distracted by her desire to provide us with ongoing commentary about her experience, she might be able to let go into the effects more easily. She reluctantly agreed to put them on her forehead so that she could flip them down over her eyes later, "if I see the need." She again kept the back of the bed upright.

Francine's high dose was unpleasant and reminded her of how much time had elapsed between her college tripping days and now. She had a busy and full life, with a lot of responsibilities, and wasn't sure about the psychic high risk involved in taking big doses of drugs anymore. As with the low dose, she kept her eyes open and talked throughout the session. One of her comments neatly summarized Francine's attitude towards the spirit molecule:

The DMT said, "Come with me, come with me," and I wasn't sure I could really afford to go.

Despite her misgivings, Francine followed through with the pindolol study without difficulty and eagerly volunteered for the psilocybin pilot work. She believed the slower progression of its effects would be more to her liking than the "nuclear cannon" of DMT.

Francine had an enormously gratifying peak experience in response to an early dose of psilocybin. She was much more cooperative with the structure of the setting that day and laughed, giggled, and exclaimed joyfully for most of the session. As the day came to a close, she summarized it for us:

It was the most unbelievable thing. I've never been that high in my life. It made 0.4 DMT look small by comparison. It was the ultimate trip. I may never want to trip again. Why would I? What would be the point? Certainly no higher dose of psilocybin would be necessary.

I needed to drive her home, as her husband could not break away from work to pick her up. It was then I learned how anxious Francine's husband was about her participation in our studies. We all three chatted briefly at their townhouse, and I left uncertain about her husband's fears. By the time I left, Francine continued looking pale and shaken, but happy.

The dose she received turned out to be less than psychedelic for the other volunteers, and I raised it by 50 percent for the next set of trials. Francine called Laura, feeling as if she needed to "keep up" with the rest of the volunteers, not wanting to be considered a "lightweight tripper." With some misgivings, I agreed to let her return.

The day got off to a rocky start, as she had moved the bed into the far corner of the room before Laura and I arrived. She didn't want to move it back into the middle, its usual position. In addition, a visiting medical student had gone in to see her before we had introduced them, expressly against my wishes. Francine was extraordinarily attentive to anonymity issues, as she was a hospital employee. I would have first cleared with her the idea of a visiting student.

Both of these irregularities—the bed placement and the student—set up high anxiety in me before we started. I nearly cancelled the study, but everyone seemed willing to carry on.

Within 15 minutes of swallowing the psilocybin capsule, Francine became restless, frightened, and anxious. She accused me of "messing" with her mind. When her panicked cell-phone call to her husband disconnected mid-conversation, she blamed my "mind waves" for the technical difficulties. Francine could tolerate only Laura in the room, and she asked if the medical student and I would step out for a while. While we were at the nurses' station deciding how to proceed, Francine's husband raced down the hall, entered Room 531, and gathered her up. They pushed their way past Laura and flew out the Research Center's double doors before I got my bearings. As her husband ran past me, he said, "I've seen her this way before."

I thought, "Now he tells me."

The security guards came too late. While peaking on psilocybin, Francine was loose in Albuquerque.

Thankfully, Francine remained under the watchful eye of her husband that day and came to no harm. Nevertheless, I needed to write up and send in reports to all the university committees and boards overseeing our research. The Food and Drug Administration and the National Institute on Drug Abuse also received copies of a narrative of the incident. I referred to Francine's session as "an unfortunate, but not unexpected adverse reaction. Psychotic breaks do happen under the influence of these drugs, and they are nearly always brief. The volunteer recompensated quickly and is showing no ill effects of her session."

Strictly speaking, this was true. Francine "felt fine" that next morning and went back to work as if nothing had happened. However, she remained convinced that leaving the Research Center against our advice, and under the influence of psilocybin, was the only thing—in fact, the courageously noble thing—to do. My "negative influence" left her little choice. Neither Laura nor I, after many months, could make even the slightest inroads into her fear and anxiety about what she began experiencing that morning.

We made some modifications in our protocols, requiring that we interview more carefully volunteers' spouses in order to learn about the nature and basis for any serious misgivings on their part. We more clearly stated the requirement that the research team give final permission to leave the hospital. We also decided to begin with the administration of a high dose of DMT in anyone interested in the psilocybin project. By doing so, we could assess more carefully their ability to handle extreme psychedelic states.

Francine's session also effectively dashed any hopes for taking the research out of the hospital.

I was deeply shaken. Francine was intelligent and experienced, and she had been through our DMT work before. On the one hand, she had warned us by saying she might never want any more psilocybin after her previous peak experience. On the other hand, I didn't want to disappoint her by refusing further participation. Her unpleasant experiences on DMT could have warned us about her inability to let go into fully psychedelic states, but it was hard to tell at the time. In addition, I chose to ignore the warning signs that morning: the peculiar bed arrangement and the visiting medical student's intrusiveness.

I began doubting my own judgment.

I also feared for giving fully psychedelic doses of psilocybin in the hospital. But if we didn't give full, active doses, what was the point? We needed to study the psychedelic, not sub-psychedelic, properties of psilocybin. Lower doses would not do, and the setting could not hold higher doses.[1]

Research team conflicts also began emerging as the study progressed. A particularly difficult one involved a part-time graduate student who joined us after we completed the first dose-response study.

I handed over to Bob much of the initial screening of prospective DMT volunteers. He returned calls, asked the first series of questions regarding suitability, and explained the studies in which the caller might participate. He then met with Laura and me to discuss whether to move the person through the next step in the screening process. If we had additional questions, Bob would follow up with them as necessary. While his role was not crucial, it had taken several months to get him up to speed, and he got to know well many of the second wave of volunteers.

A relative latecomer to the psychedelic field, Bob was like a child in a candy shop. He exuded enthusiasm about the projects and was very helpful in recruiting new subjects. He found the volunteers fascinating and wanted to spend time with them. He loved attending meetings and conferences in which well-known psychedelic research scientists reminisced about the "good old days" and the next generation of investigators planned future studies.

However, he had a difficult time knowing when to stop. One of our volunteers invited Bob over to his house to take drugs, and he couldn't pass up the opportunity. When I shared my concern about this, he looked hurt and replied, "You've been doing this for so long, I need to catch up." I advised him against any more of this type of behavior, but came up short of flatly prohibiting it.

Soon, however, an unrelated "supervisory" incident showed me that I could not afford to be so casual. This wake-up call took place in the psychiatry clinic in which I saw patients for the university.

For some years, I had been prescribing medication for Leanne, an intelligent and personable young woman with manic-depressive illness. Later, Tom, a new social-work intern, joined the staff and came under my supervision. He asked me to find him a stable and psychologically minded patient to see in psychotherapy, and I naturally thought of Leanne. They began working together, and from each of their reports, therapy was going well. A little too well, as it turned out.

Leanne and Tom started having sex a few months after beginning therapy. Neither Leanne, in our medication visits, nor Tom, in our weekly supervisory sessions, mentioned this. Within a few months, Leanne demanded that

Tom leave his wife and marry her. Tom panicked and broke off the relationship. Leanne sued Tom, the clinic, and the university. Tom then threatened to sue me for "lack of supervision" if the university didn't let him leave without serious consequences. The university, wanting to avoid a lengthy, expensive, and highly public trial, settled the case out of court, and I avoided being named in a lawsuit. Learning from this experience how liable I was for the behavior of those working under me, even if I didn't know what they were doing, I decided it was time to reign in Bob the wayward graduate student.

Crying and accusing me of being unfair, Bob did not take well to being told he could not take drugs with the volunteers. My department chairman suggested I let him go. However, our research team was small, and it would have taken months to train someone to take his place. I gave him a second chance and told him that he could continue with the research if he promised to avoid socializing with volunteers. The university attorney and my chairman recommended I make him sign a contract to that effect. This would allow me to cleanly end his relationship with the project if he slipped up again.

Considering the enthusiasm with which Bob professed his involvement in the studies, it was surprising to hear him say he "needed time to think about it." Within a week, he reluctantly agreed to sign the contract prohibiting him from inappropriate extra-research activities. However, his poor boundaries and desire to take drugs with those involved in the research spilled over into another area: wanting to take drugs with me.

Bob made the hour-long drive up to my house in the mountains behind Albuquerque one Saturday and appeared at my door unannounced. Beginning with the cheery, and unlikely, "I was in the area and thought I'd drop by," the conversation quickly turned to his interest in "maybe taking psilocybin mushrooms with you." I was surprised, and I asked him what was going on.

"I've got so much more to learn about psychedelics. I can't take them with volunteers now. But you've got so much to teach. I want to tap some of that knowledge and experience. What better way than to trip with you in your home?"

Feeling as if I were dealing with a disturbed psychiatric patient, I focused on ending the conversation and the idea as quickly as possible.

"No. That's not going to happen. You can trip with your friends, of course, but not with volunteers nor with me. What seems best, though, is that you get into some therapy to talk about this. You need to get a bit of professional distance on this, and it seems hard to do."

Bob's face turned red and he started crying again.

"I know I shouldn't have dropped by! I'm sorry. I don't know what's come over me! I guess I'm lonely. I just want to fit in."

"That's okay." I tried sounding supportive. "Have some lunch, and you can head back into town."

That wasn't the end of it. For the next several months, whenever Laura, Bob, and I would meet to discuss the research, Bob cried, or came close to tears, around the issue of taking drugs: either with the volunteers or with me. Worse, his feelings began spilling over in his dealings with prospective volunteers. People shared with me some of the comments he casually dropped while discussing the project with them:

"Rick's pretty uptight about the research, you know."

And, "It's too bad Rick keeps so much to himself about his feelings and motivations for this work."

He also wasn't getting to the volunteers important forms to sign and articles to read.

Bob had to go, and it wasn't easy telling him. He actually seemed relieved that he no longer had to labor under what he thought were such unreasonably restrictive conditions of employment. Unfortunately, he was now free to socialize and take drugs with whomever he desired. Despite his efforts to keep such activities to himself, I never stopped hearing about them.

Finally, I was having problems taking in and dealing with all that the spirit molecule was showing us it could do. I expected psychotherapeutic, near-death, and mystical experiences during our work. However, the lack of substantial change induced by them made me wonder about their validity.

I also was unprepared for the overwhelmingly frequent reports of contact with beings. They challenged my view of the brain and reality. They also stretched and frayed my ability to empathize and support our volunteers. The lack of any close psychiatric peer colleagues added to my sense of isolation and concern about how I was responding to these sessions.

The biomedical model was making it difficult to recruit volunteers, or to be encouraging about what awaited them. Long-term benefits seemed minimal, while adverse effects stood out more sharply and were accumulating. I could not comfortably accept nor incorporate the remarkably high frequency of being contact. Hoped-for colleagues did not join me or decided to compete for precious funds and collaborators. The hospital setting for a psilocybin study was impractical and possibly dangerous, thus making me pessimistic about working with full doses. Research team conflicts threatened what fragile hold I did maintain over the project.

Even Margot, my massage therapist, was worried, although I rarely spoke about my research during our sessions. She was a highly intuitive bodyworker I'd been seeing once or twice a month for years. During one particular session, she became restless and distressed while looking me over, lying on the table.

She said, "I see evil spirits hovering around you. They want to come through this plane, using you and the drugs. I'm worried. This does not look good to me."

Margot was a little New Age, even for New Mexico. I laughed and replied, "Well, Margot, I won't answer if they knock."

She was, nevertheless, accurate. Whether metaphorical, symbolic, or real, there was a tremendous amount of negativity piling up around me. What to do? I didn't have to wait much longer for the solution, nor did I directly choose it. Rather, it came my way in a frightening manner.

My former wife, Marion, suddenly developed cancer. Fortunately the tumor was localized, and the surgeon was confident none remained after the quickly scheduled operation. However, "just to be safe," the physician recommended more radical surgery, which Marion refused, preferring instead to pursue alternative medical therapies. At the same time my stepson, Marion's youngest child, had become depressed and dropped out of school while living with his father in Canada.

Marion asked if we could move to Canada to be near family while she recuperated, to help out her son, and to give me some breathing room. Uncertain as to how successfully I could commute to Albuquerque, I nevertheless agreed to the move.

Every two months I scheduled a two-week stay in New Mexico, and I tried running as many studies as we could during those visits. The wear and tear was tremendous, and I worried about local support when I was gone. No one knew the studies, nor the volunteers, as well as I did.

One of the research subjects for the dose-finding work with psilocybin began having problems. Vladan, about whose experiences we read in chapter 12, got stuck in a spiral of increasing pessimism with every psilocybin session—a "what's the point?" attitude. He never had the breakthrough he thought would come with higher doses. Instead, he became more reclusive and preoccupied. When told we wanted him to take a break from further studies, he bought a semiautomatic weapon, "just in case of Armageddon." He adamantly denied any intention of using it against us. I was not especially reassured, so I invited him to my office during one of my New Mexico trips to assess his dangerousness. I relaxed somewhat after a two-hour meeting, but Vladan did not want to give up the gun.

I obtained permission to begin an LSD study, but decided to wait. Conditions did not look promising for giving LSD at the Research Center.

Finally, my former Buddhist monastic community began criticizing my research and withdrawing their personal support at the same time. These events were the final ones that led me to discontinue the psychedelic research, and they are the focus of the next chapter.

Stepping on
Holy Toes

There generally is little support for the incorporation of spirituality, with its nonmaterial and therefore non-measurable factors, into clinical research's fold. We will see in this chapter that neither is organized religion, no matter how mystically inclined, open-minded and secure enough to seriously consider the spiritual potential of clinical research with psychedelics.

There are several places in this book where I refer to my interest in Buddhist theory and practice. In addition to theoretical and practical contributions to the research, I also received much personal support and guidance from decades of involvement with an American Zen Buddhist monastery. From the initial inspiration for the psychedelic research to the development of the rating scale and our methods of supervising sessions, my understanding of Buddhism pervaded nearly every aspect of working with the spirit molecule.

Being raised a Jew in southern California in the 1950s and 1960s, my religious training emphasized learning the Hebrew language and Jewish festivals, history, and culture. We also remembered the Holocaust and supported the newly formed Jewish state of Israel. We learned little about how to directly encounter God. This was something for the ancient patriarchs alone: Abraham, Isaac, Jacob, and Moses.

There were moments of joy in my Jewish education. Singing Hebrew folk songs and prayers in large groups was ecstatic, although I didn't use that word at the time. So were the complex swirling and whirling Israeli folk dances we learned. In addition, one of my religious school teachers did try teaching us to meditate. We closed our eyes when she did, and then looked around the room through half-shut lids to see who was peeking. Our teacher had a beatific expression on her face, sitting at her desk, fingers interlaced in front of her lap. Once or twice during this classroom meditation I glimpsed something inside that felt good, calm, and right, but I also was startled and a little uncomfortable contacting it.

I later found Eastern religious teachings and practices provided the most accessible methods to begin satisfying the desires for deeper truths that emerged during my college years. In this way I'm similar to many of my generation. These "new religions" included Zen and other forms of Buddhism, Hinduism, and Sufism. Their emphasis on mystical union with the source of all being resonated deeply with that need for ultimate truth. The personal certainty embodied in recently arrived Japanese, Indian, and Tibetan teachers, and the spiritual exercises that promised results confirmed by generations of practitioners, combined to make an irresistible package.

My introduction to the mysteries of the East came in the form of Transcendental Meditation in the early 1970s. I enjoyed the quiet and peacefulness of this practice, but the intellectual underpinnings did not appeal to me. Soon thereafter, I discovered in Buddhism both the practical and intellectual inspiration I was seeking.

Buddhism is a meditation-based religion, 2,500 years old, that in impartial, psychological, and relatively easily accessible terms describes and considers all the states of mind one could possibly imagine, whether

horrific, beatific, neutral, helpful, or harmful. In addition, Buddhism of-
fers practical, cause-and-effect moral codes that apply the insights of
meditation to daily life.

It took a few tries to find a suitable Buddhist community. Once more,
Jim Fadiman at Stanford pointed me in the right direction, this time to a
midwestern United States Zen monastery run by a rather reclusive, but
startlingly solid, Asian teacher. I attended two weekend meditation retreats there in 1974 and felt as if I had arrived home. The monks were
serene but down to earth, and we enjoyed being with each other. Most
interesting was that most of them had gained their first view of the spiritual path while on psychedelic drugs.

They did not volunteer this information, of course. But in the freewheeling early days of the temple, such informal self-disclosure was
common. It was as simple as asking, "Did you take psychedelics before
becoming a monk? How important were they in your decision?" The overwhelming majority had taken them and had experienced their first glimpse
of the enlightened state of mind with their assistance.

A five-week retreat at the monastery during a break from medical
school helped me develop a portable and efficient Buddhist practice. The
meditation was straightforward: sit comfortably, back straight, and just
sit. "Just sit" as in "just walk," "just wash the dishes," "just breathe." In
other words, focus all your attention on the task at hand. When sitting,
therefore, you just sat. No thinking, daydreaming, fidgeting, emotional
reactions, talking, or whatever else complicated the sitting process. The
regular in-and-out movement of the breath functioned as an excellent
anchor, a point upon which the wandering mind could ground and focus
its attention whenever distracting thoughts or feelings interrupted unclut-
tered awareness.

Upon returning to medical school, I reserved a room for lunchtime
meditation and there were always one or two people joining me for a half-
hour "sit." I stayed in close touch with several monks, visited the monastery
regularly, and hosted a retreat led by priests traveling to New York.

Buddhism and meditation also seemed a rich field of academic study.
I arranged to take a medical school summer elective for mental health

professionals at the Nyingma Institute, which had been established by a Tibetan Buddhist lama in the hills of Berkeley, California. During this course we learned the basic principles and practices of Buddhist psychology. It was here that I first learned about the *Abhidharma*, the Buddhist system of psychology.

Abhidharma roughly translates into "catalog of mental states." There are hundreds of *Abhidharma* texts, but the Nyingma lama was interested in sharing with us only the most basic principles.

One fundamental tenet was that the normal flow of personal experience actually was a smooth synthesis of several component parts. These facets are called the *skandhas,* or "heaps," the five "things" that make up our conscious state: form, feeling, perception, consciousness, and habitual tendencies. We spent days discussing each of these until we developed a consensus definition with which we felt comfortable and could express in familiar Western terms.

Another important point was the possibility of, and methods for, dissolving the glue that held these *skandhas* together. By deconstructing, as it were, the facade of our sense of self, Buddhists believe we can access deeper layers of reality, compassion, love, and wisdom. There was a sequence of stages in that process, and a knowledgeable teacher could help the meditator recognize and progress through those steps. Buddhism had refined these techniques over millennia, and millions of practitioners had verified and validated these methods and their results.

While these meditations were more elaborate and complicated than "just sitting," they were fascinating, and they produced the promised results. I needed to write a scientific article on my summer experience, and I used that opportunity to publish a description of the *Abhidharma* system and some of my own meditative experiences. Learning about *Abhidharma* also got me thinking about its usefulness in measuring psychedelic states.[1]

Upon graduating from medical school, I returned to California for psychiatric training. There, in Sacramento, I helped establish and administer a monastery-affiliated meditation group that met weekly and sponsored retreats led by monks. For years the group met in my house, and I had many opportunities to discuss my interests, psychedelic and otherwise, with members of the monastic community. At the monastery, I underwent a layperson's ordination into the Buddhist sect whose teachings the abbot followed, and I maintained close ties with my original monk friends, who now were becoming senior members of the priestly hierarchy.

Career and training opportunities drew me away from Sacramento after my four-year psychiatric residency at the University of California in Davis, but I returned two and a half years later to join their faculty. The local meditation group I helped establish still met, but the parent organization's structure had changed substantially. Many monks had left the fold as the teachings became increasingly focused on the teacher himself and his spiritual experiences. At the same time the abbot was becoming more reclusive, surrounding himself with trusted assistants. In addition, there now existed a hierarchy within the lay community. The atmosphere had taken a turn toward "who is in, and who is out." The informal and relaxed give-and-take no longer existed.

When I later moved to New Mexico, I considered myself loosely affiliated with the monastery's extended Buddhist community. I was not inclined to deal with the political structure now necessary to start a local meditation group, but I did seek out other local members and I meditated with them regularly in an informal setting. In addition, I remained in regular contact with several monks at the head temple, many of whom were now twenty-year acquaintances. While the monastic community as a whole had lost some of its luster, I considered it my spiritual home and was married there in 1990.

There are many ways my Buddhist training and practice affected the DMT research. One of these was in how we supervised volunteers' encounters with DMT.

Supervising psychedelic sessions usually is called "sitting." Many believe this comes from the idea of "babysitting" people who are in a highly dependent, at times confused and vulnerable state. Even more importantly, though, is "sitting" in the meditational sense. The research nurse, either Cindy or Laura, and I did our best to practice "just sitting" while being with our volunteers: watching the breath, being alert, eyes gazing straight ahead, ready to respond, keeping a positive and aware attitude, letting the research subject's experience unfold without unnecessary interference.[2]

My understanding of meditation also helped me guide people through the stages of the DMT experience. For example, I applied the *Abhidharma's* model of mind when coaching volunteers not to get swept away by the onslaught of colors, or to investigate the space within the grains of wood in the door if they kept their eyes open. Suggesting volunteers let go, focus on the breath and body sensations, keep an open but fluid mind to whatever came their way—all of these were tools I had acquired during decades of meditation practice and study.

Another example of how psychedelics and Buddhist meditation met was in the development of our rating scale.

Previous paper-and-pencil psychological questionnaires that measured psychedelic drug effects had serious shortcomings. They assumed that psychedelics were "psychotomimetic" or "schizotoxic," and therefore they emphasized unpleasant experiences. Many of these scales were developed using volunteers, sometimes ex-narcotic-addict prisoners, who were not told what drugs they were given, or what the effects might be.

To offer an alternative to these tools for measuring the psychedelic experience, I used an *Abhidharma-* and *skandha*-based method of characterizing mental states. This purely descriptive model meshed well with what's known as the "mental-status" approach to interviewing psychiatric patients: You talk with someone and gently investigate the quality of their basic mental functions, such as mood, thinking, and perceptions.

The familiar *Abhidharma* terms "form," "feeling," "perception," "consciousness," and "habitual tendencies" became the framework or structure within which the rating scale's questions emerged, and how we classified replies to those questions. However, instead of calling them *skandhas*, "clinical clusters" seemed more appropriate and palatable for a Western scientific audience.

We gave and analyzed this new questionnaire, the Hallucinogen Rating Scale, or HRS, at the end of every DMT session for the entire project.

The results were remarkable.

It is well-known in clinical psychopharmacology that a good questionnaire is more sensitive than any biological factor in assessing drug effects. In other words, a well-designed rating scale is better than measurements of blood pressure, heart rate, or hormone levels in distinguishing doses of a drug, or different types of drugs, from each other. I hoped that the HRS would follow in that tradition, and this it did without difficulty. We were better able to separate responses to various doses of DMT, or the effects of combining DMT with other drugs, using HRS scores than by measuring changes in any biological variable, including all the cardiovascular and blood hormone data. However, it also validated the wisdom and strength of the Buddhist approach to mental states.

Clifford Qualls, Ph.D., the Research Center biostatistician, and I grouped together HRS questions using the "clinical cluster" or *skandha* method and compared this method of analysis to a large number of alternative purely statistical models. The *Abhidharma's* technique was as good as, if not superior to, ones developed solely upon mathematical considerations. Since the computer-derived classification of results was no better than the clinical cluster one, and since using the *skandhas* made more sense intuitively, the Buddhist classification system won out. Other groups have since used the HRS and confirmed its usefulness in measuring other altered states of consciousness, drug-induced and otherwise.[3]

Buddhism also helped me make sense of people's DMT sessions. Its farreaching perspective includes all experiences: spiritual, near-death, and even nonmaterial or invisible realms. However, I did come up against two serious limitations in my lack of Buddhist education.

How was I to respond to a volunteer who spoke as if she or he just had undergone a drug-induced spiritual experience? Was it a "real" enlightenment or not? As detailed in chapter 16, "Mystical States," these sessions certainly left me feeling as if something deeply profound had happened. And there was no question on the volunteers' part that they had undergone the deepest and most profound experience of their lives. However, it was beyond my training and expertise to determine the validity or "certifiability" of a volunteer's understanding with anything other than psychiatric models of interpretation.

Another problem was how to relate what I knew about Buddhist approaches to nonmaterial beings with what our volunteers were reporting. For example, Tibetan and Japanese versions of Buddhism possess a full roster of demons, gods, and angels. I understood these encounters to symbolically represent certain qualities of ourselves, not autonomous noncorporeal life forms.

When volunteers began reporting contact, my first reaction was, "Oh, this is something they talk about in Buddhism. They are just aspects of our own minds."

These encounters got stranger, however, and the beings started testing, probing, inserting things into, eating, and raping our volunteers. A Buddhist framework seemed less capable of explaining these types of experiences. Generically I could apply the inherent skepticism of Buddhism in taking anything as "real" or "special" about these stories. That is, it was "just meeting beings." These apparent life forms were not necessarily any wiser or more trustworthy than anything else we might meet in our lives or minds.

Nevertheless, I needed some guidance, both for the spiritual experience and the "contact" aspects of our work. I began sharing our findings, and my questions, with trusted monk friends. The one to whom I turned most often was Venerable Margaret, a Buddhist priest I met in 1974 during my first stay at the monastery.[4]

A clinical psychologist by training, Margaret became a Buddhist monk after realizing, "I didn't want to be let loose on the world the way I was." She wanted to experience her own mental and spiritual health before trying to help others. She loved monastic life, however, and stayed on. Margaret and I spoke the same language, shared the same concerns, and viewed the human condition through similarly trained clinical eyes.

Before beginning the actual DMT studies, I happened to spend a few days at the monastery. My two-year journey through the regulatory labyrinth, seeking permission and funding to begin giving DMT, was drawing to a close. Margaret had risen to chief assistant to the abbot, and her time was heavily scheduled. However, we found an opportunity to meet and I updated her on my personal and professional life. The conversation moved into my interest in giving DMT to human research subjects. Sharing with her my belief that the pineal gland might make DMT at mystical moments in our lives, I speculated about its possible role in death and near-death states.

The lanky and shaven-headed woman monk touched the tips of her fingers together in front of her mouth, tenting them in and out. Her intensely blue eyes narrowed, and she looked over my shoulder, meeting the white wall with her gaze.

She said quietly, "What you are suggesting is something that only one out of a million people could do."

I took this intentionally unclear remark as encouragement to go deeper with the topic. Wondering about the role of psychedelics in spiritual development, I commented on how many of the now-senior monks had gotten their first sighting of the spiritual path from LSD and other drugs.

Margaret laughed, saying, "You know, I honestly can't say if my LSD trips helped or hurt my spiritual practice!"

"Hard to tell, isn't it?" I replied.

"Indeed."

She looked at her watch, picked up her tea cup, and graciously excused herself.

The next year, 1990, I was married at the monastery. At separate meetings before the ceremony, I chatted with two other monk friends, now some of the highest ranking officers in the order. Both of them had taken psychedelic drugs in college with a fellow who later became a close friend of mine in New Mexico. This mutual acquaintance was well-known for using MDMA in a psychotherapeutic setting. They both asked about their friend and his MDMA research and were in kind fascinated by my plans to study DMT.

After wrapping up the dose-response study in 1992, I wrote a long letter to Margaret describing the full range of the stories volunteers shared with us, including near-death, enlightenment, and being contact. I also shared with her my feelings that the setting was too neutral, and our volunteers too familiar with psychedelics, for any real beneficial effects to result. I raised the issue of helping people more directly, along the lines of a psilocybin-assisted psychotherapy project with the terminally ill.

I was drawn to a terminal illness study because of the promising work in this area performed during the first wave of psychedelic clinical research in the 1960s. In addition, its emphasis on the positive effects of spiritual and near-death experiences possible with psychedelics appealed to my deeper interest in these drugs.

Margaret replied, "Most interesting! But to what purpose? Maybe future 'helping' work will shed some light on that." She also wondered about the risk-to-benefit ratio and advised performing such a study only if I was sure there were extremely few risks and an equally high likelihood of success. Insightfully, she also asked me to consider the lack of time available to undo any harm incurred from a painful or disturbing psilocybin session.

The years passed quickly, and by the end of 1994 my questions grew regarding the utility of my psychedelic research. Adverse effects accumulated, and long-term benefit was difficult to assess. In addition, the constant exposure to psychedelicized volunteers was beginning to exhaust me. I shared these developments with Margaret.

As always, she supported whatever seemed most useful for my own spiritual growth. If it involved giving up the research, she understood. However, she encouraged me to look for someone to whom I might transfer the project so the work I had begun would not end in my absence.

The additional circumstances described in the last chapter led to my moving to Canada, but I commuted to Albuquerque in order to continue running studies. After relocating, I met the members of the local monastery-affiliated meditation group and started sitting with them. There existed a major branch of the order in a nearby U.S. state across the border, and their priest scheduled a retreat in our community. Venerable Gwendolyn arrived, and the weekend workshop began.

Gwendolyn had entered the head temple directly from her parents' home. She had had a series of extraordinarily profound spiritual experiences at the monastery and was a highly ranked teacher. Nevertheless, she was not especially wise in the ways of the world, and running an urban meditation center was a significant challenge to her social skills.

During a pastoral counseling session with Gwendolyn, I let her know of the New Mexico research and some of my growing ambivalence toward it. I appreciated the opportunity to air my story to a monk who knew nothing about me, and to listen to her fresh perspective.

I was surprised to hear Gwendolyn's voice on the phone a week later.

"I was sick for three days after talking with you, it upset me so. I called the abbot, who as you know is near death. This is the first issue he's taken a personal interest in for over a year. He and I talked, as I did with other senior monks. We have decided you must stop your research immediately. I'll write you this week a more formal letter."

I replied, "Let me think about it."

Two weeks later, a letter came, not from Gwendolyn, but from Margaret. It began with, "I hope what I heard third-hand isn't true. But if it is, let me say this." With that introduction, she began an indictment of my research: past, present, and planned:

"Your psychedelic research is ultimately futile, devoid of real benefit to humanity, and dangerous;

"The idea of administering psychedelics to the terminally ill is to me appallingly dangerous. It comes about as close to 'playing God' as anything I've seen in the mental health professions;

"An attempt to induce enlightenment experiences by chemical means can never, will never, succeed. What it will do is badly confuse people and result in serious consequences for you."

Gwendolyn's letter arrived next.

"[Your research] constitutes wrong livelihood according to the Buddha's teachings;

"That DMT might elicit enlightenment experiences is delusional and contrary to the teachings of the Buddha;

"Hallucinogens disorder and confuse the mind, impede religious training, and can be a cause of rebirth into realms of confusion and suffering;

"This is the teaching and viewpoint of myself, [the abbot], [the order], and the whole of Buddhism.

"We urge you to cease all such experiments."

I reminded these monks of the years of dialogue I'd had with them regarding my interest in and performance of psychedelic research. I also pointed out the continuous interest in my work by members of the community, and the absence of any prior recommendations to avoid or stop it. If anything, there was enthusiasm and encouragement to use these interests as grist for going deeply into my own spiritual relationship to the outside world. I recalled the many conversations I'd had with monks who'd validated the importance of their psychedelic experiences as leading to their first inklings of enlightenment.

Additionally, I was eager to discuss some of their concerns. These included the obvious problems associated with thinking that certain knowledge was accessible only with an outside agent; that is, a drug. I also accepted the theoretical possibility raised by Gwendolyn that someone might mistake a real enlightenment experience for a psychedelic "flashback."

However, none of these attempts at enlarging the dialogue met with any success.

What was going on?

The abbot was dying, and he was making sure the teachings he left behind were as unsullied by controversy as possible. In addition, senior monks were lobbying for elected posts that would determine the future of the community. Who was the most zealous defender of the teaching? Those whose positive psychedelic experiences had led them to Buddhism in the first place had to remain silent, and close rank behind those without such backgrounds. Psychedelics could not become a divisive issue at this crucial moment in the monastery's existence.

And then the Fall 1996 issue of *Tricycle, The Buddhist Review* came out with my article calling for a discussion of integrating psychedelics into Buddhist practice.

In that article I presented Elena's first high-dose session, which we've read in chapter 16, "Mystical States." Her experience served as an example of the type of spiritual breakthrough possible with DMT in someone open to them—that is, a person with a serious meditation practice, solid psychological mindedness, and a deep reverence and respect for drugs like DMT. I also raised the concern that isolated experiences, occurring without any sort of spiritual or therapeutic context, were not especially effective in producing long-term serious change in our volunteers. I therefore concluded with the following:

"I believe there are ways in which Buddhism and the psychedelic community might benefit from an open, frank exchange of ideas, practices, and ethics. For the psychedelic community, the ethical, disciplined structuring of life, experience, and relationship provided by thousands of years of Buddhist communal tradition have much to offer. This well-developed tradition could infuse meaning and consistency into isolated, disjointed, and poorly integrated psychedelic experiences. The wisdom of the psychedelic experience, without the accompanying and necessary love and compassion cultivated in a daily practice, may otherwise be frittered away in an excess of narcissism and self-indulgence. While this is also possible within a Buddhist meditative tradition, it is less likely with the checks and balances in place within a dynamic community of practitioners.

"On the other hand, dedicated Buddhist practitioners with little success in their meditation, but well along in moral and intellectual development, might benefit from a carefully timed, prepared, supervised, and followed-up psychedelic session to accelerate their practice. Psychedelics, if anything, provide a view. And a view, to one so inclined, can inspire the long hard work required to make that view a living reality."[5]

This article sealed my fate within the monastic community. My life-long affiliation with the order would implicate it as contributing to these ideas. Gwendolyn sent copies of the *Tricycle* article to members of my new meditation group as well as to other groups and the monastery. In it she scribbled comments she remembered I made during what I believed was our confidential pastoral counseling session. She wrote to the local congregation, telling them not to enter my house because there might be psychedelic drugs kept in it.

Her behavior brought these issues to the boiling point. I lodged a formal complaint against this breach of confidence. As much as calling Gwendolyn's behavior into question, I wanted a definitive statement from the order regarding their attitude about my research. They complied on both counts.

The monastic review agreed she had indeed broken confidence, but it was for a "greater good." That is, it was done to "prevent mistakes from being made in the name of Buddhism." One could not be a proper Buddhist and consider psychedelics to play any part in it.

There was little I could do. Holiness had won out over truth. This particular brand of Buddhism was no different from any other organization whose survival depended upon a uniformly accepted platform of ideas. Only they could determine what were permissible questions, and what were not.

Later I learned that the monastic community had elected Margaret head of the order. The two monks who had taken psychedelics years before with my New Mexico friend also did well in the elections. One was elected abbot of the monastery, the other his chief assistant. So political ambitions also took on greater importance than a truthful dialogue. It was unlikely that the organization could admit and openly discuss that their three leading teachers were former LSD users, or that they had decided to enter a monastic life after drug-induced inspiration.

Although I could see beyond the hypocrisy that motivated much of the monastery's repudiation of my work, it took its toll. Combined with the events and circumstances I described in the last chapter, my energy to continue with the research flagged considerably. After completing two long-distance research trips to Albuquerque, the extra pressure exerted by my spiritual community broke down the last remnant of my desire to continue. It was time to stop.

I resigned from the university and returned the drugs and the last year's worth of grant money to the National Institute on Drug Abuse. I wrote closing summaries on all of the projects and sent copies to the boards and committees who had been working with me for the past seven years. The pharmacy weighed all our drugs, packed them up, and mailed them to a secure facility near Washington, D.C. The supplies of DMT, psilocybin, and LSD remain there to this day.

■ Part VI ■

What Could and Might Be

DMT:
The Spirit Molecule

It is almost inconceivable that a chemical as simple as DMT could provide access to such an amazingly varied array of experiences, from the least dramatic to the most unimaginably earth-shattering. From psychological insights to encounters with aliens. Abject terror or nearly unbearable bliss. Near-death and rebirth. Enlightenment. All of these from a naturally occurring chemical cousin of serotonin, a widespread and essential brain neurotransmitter.

It is just as fascinating to ponder why Nature, or God, made DMT. What is the biological or evolutionary advantage to having various plants and our bodies synthesize the spirit molecule? If DMT is indeed released at particularly stressful times in our lives, is that a coincidence, or is it intended? If it is intended, for what purpose?

In the case reports, we've seen how strikingly similar volunteers' experiences are to naturally occurring psychedelic states of consciousness. It's difficult to ignore the overlap of research subjects' descriptions of high-dose DMT sessions with those from people who have undergone spontaneous near-death, spiritual, and mystical states. While I was not expecting contact with nonmaterial beings to be especially common before starting our work, the resemblance between those occurring "in the field" and in Room 531 is also undeniable.

The similarities between naturally occurring and DMT-induced phenomena support my suggestion that spontaneously occurring "psychedelic" experiences are mediated by elevated levels of *endogenous* DMT. In chapter 4, "The Psychedelic Pineal," I presented a series of biological scenarios in which the pineal may synthesize DMT, and I speculated about the metaphysical and spiritual implications of these possibilities.

How then might this spirit molecule, whether produced from the inside through these presumed biological pathways, or taken from outside as in our studies, modify our perceptions so radically? In this chapter we will give our imaginations free rein to consider any and all possibilities.

Most of us, including the most hard-nosed neuroscientists and non-materialistic mystics, accept that the brain is a machine, the instrument of consciousness. It is a bodily organ made up of cells and tissues, proteins, fats, and carbohydrates. It processes raw sensory data delivered by the sense organs using electricity and chemicals.

If we accept the "receiver of reality" model for brain function, let's compare it to another receiver with which we're all familiar: the television. By making the analogy of the brain to the TV, it's possible to think of how altered states of consciousness, including psychedelic ones brought about by DMT, relate to the brain as a sophisticated receiver.

The simplest and most familiar levels of change to which the spirit molecule provides access are the personal and psychological. These effects may be like fine-tuning the television image, adjusting the contrast, brightness, and color scheme. These "images" consists of feelings, memories, and sensations that are not at all unusual or unsuspected. There is nothing especially new, but what is there is now seen much more clearly and in finer detail.

Low doses of DMT brought about these types of responses in our volunteers. They sometimes also occurred at higher doses in those whose personal needs and makeup required a deeper reworking of their own lives and relationships.

In performing these consciousness adjustments, DMT does not differ much from other drugs or processes used in the psychotherapeutic process. Stimulants, especially the amphetamines and amphetamine-like drugs like MDMA, enhance mental processes in a potentially helpful way. They make it easier to remember and think. By magnifying and clarifying the feelings attached to those memories and thoughts, they make it possible for us to face and accept those emotions, and move on.

Many of the same mechanisms apply to a deep psychotherapeutic setting. The persistence and support of the therapist in dredging up painful memories and managing the powerful emotions they evoke have similarly beneficial effects. In our DMT work, we saw drug-induced effects on the normal everyday mind combine with supportive and encouraging attitudes on our part to produce new and powerfully felt personal insights.

For example, Stan could feel more acutely and directly the anxiety and stress of his divorce and its effect on his daughter. Marsha, through her dreamlike sessions in which she saw caricatures of Anglo beauty, faced the pain of her husband's difficulty accepting who she really was—physically and culturally. And Cassandra finally felt the relationship between her brutal rape and the abdominal pain she carried around with her for so many years, and thereby began to release it.

There also may be biological components to some of the personal clearing, therapeutic, and healing effects we saw in these types of sessions.

For example, the euphoria brought on by DMT helped volunteers more unflinchingly look at their lives and conflicts. These ecstatic feelings may be, in part, related to the powerful DMT-induced surge of the morphinelike brain chemical beta-endorphin. DMT also stimulated a massive rise in the brain hormones vasopressin and prolactin. Scientists believe these compounds are important in feelings of bonding, attachment, and comfort with other members of the species. Perhaps the elevations in these brain chemicals made it easier for our volunteers to trust us, relax into the drug effects, and share powerfully personal issues in ways that previously were impossible.

What happens when the spirit molecule pulls and pushes us beyond the physical and emotional levels of awareness? We enter into invisible realms, ones we cannot normally sense and whose presence we can scarcely imagine. Even more surprising, these realms appear to be inhabited.

At a certain point, I decided to accept at face value volunteers' reports. This thought experiment replaced my original tendency to explain away, interpret, or reduce their experiences into something else, such as a disordered brain's hallucinations, dreams, or psychological symbolism. Now, after several years of additional study and reflection, I think it's worth considering seriously whether it's possible that these experiences indeed were exactly what they seemed to be.[1]

I have struggled personally and professionally with developing the following radical explanations for our volunteers' apparent contact with nonmaterial beings. Even after stating them, I remain skeptical about their merit. Why couldn't I stick with tried and true biological or more traditional psychological models?

At a brain science level, maybe what our volunteers encountered was a vivid hallucinatory experience, resulting from DMT activation of brain centers responsible for vision, emotion, and thought. After all, people dream and are completely swept up in the reality of the experience at the time. The rapid eye movements that sometimes took place in our subjects may have indicated the presence of a "waking" dream state.

However, volunteers were convinced that there were differences between what they experienced during DMT-induced contact with beings and their typical dreams. Observing the same things with eyes opened or closed, in an alert, awake state of consciousness, also made it difficult for them to accept that it was "just a dream." Neither did I feel the same way listening to their stories of encounters as I do when one normally relates a dream to me in psychotherapy. Our volunteers' reports were so clear, convincing, and "real" that I repeatedly thought, "This sounds like nothing I've ever heard about in my therapy patients' dream life. It is much more bizarre, well-remembered, and internally consistent."

In addition, a biological explanation along the lines of a waking dream or hallucination usually brought on a certain resistance within the volunteer. A subtle friction might develop between us that limited the depth of their sharing and disclosure that was so valuable in our work together. A research subject might say in so many words, "No, that wasn't a dream, or a hallucination. It was real. I can tell the difference. And if that's what you think it is, then I'll keep the strangest aspects of my session to myself!"

Even more prone to cause a volunteer to dismiss my interpretations as inaccurate or inappropriate was any attempt to use psychological explanatory models. Freudian psychoanalytic systems would understand the experience of contact with beings as an expression of unconscious conflicts over aggressive, sexual, or dependency impulses. There were certainly times I used this approach in reacting to particular dreamlike sessions. However, I could not in good conscience suggest that any repressed unconscious infantile drives were behind the experimental manipulations by, or communication with, these beings.

Jungian psychology includes a broader perspective on the language of the unconscious, and builds upon and incorporates the fields of mythology, art, and religion more than the Freudian school usually does. Nevertheless, it is a psychological model, not a physical or biological one. For example, Jung referred to the image of "unidentified flying objects" as a yearning for wholeness as represented by the circle. Responding to beings as mental constructs or projections, no matter how large the scale, continues to convert the experience into "something else." It does not address the overwhelming and convincing sense of certainty felt by the person having the experience.

Beyond these intellectual concerns, I was continually faced with the emotional challenge of the developing relationship between the volunteers' experiences and my ability to respond to them. My study, background, and experience meshed well with research subjects' descriptions of personal and transpersonal sessions, such as "feeling and thinking," near-death and rebirth, and mystical states. I understood these experiences, volunteers felt I was appropriately tracking and responding to them, and there was little conflict.

However, whenever I tried to react to being-contact sessions with anything I knew or believed previously, it just didn't work. I was stuck. So, I decided to engage in the thought-experiment to which I refer at the end of chapter 13, Contact Through the Veil: 1. That is, I tried responding to volunteers' reports of contact with beings *as if they were true*. At first, this involved simply listening, and asking for clarification. Later on, as more tales accumulated, I could refer to other people's accounts in an empathic manner that made it easier for volunteers to feel I understood and accepted what they had to say. That way they could share with me their most unusual and almost embarrassingly unexpected encounters.

Therefore, let's consider the proposal that when our volunteers journeyed to the further bounds of DMT's reach, when they felt as if they were *somewhere else*, they were indeed perceiving different levels of reality. The alternative levels are as real as this one. It's just that we cannot perceive them most of the time.

In making this suggestion, I'm not discarding the brain-chemistry and psychological models. Rather, I wish to add to the options we entertain in attempting to develop explanations that are helpful to volunteers, intellectually satisfying to researchers, and perhaps even testable using methods not yet invented but theoretically possible.

Returning to the TV analogy, these cases suggest that, rather than merely adjusting the brightness, contrast, and color of the previous program, we have changed the channel. No longer is the show we are watching everyday reality, Channel Normal.

DMT provides regular, repeated, and reliable access to "other" channels. The other planes of existence are always there. In fact, they are right here, transmitting all the time! But we cannot perceive them because we are not designed to do so; our hard-wiring keeps us tuned in to

Channel Normal. It takes only a second or two—the few heartbeats the spirit molecule requires to make its way to the brain—to change the channel, to open our mind to these other planes of existence.[2]

How might this happen?

I claim little understanding of the physics underlying theories of parallel universes and dark matter. What I do know, however, causes me to consider them as possible places where DMT might lead us, once we have rushed past the personal.

Theoretical physicists propose the existence of parallel universes based upon the phenomenon of *interference*. One of the simplest demonstrations of interference is what happens to a light beam passing through narrow holes or slits in cardboard. Various rings and colored edges appear on the screen on which the light lands, not the simple outlines of the cardboard one would expect. Scientists conclude from this and more complex experiments that there are "invisible" light particles that interfere with those we can see, deflecting light in unexpected ways.

Parallel universes interact with each other when interference happens. There are, theoretically, an inconceivably large number of parallel universes, or "multiverses," each similar to this one and possessing the same laws of physics. Thus, there would not necessarily be anything especially odd or exotic about these different realms. However, what makes them parallel is that the particles composing them are located in different positions in each universe.

DMT may allow our receiver brain to sense these multiverses.

British scientist David Deutsch, author of *The Fabric of Reality*, is a leading theorist in this field.[3] Deutsch and I have corresponded about whether DMT could modify brain function so as to provide access to or awareness of parallel universes. He doubted that this was possible, because it would require "quantum computing." Quantum computing, according to Deutsch, "would be capable of distributing components of a complex task among vast numbers of parallel universes, and then sharing the results." Thus, its potential power is unimaginably great. One of the conditions necessary for quantum computing is a temperature near absolute zero, as cold as deep space. Thus, prolonged contact between universes is unlikely in a biological system.

Nevertheless, physicists once believed that superconductivity—when electricity passes through wires or other material with almost no resistance—could occur only at similarly low temperatures. Over the last ten to fifteen years, however, chemists have developed new materials that allow superconductivity at higher and higher temperatures. In fact, it is conceivable that superconductivity may one day actually occur at room temperature.

I asked Deutsch if the future of quantum computing might follow a similar trajectory. While he considered this a "reasonably good" analogy, he held that the complexity of quantum computing was much greater than that of superconductivity: "A room-temperature quantum computer would be an enormously more surprising thing than room-temperature superconductivity."[4]

Because I know so little about theoretical physics, there are fewer constraints reining me in regarding such speculations. That the analogy between superconductivity and quantum computing is "reasonably good" encourages me to take the next step in theorizing about DMT and the brain.

In such a scenario, DMT is the key ingredient changing the brain's physical properties in such a way that quantum computing may occur at body temperature. If this were the case, "seeing into" parallel universes is a possible outcome.

Along these lines, however, Deutsch did not think that glimpsing parallel universes would be particularly strange. He said, "Even if there *were* quantum computation in the brain, it would definitely not feel, subjectively, like 'seeing into quantum realms' [my phrase]. It would not feel special at all at the time. Just as in any other interference experiment, one would have to work backward from the logic, statistics, and complexity of the *outcome* of one's thoughts to infer that one must have been 'thinking in a quantum manner' at an earlier time to achieve that outcome."[5]

Deutsch's comment about how normal a parallel universe might seem reminds me of some of the stories we did hear about in chapter 12, "Unseen Worlds": Encounters with relatively normal-appearing, everyday existences that had no relationship at all to what was occurring at the Research Center. People, scenes, and interactions that to all intents and purposes appeared to be going on *parallel* to this here-and-now existence.

Consider, for example, Sean's landing in the middle of an remarkably ordinary family scene in what seemed to be rural Mexico, and Heather's meeting with the Spanish-speaking woman who repeatedly threw a white blanket in front of her. Many volunteers also found themselves in empty rooms, halls, or apartments that seemed similar to this world, but also different.

On the other hand, I wonder if parallel universes that formed, like ours, billions of years ago would appear especially familiar to us. For while the same laws of physics, and therefore biology, would hold sway in our world and theirs, the organisms and the technologies they developed might have taken fantastically different turns. Reptilian, insectlike, and unrecognizable shapes possessing intelligence should not be unexpected, nor should be highly advanced technology of space travel, supercomputation, and a blending of biology and technology, such as those reported by many of our volunteers.

The strangest realms to which DMT might lead are those that exist within the mysterious realms of dark matter. There, which may indeed *be* here, no one knows what we will find.

Dark matter comprises at least 95 percent of this universe's mass. In other words, nearly all of the matter in the universe is invisible. We cannot see it. It neither generates nor reflects radiation of any type, visible or otherwise. The only way we know it is there is by its gravitational effects. It *must* exist by virtue of the fact that the visible universe maintains its particular shape. Without this mass, there would not be enough gravity to hold the universe together—it would fly apart.

Scientists have nominated several candidates for the "stuff" that comprises dark matter. "Normal" matter that radiates little or no light—planets, dead or unborn stars, and black holes—may account for about 20 percent of dark matter.

However, it's likely that most, if not all, dark matter consists of particles quite different from our familiar protons, electrons, and neutrons. These "black" particles may obey entirely different laws of physics, unlike those in parallel universes. Finding ourselves in a world composed of them, we most likely would not recognize much.

The leading candidates for being the building blocks of dark matter are WIMPS, or "weakly interacting massive particles." They are called massive only in a relative sense, meaning they are larger than a proton or a hydrogen atom.

Recent thinking about WIMPS suggests their strange nature, one that immediately causes us to hearken back to many of our volunteers' reports: "If WIMPS were indeed created in the Big Bang, we will be surrounded by them because of their gravitational interaction with the visible matter in the universe. Indeed, as you read this article there could be a billion WIMPS streaming through your body every second, travelling at a million kilometers per hour. However, as WIMPS only interact weakly with matter, most will pass straight through you with no hindrance."[6]

Science agencies in the United States and other nations are spending billions of dollars on WIMPS sensors buried deep in the earth. They are looking for the occasional flash of light that indicates a rare collision of a dark-matter particle with one of regular matter. These sensitive machines require such subterranean depths so as to block out other sources of radiation.

Maybe we do not need such expensive detectors. It may be that DMT alters the characteristics of our brains so that it is possible to perceive WIMPS interacting with normal matter.

It is difficult to imagine what a dark-matter world might look like, let alone how its residents might appear. Maybe some of what several volunteers described as a "visualization of information" in chapter 12 is a variety of dark-matter "life": moving hieroglyphics pregnant with meaning, numbers and words floating by, imparting information.

Either of these invisible levels of existence, parallel universes or dark matter, are present at the same time as this reality. Thus, they both are options we must consider for where DMT takes us when our consciousness is no longer in this plane of experience. The immediacy of the transition makes appealing these two alternate viewpoints regarding the incredibly unusual places our volunteers describe. This is because they are as much here as there. So the question about "inside" versus "outside," as many volunteers posed it, really no longer has any meaning.

The concept of these different levels of reality permeating and suffusing ours leads us next to the surprisingly common report by the volunteers that "They were expecting me," "They welcomed me back." The beings are at home working in this environment, and "it's business as usual" for them. We, on the other hand, can only gape slack-jawed in awe, barely able to respond.

Since we usually do not see or feel these beings' presence at other times, it's worth wondering how they know when to anticipate our arrival. Perhaps before we see them our presence is less real for these beings, too. They might sense us, but not especially clearly or in a way that allows interaction with us. It is as if they see us, but only our images, as in a mirror or through a window. Thus, they could be ready, but not be able to act upon us until we step through the door or walk around to their side of the window.

Think of an instrument that requires an extremely hot temperature to record and send information. While at room temperature, not functioning, it is a dusty gray color and appears nearly invisible as it blends into the background. When it reaches its operating temperature, in addition to being able to perform its new receiving and transmitting functions, it now glows bright red and stands out quite clearly. Perhaps by changing our consciousness in such a way that we perceive denizens of alternate planes of existence, DMT modifies the "appearance" of our consciousness, too. Thus we become real for the beings once they become real for us.

How might these beings be even dimly aware of our presence, if we normally don't have an inkling of theirs? Once more, we're treading on extraordinarily thin ice by even thinking about explanations for this phenomenon. The mere need to attempt an understanding shows us how far afield our thinking has come. Nevertheless, we can take another small step in the suspension of disbelief, and consider this question.

Perhaps we are not "dark" for the denizens of dark matter, or "parallel" to those intelligent beings who have mastered quantum computing. We are limited to inferring these alternative realities exist by employing powerful mathematical treatment of massive amounts of experimental data. It may be that those who have evolved in different universes, or according to their own unique laws of physics, actually can observe us directly with their own senses or by using particular types of technology.

We must ask the next question that naturally follows. Once we are "there" and the beings and we have made contact, with what body do they interact? As we have heard, all manner of manipulations took place: adjustments, implants, pleasant and fearful sexual or physical contact. It's not an especially difficult leap to accept consciousness-to-consciousness exchanges in dark matter or parallel universes. More problematic is imagining how changes in our ability to receive new levels of reality affect our "bodies." Nevertheless, I think we need to consider this, if only in a preliminary manner.

While we are watching, or rather are existing in, Channel Normal, our body is solid, has discrete boundaries, and responds to gravity. While we are perceiving, or established in, Channel Dark Matter, we may be experiencing our body using WIMPS rather than visible light and gravity. With our brain receiving such new and different levels of reality, our body also no longer appears the same. Just as the certainty of what we see, hear, and know is unquestionably true in the DMT state, so too does the nature of our physical self assume a radically different, but similarly real, nature.

Sight and sound play such an inordinately important role in our normal awareness, and we notice our new location first with these senses. However, touch, body sensation, and matter also may assume entirely different capabilities. Using the gray and red instrument analogy above, we can just as easily substitute "insubstantial" for gray, and "palpable" or "solid" for red.

Once the dark-matter beings and we are perceiving each other in the same medium, using WIMPS, they may begin to work on our dark-matter bodies: adjusting Sean's ear, placing an implant under the skin of Ben's forearm, inserting a probe into Jim's eye, reprogramming Jeremiah's brain.

Those interventions take place using "things" made of dark matter (or existing in parallel universes). Because of this, there is no "physical evidence" of these interventions back in Channel Normal. They don't use the material of this universe. Nevertheless, these interventions did take place.[7]

These speculations regarding unseen worlds and their residents return us to alien abduction experiences. In fact, this discussion could just as well have been about those experiences and how they happen. This striking similarity is at the basis of the hypothesis that the alien abduction experience is related to abnormally elevated levels of brain DMT.

In chapter 4, "The Psychedelic Pineal," I proposed a pineal-DMT link for the pivotal experiences of birth, near-death, mystical states, and death. I had little interest in or knowledge about alien encounters. The results of the DMT study challenged my ignorance and require that I now include "contact" as another phenomenon mediated by extraordinarily high levels of brain DMT.

In his work with naturally occurring alien encounters, John Mack refers to how often these experiences occur at times of personal crisis, trauma, and loss. Perhaps in these individuals, stress and pain overcome the pineal's ability to prevent excessive DMT release and trigger access to these unusual experiences. In addition, many abductees have a history of these encounters that dates back to childhood. Such individuals may possess especially active DMT-production capacities due to a biological hard-wiring predisposition, possibly combined with chronic or repeated overwhelming stress. We previously discussed how some of the tendencies for excessive DMT formation might manifest using specific enzymes or enzyme inhibitors.

Mack also notes that many abductions from people's homes take place in the early morning hours. The pineal gland is most active at this time. Might early morning DMT production open the portals to alien encounters in these predisposed individuals?

It's fascinating to note that Mack has recently suggested that "reconnection with spirituality" is at the heart of the abduction phenomenon. Similarly, some of our DMT-induced being contacts, for example, those of Cassandra, Sean, and Willow, demonstrated a transition from surprise and shock at the presence of intelligent beings to a greater depth of spiritual and psychological equilibrium.

These mystical experiences are the last set of encounters to which the spirit molecule may lead. They were the ultimate goals of many volunteers who participated in our research. Why, then, did so many of our research subjects instead find themselves in unexpected unseen worlds?

It may be that the raw, unbridled power of DMT caused our research subjects to overshoot, or miss, their target. It reminds me of the first time we get in the saddle of a powerful motorcycle. The thrust is so unimaginably forceful that we often fly off the back of the vehicle or head straight into a ditch. Only by learning how to deal with its strength can we harness the machine and go straight ahead to our goal.

In a similar vein, I believe research subjects with primarily contact experiences would have gone beyond that level and reached the transpersonal if given adequate time and practice. Sean's and Cassandra's cases support this theory: They moved on from contact with beings to mystical and healing experiences with repeated exposure to high doses of DMT in the tolerance study.

Another explanation is less sanguine. That is, high doses of IV DMT thrust people into being-inhabited planes of reality because that is what it does. Give enough DMT to people, and this is what happens.

I'm reminded of Jeremiah, in chapter 13, "Contact Through the Veil: 1," when he was swept into the alien laboratory-nursery. He attempted to steer the sheer intensity of the experience into a spiritual encounter by "opening to love." However, he immediately realized it was impossible to do so. Maybe contact through the veil is the *real* ultimate function of DMT, rather than initiating mystical awareness. If the sheer numbers of volunteers' reports are any indication of the truth of this suggestion, we must consider it likely.

In the case of near-death and mystical states, let's consider that DMT does more than just change channels, providing us with a view of another channel's program. I suggest this because of the empty, or contentless, nature of the peak mystical experience. There is no sound, touch, vision, smell, or taste. No thoughts or words, and no time. Simultaneously there is an indescribable completeness, power, and understanding.

In between TV channels is "snow," the white noise and images associated with what is "between" the various stations' programming material. What is there if we look and listen carefully? It is the very nature of the activated television itself, electricity coursing through it, energizing and driving it to display something, but that something seems like nothing to the pattern-seeking everyday mind.

In this case, the best analogy might be that DMT has reconfigured the brain's receptive qualities to now stop receiving "outside" information. It is only aware of its own existence, its own intrinsic nature. It displays its own consciousness or resonating frequencies, which have no particular content. Nevertheless, it is the ground upon which all of the programs depend for support—the space that the channels fill.

This space between channels, or the absence of channels, is not empty; rather, it is itself full. The content of the programs replaces this perfect emptiness with their busy fullness. Neither is its nature necessarily "potential." Rather, it is complete unto itself. It needs nothing to exist as it is. But it needs something in order to take shape or form, to manifest.

For some volunteers, DMT's ripping away of consciousness from the body was the stimulus to seek that space between the various levels of perceived reality. They went straight to that empty totality underlying their sense of themselves and the outside world, no longer supported by the body. As Freud commented years ago, "The ego is first and foremost a body-ego." With no body, what's left? These research subjects, like Carlos and Willow, experienced mystical consciousness by virtue of leaving their bodies behind.

Other volunteers found their way to their essential nature through a more direct use of their own will. Sean gave himself permission to go further and deeper into the unknown. Elena disengaged from the wild display of psychedelic colors that obscured their formless foundation. Both succeeded in pulling back and moving forward with just the exquisite knife-edge balance required to make that daring leap into the space between thought, perception, and feeling. The spirit molecule led them to the edge, but it was up to them to take the final step.

Now that we've covered some of the ways in which naturally occurring or outside-administered DMT may provide us with access to such remarkable and astonishing experiences, let's consider the evolutionary significance of naturally produced DMT. In other words, why is there DMT in all of our bodies? Is it a coincidence? Or is it for a purpose?

From the perspective of plants, mushrooms, and animals that contain DMT, it is reasonable to propose that other species, especially humans, would seek and protect them. Those who smoke, drink, or eat DMT-rich life-forms experience highly desirable transport to worlds beyond the imagination. Those psychedelic experience–inducing species would rank high on a list of essential renewable resources, and their survival becomes important to their neighbors.

But then why do humans produce DMT? To date we have discovered no life-form that smokes, eats, or drinks human pineal glands, so we must discard the hypothesis that DMT somehow ensured our physical survival.

Perhaps our ancient ancestors who produced DMT possessed some adaptive advantage over those who did not. Maybe their access to different states of consciousness provided superior problem-solving abilities compared to DMT-less members of our species. Those who had the capacity to synthesize DMT eventually replaced those who did not.

While there is some appeal to this argument, the presence of DMT in so many other readily available forms weakens it to some extent. That is, if someone could not make their own DMT by, for example, deep meditation, there are plenty of plants full of DMT much easier to use than austere spiritual practices. This would certainly be the case for people who live in a DMT-rich environment, such as Latin America.

A more fruitful line of reasoning emerges from the implications of DMT release at death and near-death conditions. These are the times in which the life-force or spirit moves into, out of, and through our bodies. We discussed the biological mechanisms of this proposal in chapter 4. Here, let's use those ideas to investigate their possible significance.

At first glance there seems little evolutionary advantage to the individual or the species in releasing enlightening chemicals as we die. However, Karl Jansen, a British psychiatrist, proposes that one particular type of near-death brain chemicals does indeed confer benefit to the nearly dead. This is because of their "neuroprotective" properties.

In the presence of ketamine, strokes and other acute forms of brain injury are less destructive. Animal data suggest that ketamine-like substances exist in the brain. Thus, during near-death experiences the brain may release these substances in order to minimize brain damage in case that individual survives. The nature of the near-death experience is due to the psychedelic "side effects" of ketamine.[8]

However, there remains the question of why ketamine has psychedelic, rather than, say, tranquilizing, effects. While the release of neuroprotective compounds near death certainly is a useful response, the psychedelic side effects are not as obviously beneficial. We must therefore wonder, are these spiritual properties a coincidence, or do they have a purpose?

I suggest that near-death chemicals released by the brain are psychedelic for this reason: They must be. It is similar to asking why there is silicon in computer chips. Silicon works. It does the job. Near-death brain products are psychedelic because those are the properties consciousness requires at that time.

Psychedelic compounds released near death mediate consciousness exiting the body. This is their function and this is what they do. DMT is a spirit molecule, just as silicon is a chip molecule. Rather than just causing the mind to feel as if it were leaving the body, DMT release is the means by which the mind senses the departure of the life-force from it, the content of consciousness as it leaves the body.

These theories refer solely to DMT's role in unusual states of consciousness. However, might DMT exert an effect on our normal everyday awareness? The fact that the brain actively transports the spirit molecule across the blood-brain barrier suggests this might be the case.

In chapter 2, "What DMT Is," I pointed out that the brain seems to "hunger" for DMT; it expends precious energy actively transporting the drug from the blood into its inner recesses. It is as if DMT were necessary for normal brain function.

Perhaps just the right amount of DMT is involved in the brain's maintenance of the correct receiving properties. That is, it keeps our brains tuned in to Channel Normal. Too much and all manner of unusual and unexpected programs appear on the mind's screen. Too little, and our view of the world dims and flattens.

In fact, these types of numbing, vitality-draining effects are what normal volunteers describe when they take antipsychotic drugs. These drugs may block the effects of endogenous DMT. Perhaps we see and feel what we do on this level of existence because of just the right amount of endogenous DMT. It is an essential component maintaining our brain's awareness of everyday reality. In a way, we might consider DMT to be a "reality thermostat" keeping us in a narrow band of awareness so as to ensure our survival.

When all the speculation, no matter how exciting, stimulating, and revolutionary, is over and done, what are we left with? Even if it turns out that what I've proposed is one day proven true, what do we truly gain from DMT? Once more, we return to "if so, so what?" To what purpose? As the New Mexico research drew to its complicated ending, I began to work through the deepest question that I brought to the studies.

In the beginning of this chapter, I raised the issue of how difficult it is to accept the existence and effects of the spirit molecule in our bodies. In a similar way, can we accept the conclusion I have finally reached? That is, that the nature of DMT is essentially neutral and value-free?

The spirit molecule is neither good nor bad, beneficial nor harmful, in and of itself. Rather, set and setting establish the context and the quality of the experiences to which DMT leads us. Who we are and what we bring to the sessions and to our lives ultimately mean more than the drug experience itself.

Nevertheless, DMT and other psychedelics will never disappear, especially those we make in our own brains every minute of the day. We must

take into account all of their complex and mysterious power in any reck-
oning of human consciousness. So, this one "neither-nor" answer does
not mean that there aren't many unqualified "yes's" to important questions about the best use of these drugs. The set and setting we used in
New Mexico provided a tremendous amount of information about what is
and isn't possible with the assistance of the spirit molecule. Now it is time
to turn to what to do with that knowledge. Is it possible to convert that
information to good use?

The Futures of
Psychedelic Research

This closing chapter discusses possible futures for using and studying DMT and other psychedelic drugs. These scenarios assume a willingness to enlarge the scope of discussion about psychedelic drugs, much as Willis Harman yearned for during our walk along the California coast years ago. Well-informed opinion shapers and decision makers will best determine how accessible and acceptable these drugs become. The most fruitful applications will emerge only if we can set aside the fear, ignorance, and stigma associated with the psychedelics. We also must avoid the naïve and wishful thinking that mars the arguments of some advocates for their use.

These proposals are based upon years of intensive reflection and discussion over the events at the University of New Mexico. While the overall picture this chapter will paint may look overly optimistic, it is, on the contrary, more realistic than my original research designs. This is because it is based upon anticipating and dealing with most of the implicit assumptions about working with psychedelics that inevitably lead to negative outcomes and premature closure.

One of the most important of these is that psychedelic drugs are inherently beneficial. All that's necessary for a positive outcome is to take them.

Another is that psychedelics are "only" drugs. That is, their effects are independent of the environment in which people take them, and of the goals, expectations, and models held by those who give them.

We have rediscovered for ourselves in the DMT research that neither of these common beliefs is true. Thus the model I will present avoids these two most basic and pernicious fallacies regarding working with psychedelic drugs.

Before peering into the future, let's take a brief look at the present research situation. It will be a quick glance.

Several human psychedelic research projects using mescaline, psilocybin, ketamine, and MDMA are active in the United States and Europe. No one is studying DMT. All these projects use the "psychotomimetic" model, comparing psychedelics' effects to symptoms of schizophrenia. These are pharmacology and brain physiology studies.

Two psychedelic psychotherapy programs are underway. One, in the Caribbean, is an ibogaine treatment program for substance abuse; the other, based out of St. Petersburg, Russia, is studying ketamine-assisted psychotherapy, also for drug abuse.

I see many forks in the road when imagining future work with DMT and other psychedelic drugs. One of the major branches divides into "research" versus "use." Some wonder if "psychedelic" and "research" are two words that even belong anywhere near each other. Let's first address this concern.

In the research setting there is the expectation of getting data from your subjects. This affects the relationship between those who administer and those who receive psychedelics. Volunteers know they need to give something to the project, and scientists want something from them. For the person under the influence, just having his or her trip is not enough.

For the investigator, helping that person have the best possible outcome isn't fully adequate, either. This sets up expectations, with the inevitable possibility of disappointment, resentment, and miscommunication. The interpersonal setting is fundamentally altered.

There are several alternatives to this model, all of which are much more popular than the research one. However, popular doesn't necessarily mean "best." And the argument against the research model often is just that: there are better ways to experience these drugs.

Indigenous cultures continue using psychedelic plants much as they have done for thousands of years. Members of African churches in Gabon take ibogaine to contact their ancestors; in Latin America, the DMT-containing brew *ayahuasca* provides the soul access to other worlds; and in North America, peyote opens spiritual realms for healing and guidance.

Modern Western use of psychedelics in non-research settings continues to grow. Many people take psychedelics, by themselves or in intimate group settings. In these cases of "popular" use, psychedelics might be used to gain different perspectives on the self, our relationships, or the natural world. Some use them at large communal gatherings, indoors or outdoors, with or without music and dazzling light shows. A small number of psychedelic therapists administer these drugs in individual or group therapy. Pockets of religious use also exist—for example, *ayahuasca*-using churches are spreading to North America and Europe. In all these cases, the illegality of psychedelics' use stunts open dialogue about their effects in these settings.

There is nothing wrong with any of these models, but it's important not to confuse or interchange them with the research format. Research may one day lead to ways of using psychedelics that don't require obtaining data from participants and adhering to relatively rigid rules of interaction. In the same way, new medications and therapy techniques, if shown helpful in research, make their way into everyday professional and social interactions.

Much of this conflict seems to come from muddled thinking regarding the underlying motives for using psychedelics. Thus, the answer to the question "What is the best way to take psychedelics?" is "It depends."

If you want to have fun, take them alone or with friends and spend the day in a beautiful setting. If you want to learn something about yourself and your relationships, take them with a therapist. If you want to feel part of humanity, take them at a concert, rave, or other large gathering. If you want to experience a deeper relationship with the divine and its creations, take them with a religious teacher, community, or in Nature. If you want to contribute to the research endeavor, volunteer for a scientific study. These categories are somewhat arbitrary, and all sorts of effects might occur in any one of these possible settings; spiritual experiences may occur in a research study, for example, and psychotherapeutic ones in a religious context.

However, trouble and conflict emerge when trying to blend different models because of confusion regarding authority and permissible behavior. This was the most obvious to me when dealing with the friction between the wide-open, rough-and-tumble, trial-and-error methods of science and my Buddhist community's competing priorities of faith, discipleship, and doctrine.[1]

We need an open dialogue about how best to employ these drugs in our lives and society. Because legitimate research is significantly more likely to provide a context for that level of discussion than any other type of use, I will limit this discussion to a research viewpoint.

At the research level, we can divide projects into those that *could* be done as opposed to ones that *should* take place. That is, while there are numerous possible questions we can ask and study, doing so may be misleading or dangerous. Those dangers may affect us directly or indirectly. They also may be dangerous to other living things.

The overarching concern I have about the use of psychedelic drugs has to do with applying them in the service of being helpful, rather than in being smart. Knowing how enlightenment "works," near-death states occur, or alien abductions take place is not as useful as learning to be more kind, wise, and compassionate. That is, the biomedical model, "taking it apart and seeing how it works," may be antithetical to the most fruitful applications of the psychedelic drugs.

I come to this conclusion with a certain amount of irony, as many of the studies I will suggest are ones that I conceived some years before actually performing the research. Now that this stage of my involvement with psychedelics is over, I don't necessarily feel they are as important as I once did, nor that I would want to do them myself.

Let's examine the range of research studies possible with these drugs, and their potential benefits, limitations, and drawbacks.

Mechanisms-of-action projects will provide increasingly refined determination of the types of neurotransmitter receptors involved in psychedelic effects. Modern brain-imaging technologies also will allow us to localize brain sites affected by these drugs.

However, while it may be possible to relate specific changes in brain physiology to certain subjective effects, we are far from knowing how one translates into the other. This, of course, is the holy grail of clinical neuroscience, but it may be an unattainable goal, similar to finding the center of an onion: we can pull back deeper and deeper layers, but the center eludes us.

Nevertheless, we will discover theoretically and clinically important information. A more sophisticated understanding of thinking, perception, and emotion may lead to new treatments for patients for whom brain damage or psychotic illness limits their ability to process information. It's also important to be able to reverse acute negative effects of psychedelics in an emergency setting. Finally, we may be able to develop new psychedelic compounds with unique properties.

This type of research is heavily dependent upon animal studies. We should balance our "need to know" with basic tenets of compassion for non-human animals. This pertains even more to those interested in psychedelics for therapeutic and spiritual purposes. Is it "spiritual" to kill countless laboratory animals so as to enhance our religious ecstasy or creative process?

We already know a great deal about how these drugs work. Primarily focusing on mechanism of action or new drug development may lull us into believing that we are studying psychedelics in the best or most important manner. Perhaps we can spend as much time and energy learning how best to use the drugs we already have as we now do studying how they exert their effects, or designing new agents.

We can investigate even the most unusual and controversial experiences to which the spirit molecule leads us by breaking them down into smaller component parts. No matter how exotic, however, these remain mechanism-of-action studies. We should remember the "if so, so what?" mantra as we probe, analyze, and experiment within even these lines of inquiry. How is what we learn helping us?

I hope to have convincingly argued that naturally occurring psyche-delic states, such as contact with nonmaterial beings, and near-death and mystical experiences, resemble those induced by outside-administered DMT in our volunteers. Many of the following series of studies build upon these similarities.

The first step is to examine the role of endogenous DMT in mediating the naturally occurring psychedelic states under discussion. We could begin by investigating the role of the pineal gland in producing endog-enous DMT.

There are many non-invasive ways of studying pineal physiology in the living person using modern brain-imaging techniques. If the spirit gland is more active during dreams, deep meditation, or alien abduction experiences, this would be evidence for its role in their occurrence. In addition, we could use these technologies to determine if psychedelic drugs directly affect the pineal gland.

We might remove pineal glands from dying animals at various time points after death. If there were measurable amounts of DMT in them, it would support something similar happening in humans. Human pineal re-lease of DMT near, at, or after death would strengthen the hypothesis that the spirit molecule accompanies consciousness's departure from the body.

Elevated DMT levels in body fluids during dreams and childbirth would suggest a relationship between endogenous DMT and these pro-found shifts in consciousness. Even more compelling would be to find high DMT levels in people in the midst of a near-death, mystical, or ab-duction experience.

We could explore further the hypothesis that Cesarean-born infants are not exposed to a primordial "high-dose DMT session" at birth. In chapter 4 I propose that DMT's absence in their deliveries is responsible for some of the psychological and spiritual difficulties Cesarean-born adults encounter later in life. Different responses to DMT in Cesarean-born adults compared to those born vaginally would support this idea. Controlled exposure to DMT in Cesarean-born adults might allow them to partake of the subjective experience of a normal vaginal birth, and therefore may be remedial.

Another series of experiments would give DMT to those who have undergone spontaneous psychedelic experiences, and then ask them to compare the two experiences. Substantial similarity would support a role for endogenous DMT in the original, naturally occurring event. Outside-administered DMT might then provide more controlled access to those states for us to study and utilize more effectively.

The simplest of these projects would be to investigate the relationship between DMT and rapid eye movement, or dream, sleep. If giving DMT during sleep caused the immediate onset of typical dreams, this would support a role for naturally produced DMT in this common altered state.

If administering DMT reproduced part or all of a particular person's previous spontaneous near-death, enlightenment, or abduction experience, we'd be on firmer ground proposing a role for natural DMT in these experiences.

We began approaching the issue of natural and drug-induced enlightenment with one of our volunteers, Sophie, a forty-two-year-old former nun. She had had a mystical experience during a retreat at her nunnery that the abbess confirmed as genuine. She demonstrated a minimal response to her high doses of DMT, an exciting initial confirmation of my hypothesis. That is, if DMT were involved in her mystical experience, perhaps her brain had learned to deal with naturally occurring elevated levels by reducing its sensitivity to the spirit molecule. This would be something like tolerance.

However, the next volunteer who demonstrated even less of a response to 0.4 mg/kg DMT seriously challenged this theory. Charles, a thirty-four-year-old bartender, had never meditated a day in his life. In his case, we proposed a hard-wiring, genetic predisposition to his mild DMT response. He was born that way.

I therefore needed to be more modest in attributing Sophie's minimal reaction to her prior mystical experience. Of course, it's possible that each hypothesis was true for the particular individual, but there would be a certain intellectual dishonesty in using the data in such a self-serving manner.[2]

While the above projects would go a long way toward legitimizing the study of highly unusual states of mind, they no longer hold the appeal for me they once did. I am now less interested in the "how" than in the "if so, so what?" Whether what we learn is ultimately helpful depends upon how we use that information.

I believe the best research use of psychedelics is to treat uniquely human disorders and to enhance distinctly human characteristics. Let's then visualize an optimal setting for administering and taking psychedelic drugs that accepts these challenges.

Such a center would exist in a beautiful natural setting but would possess all the required medical facilities for emergency backup. There would be examples of exquisite art and architecture that could provide inspiration for those participating in the research protocols. Research scientists and staff would possess psychotherapeutic, psychedelic, and spiritual training and would work under medical direction. Protocols would occur in the fields of psychotherapy, creativity, spirituality, and the dying process. There would be studies, too, of the being-contact phenomenon and its relationship to parallel universes and dark matter.

Time and again we saw how the Research Center environment negatively impacted our DMT sessions. The clinical environment was even more problematic for the longer psilocybin sessions. While a more pleasant setting is essential, one of great beauty is even better suited to guide and support research subjects during their highly suggestible and vulnerable experiences. Nevertheless, there are potentially dangerous adverse physical, especially cardiovascular, effects of psychedelics, and equipment and staff must exist to respond to them.

Medical doctors' training and experience provide them unique abilities to appreciate, understand, and respond to the whole human organism's reaction to medications. Therefore, the law places the privilege and responsibility of using drugs in the hands of physicians. Within the field of medicine, psychiatrists receive the most exhaustive training in dealing with human behavior and its relationship to the physical body. However, traditional psychiatric medical training ought to be only the preliminary requirement for being able to administer psychedelic drugs to another human being. One of the most important additional qualifications should be having taken psychedelics oneself.

In the 1950s and 1960s self-experimentation was a generally recognized tool in psychopharmacology. Similarly, and in contrast to contemporary American protocol, European psychedelic researchers must "go first" in their studies. This approach increases the quality of informed consent provided by the investigator, provides pilot data for further refinement of hypotheses and techniques, and enhances researchers' empathy with volunteers' experiences. Future North American studies should request permission from regulatory boards to follow our European colleagues in this extraordinarily important matter.[3]

In addition to "having been there oneself," a researcher who plans on administering psychedelics to others must clearly examine his or her motivations to do so. Formal supervised training in self-examination is necessary for anyone in the powerful position of giving people psychedelic drugs. While there are many such systems, I believe the psychoanalytic model is the most thorough and comprehensive. It explores important childhood experiences in the context of developing and working through a close relationship with a therapist. It also examines unconscious motivations and urges affecting our behavior and feelings. This inner psychological work is crucial in helping us relate to our research subjects whose interpersonal needs and fears are magnified powerfully while under a psychedelic's spell.

Understanding religious sensibilities in as deep a manner as possible also is necessary for being fully supportive and understanding while supervising psychedelic sessions. This does not mean simply having spiritual or religious experiences oneself, with or without a psychedelic. Rather, it ought to include training and background in religious sensibilities. Education in theology, ethics, and ritual additionally will help in empathizing with and understanding important aspects of the full psychedelic experience.

Before performing the DMT research, I never would have suggested that familiarity with alien abduction phenomena would be important in providing the best possible supervision for sessions. However, I do now. I also believe it's helpful to know something about current theories regarding "invisible realms," like dark matter and parallel universes.

Equipped with these types of training and experience, research scientists and staff will be ready to understand, accept, and react to nearly everything that might come up during deep psychedelic sessions.

Ongoing studies at this ideal research site could generate an exhaustive dose-response database for old and new psychedelic drugs. By standardizing and optimizing the setting, we will learn what really is possible with particular doses of individual drugs.

In addition, there's a lot to be learned from small doses of psychedelics. These "little trips" receive scant attention, but they can have highly desirable effects. For example, many of the early psychedelic psychotherapy researchers preferred treating patients with low doses in "psycholytic," or "mind-loosening," psychotherapy because they were easier to use and patients better retained therapeutic effects.

Over a cup of tea one summer day at his house in Switzerland, Albert Hofmann, who discovered LSD, shared with me his fondness for low doses of this drug. He and others have described a quickening of thought, brightening of perception, and elevation in mood that contribute to subtle but profound effects on mental function. Side effects are nearly nonexistent.

Psychedelics may help treat our most troubling psychiatric and psychological problems. Our proposed psychedelic research center would focus much of its work in this area. However, we must be ready for the potentially clashing views of healing that will surface in the design and interpretation of such research.

For example, there are several reports in the psychiatric literature describing relief of symptoms in patients with obsessive-compulsive disorder, or OCD, after taking psilocybin-containing mushrooms. The OCD syndrome consists of irresistible urges to repeat useless behavior and thoughts that consume distressing amounts of time and energy. That serotonin-active drugs like Prozac help patients with OCD has focused attention on this neurotransmitter. Researchers now plan to give psilocybin in an attempt to treat patients with OCD, using serotonin-receptor physiology as their underlying model. No recourse to psychological processes really is necessary, although it may prove crucial to a fuller understanding of its beneficial effects.

We also might treat conditions with deficits in psychological, rather than only neurotransmitter, health, such as post-traumatic stress disorder, drug and alcohol abuse, and the anguish and suffering associated with terminal illness.

Post-traumatic stress disorder causes feeling of being trapped in the past, endlessly rushing backward on a time machine toward horrible events. Childhood physical and sexual abuse and exposure to natural and man-made catastrophes are ever-increasing concerns in our society. Early studies by psychedelic psychotherapy researchers explored these drugs' use in post-traumatic conditions. Up until his recent death, the Dutch psychiatrist Jan Bastiaans used psychedelic drugs to treat successfully many difficult cases of concentration-camp survivor syndrome.[4]

Many people abuse drugs and alcohol in an attempt to resolve similarly painful memories and emotions. Soon, however, complications of substance abuse become more troubling than the initial problems. It's been shown that membership in the peyote-using Native American Church reduces the incidence of alcoholism. Similar effects on alcohol and cocaine dependence seem to occur in members of *ayahuasca*-using churches in Brazil.[5]

Finally, negative reactions to the pain and deterioration of terminal illness trigger a vast array of unresolved feelings. The growing number of aging and dying "baby-boomers" as well as AIDS and other epidemics give great poignancy to a desire for a comfortable and "good" death.

Several early studies demonstrated promising results using high-dose psychedelic therapy sessions.

The implications of our research with DMT may make work with the dying perhaps even more compelling. If DMT is released at the time of death, then administering it to the living would provide a "dry run" for the real thing. The letting go, the experience of consciousness existing independently of the body, encountering a loving and powerful presence in that state—all seemed to provide a powerful intimation of what happens as the body drops away.

However, we are treading in sensitive waters when considering work with the dying. If a patient has frightening encounters with their own psyche or nonmaterial realms, there may be precious little time to set things straight. Furthermore, what if there is nothing at all similar between the experience of dying and a high dose of DMT? The shock, disorientation, and fear could make the dying process more difficult than would otherwise have been the case.

In addition to the treatment of clinical disorders, psychedelics could be used to enhance characteristics of our normal state of being, such as creativity, problem-solving abilities, spirituality, and so on. The research institute I envision will carefully and responsibly take the lead in such studies. This work may ultimately serve more people, and have greater overall impact, than strictly pathology-based therapy projects.

We are seeing an ever-increasing availability of relatively side-effect-free antidepressants, sexual performance enhancers, stimulants, and mood stabilizers. These new, easy-to-take chemical agents are forcing us to reevaluate the risks and benefits involved in making us better than average. Why not use psychedelics, too, for indications other than treating the sick?

DMT elicited ideas, feelings, thoughts, and images our volunteers said they never could have imagined. Psychedelics stimulate the imagination, and thus they are logical tools to enhance creativity. The problems facing our society and planet require the use of novel ideas as much as new and more powerful technology. It's impossible to overstate the urgent need to improve our imaginative abilities. Psychedelics may provide a powerful tool for doing so.

I've mentioned previously Harman's and Fadiman's 1960s studies of psychedelics' positive effects on problem solving. Research subjects, all professionals in their fields, found that many of these psychedelically enhanced solutions were quite effective. There currently are many well-characterized ways of measuring creativity, including artistic, scientific, psychological, spiritual, and emotional. It would be relatively straightforward to renew research into psychedelics' effects on this crucial human quality.

Many definitions of imagination refer to the divine nature of this attribute. To conceive of and produce something new allows us to share in some of God's creative power. Our imagination extends us by thought into places where nothing previously existed. We therefore return to the role of psychedelics in spirituality.

As I suggested in chapter 20, "Stepping on Holy Toes," there is a rational course of action for melding psychedelics within a spiritual discipline. If a religious aspirant lacks firsthand knowledge of the sublime states that trickle down through scripture, ritual, and discipleship, carefully guided, supervised, and followed-up psychedelic sessions may spur him or her on within the chosen faith. This type of work also may help develop a more broad-minded and universal approach to the spiritual.

We may quibble about what is biological, psychological, or spiritual. Resolving inner conflicts, ending damaging relationships with people or substances, and stimulating the imagination all can be held and supported using these three models. However, we are pressed far beyond our comfort zone as clinician-researchers when dealing with psychedelic subjects who return telling tales of contact and interactions with seemingly autonomous nonmaterial entities. How, then, do we study these "transdimensional" properties of DMT?

We must begin by assuming that these types of experiences are "possibly real." In other words, they may indicate "what it's like" in alternate realities. The earliest attempts at systematically investigating these contacts should determine the consistency and stability of the beings. With lessening shock at their presence, is it possible to prolong, expand, and deepen our interactions with them? Do people encountering beings possessing similar appearances, behaviors, and "locale" also report the exchange of comparable messages and information?

Not only research would take place at such an institution. Experimental studies first would establish the best use of psychedelics for particular indications: therapeutic, creative, or spiritual. As in any other comparable setting where innovative treatments take place, greater numbers of people then would receive these specialized services. During their stay, there would be less data gathering and more emphasis on outcome measures for follow-up purposes.

A natural consequence of the expertise available at this institute is that education and training also would be a prominent activity. There would be ongoing opportunities for learning from experts in all the fields that might inform, and be enhanced, by the psychedelic experience. Finally, the research center would house an exhaustive library and archival service and could serve as a clearinghouse for all manner of educational materials.

Epilogue

While professionally and personally grueling, the University of New Mexico psychedelic drug research was undoubtedly the most inspiring and remarkable time in my life. The resumption of this work in the United States was my lifelong dream, and I'm glad to have been in the right place at the right time to do it.

As a clinical research scientist with extensive psychotherapeutic and spiritual training and experience, I believed I was qualified to initiate this American renewal of human psychedelic research. In some ways I was, and in others I wasn't, ready for where the spirit molecule would lead us. We succeeded in opening a door that had remained tightly locked for a generation. However, the box, like Pandora's, once opened, let out a force with its own agenda and language. It was a power that healed, hurt, startled, and was indifferent in wild and unpredictable ways. At every turn, I heard it call out in a voice that was tender, challenging, engaging, and frightening. But the question never changed.

This is the same question that Saul, a volunteer whom we've not yet met, encountered on his first high-dose DMT session. Let's close with his story.

A thirty-four-year-old married psychologist, Saul was wiry and energetic, with a wry sense of humor and an intense gaze. He had taken psychedelics about forty times and had been practicing meditation for nearly twenty years. (I did my best to recruit research subjects with a background in meditation. They seemed more able to deal with the initial anxiety of the DMT rush and also helped me compare meditation and drug-induced states of mind.) Saul volunteered for the dose-response study because "I've heard about DMT and have always wanted to try it. Plus, I like the idea of being able to try it in the hospital under medical supervision."

Saul's low dose was mild, and he returned the following day for his 0.4 mg/kg session.

Saul liked to write, and while my notes are rather complete, a letter he later sent to me does an even better job of describing his experience that day:

The empty space in the room began sparkling. Large crystalline prisms appeared, a wild display of lights shooting off into all directions. More complicated and beautiful geometric patterns overlaid my visual field. My body felt cool and light. Was I about to faint? I closed my eyes, sighing, and thought, "My God!"

I heard absolutely nothing, but my mind was completely full of some sort of sound, like the aftereffects of a large ringing bell. I didn't know if I was breathing. I trusted things would be fine and let go of that thought before panic could set in.

The ecstasy was so great that my body could not contain it. Almost out of necessity, I felt my awareness rush out, leaving its physical container behind.

Out of the raging colossal waterfall of flaming color expanding into my visual field, the roaring silence, and an unspeakable joy, they stepped, or rather, emerged. Welcoming, curious, they almost sang, "Now do you see?" I felt their question pour into and fill every possible corner of my awareness: "Now do you see? Now do you see?" Trilling, sing-song voices, exerting enormous pressure on my mind.

There was no need to answer. It was as if someone had asked me, on a blazing cloudless midsummer afternoon in the New Mexico desert, "Is it bright? Is it bright?" The question and the answer are identical. Added to my "Yes!" was a deeper "Of course!" And finally, an intensely poignant "At last!"

I "stared" with my inner eyes, and we appraised each other. As they disappeared back into the torrent of color, now beginning to fade, I could hear some sounds in the room. I knew I was coming down. I felt my breathing, my face, my fingers, and I was dimly aware of an encroaching darkness. Were there flames, smoke, dust, battling troops, enormous suffering? I opened my eyes.

Notes

Dedication

1. Jean Toomer and Rudolph P. Byrd, *Essentials* (Athens: University of Georgia Press, 1991), 27.

Acknowledgments

1. National Institutes of Health grants funded the melatonin project (RR00997-10), the DMT and psilocybin studies (R03 DA06524 and R01 DA08096), and general operations of the Clinical Research Center (M01 RR00997).

Prologue

1. The most direct way to get DMT into the brain, of course, is to inject it straight into this sensitive organ. I know of no studies in which researchers gave psychedelic drugs to humans in this manner. However, there is a report describing direct administration of LSD into the cerebrospinal fluid using a spinal tap. Since the cerebrospinal fluid bathes the brain, it allows direct access to it. In this case, LSD effects began "almost instantly." See Paul Hoch, "Studies in Routes of Administration and Counteracting Drugs," in *Lysergic Acid Diethylamide and Mescaline in Experimental Psychiatry*, edited by Louis Cholden (New York: Grune & Stratton, 1956), 8–12.

2. There were people who had used IV DMT in non-research, or recreational, settings. One of the men I interviewed in the process of developing the rating scale took it this way in the 1960s. His opinion was that it was "just slightly faster" than smoking it.

3. William J. Turner Jr. and Sidney Merlis, "Effect of Some Indolealkylamines on Man," *Archives of Neurology and Psychiatry* 81 (1959): 121–29.

Chapter 1

1. For reviews of historical data regarding naturally occurring psychedelics' importance, see Marlene Dobkin de Rios, *Hallucinogens: Cross-Cultural Perspectives* (Albuquerque, NM: University of New Mexico Press, 1984); and Peter Furst, *Flesh of the Gods: The Ritual Use of Hallucinogens* (New York: Waveland, 1990).

For more speculative musings regarding these issues, see Ronald Siegel, *Intoxication: Life in Pursuit of Artificial Paradise* (New York: EP Dutton, 1989); Terence McKenna, *Food of the Gods* (New York: Bantam, 1993); and Paul Devereux, *The Long Trip: A Prehistory of Psychedelia* (New York: Penguin, 1997).

Wasson's work is the most exhaustive regarding early spiritual functions of psychedelic natural substances—see R. Gordon Wasson, Carl A. P. Ruck, and Stella Krammrisch, *Persephone's Quest: Entheogens and the Origins of Religion* (New Haven, CT: Yale University Press, 1988).

For in-depth discussions of specific plants and their roles in aboriginal societies, see Richard E. Schultes and Albert Hofmann, *Plants of the Gods* (New York: McGraw Hill, 1979). For the chemistry of those plants, see Richard E. Schultes and Albert Hofmann, *The Botany and Chemistry of Hallucinogens*, 2nd ed. (Springfield, IL: Charles C. Thomas, 1980); and Jonathan Ott, *Pharmacotheon* (Kennewick, WA: Natural Products Co., 1993). Albert Hofmann's tale of discovering LSD never fails to delight—*LSD: My Problem Child* (New York: McGraw Hill, 1980).

2. Neurotransmitters allow chemical communication among nerve cells in the brain. A transmitting cell releases a neurotransmitter, which then attaches to specialized receptor sites on the receiving cell. This docking of transmitter to receptor begins a sequence of events ending in the release of the receiving cell's own neurotransmitter, and the process continues down the line. Other well-known neurotransmitters include norepinephrine (noradrenaline), acetylcholine, and dopamine.

3. For a sense of the vast amount of information accumulated during those years, see Abram Hoffer and Humphrey Osmond, *The Hallucinogens* (New York: Academic Press, 1967). Remarkably, almost forty years after its publication, this remains the best available textbook on these drugs.

4. For an excellent review of the scientific basis for psychedelic-assisted psychotherapy, see Walter N. Pahnke, Albert A. Kurland, Sanford Unger, Charles Savage, and Stanislav Grof, "The Experimental Use of Psychedelic (LSD) Psychotherapy," *Journal of the American Medical Association* 212 (1970): 1856–63.

5. Aldous Huxley, *Doors of Perception and Heaven and Hell* (New York: HarperCollins, 1990).

6. Historians often contrast Leary's freewheeling take-all-comers approach to the use of psychedelics with Huxley's view that their use must be limited to a small elite of leaders and artists. The fact remains, however, that without the relatively lawless approach of Leary (see Timothy Leary, *Flashbacks* [New York: JP Tarcher, 1997]) and Ken Kesey (see Paul Perry, *On the Bus* [St. Paul, MN: Thunder's Mouth Press, 1997]), it is unlikely many of us would have had the opportunity to encounter these drugs.

7. Rick J. Strassman, "Adverse Reactions to Psychedelic Drugs. A Review of the Literature," *Journal of Nervous and Mental Disease* 172 (1984): 577–95.

8. Later revelations of CIA involvement in dosing unsuspecting citizens and Army recruits with LSD and other psychedelics added shame and embarrassment to this already painful assortment of feelings. See Martin A. Lee and Bruce Shlain, *Acid Dreams: The Complete Social History of LSD, the CIA, the Sixties, and Beyond* (New York: Grove Press, 1986); and Jay Stevens, *Storming Heaven: LSD and the American Dream* (New York: Grove Press, 1998), for thorough reviews of this remarkable chapter in American domestic national security operations.

9. Stanley Schachter and Jerome E. Singer, "Cognitive, Social, and Physiological Determinants of Emotional State," *Psychological Review* 69 (1962): 379–99.

10. In addition to spawning so many names, psychedelics have inspired quite a following. I know of no other drugs, except perhaps marijuana, with as many organizations dedicated to educating about them, and promoting their use. There are dozens of psychedelic organizations with thousands of dues-paying members. They publish magazines, newsletters, journals, and Web sites. They organize and sponsor conferences and publish and distribute books. The late Dr. Freedman from UCLA, an early LSD researcher and a driving force behind my study, coined the term *cultogen*, referring to this zeal with which advocates and enemies of their use rushed in with simple, one-sided descriptions of their effects. Opiate, cocaine, or solvent users don't organize in such an effective manner. What is so unique about psychedelics that they provoke such evangelical responses?

11. Drugs from other chemical families also may be psychedelic, but only within a narrow dose range. For example, compounds in the nightshade family of plants, such as jimsonweed, cause hallucinations and altered thinking processes. However, they do so in the context of a confused, delirious state, with dangerous disturbances of cardiac function and temperature control. Oftentimes one remembers little, and serious toxicity, including death, may result from taking "a little too much." On the other hand, there are no cases of psychedelic drugs being directly fatal.

Drugs like ketamine ("K" or "special K") and phencyclidine (PCP or "angel dust") also produce psychedelic effects. However, they first saw use as general anesthetic agents and cause unconsciousness at higher doses. The "classical" psychedelic drugs such as LSD or mescaline don't cause general anesthesia.

In addition, ketamine, PCP, and nightshade-based drugs exert their psychoactive effects through pharmacological mechanisms different from those of LSD, psilocybin, and DMT. For our purposes I will limit my discussion of "psychedelics" to those with similar structures and pharmacological properties. For a review of any and all substances with psychedelic properties, see Peter Stafford, *Psychedelics Encyclopedia* (Berkeley, CA: Ronin Press, 1992).

12. Methyl groups, which consist of a carbon and three hydrogens, are themselves the simplest possible addition to an organic molecule.

13. 5-MeO-DMT is the active ingredient in the secretion from the venom glands of the Sonoran desert toad, *Bufo alvarius*. The drug is not obtained by licking these toads, as inaccurate media reports would have it. Rather, intrepid users catch a toad and painlessly "milk" the venom onto a glass slide. They release the toad, dry the secretions, and smoke them in a pipe. See Wade Davis and Andrew T. Weil, "Identity of a New World Psychoactive Toad," *Ancient Mesoamerican* (1988): 51–59.

Chapter 2

1. Alexander Shulgin and Ann Shulgin, *TIHKAL* (Berkeley,CA: Transform Press, 1997), 247–84.

2. R. H. F. Manske, "A Synthesis of the Methyl-Tryptamines and Some Derivatives," *Canadian Journal of Research* 5 (1931): 592–600.

3. O. Gonçalves de Lima, "Observaçoes Sôbre o Vihno da Jurema Utilazado Pelos Indios Pancarú de Tacaratú (Pernambuco)," *Arquiv. Inst. Pesquisas Agron.*4 (1946): 45–80; and M. S. Fish, N. M. Johnson, and E. C. Horning, "Piptadenia Alkaloids. Indole Bases of P. Peregrina (L.) Benth. and Related Species," *Journal of the American Chemical Society* 77 (1955): 5892–95.

4. Stephen Szára, "The Social Chemistry of Discovery: The DMT Story," *Social Pharmacology* 3 (1989): 237–48.

5. Stephen Szára, "The Comparison of the Psychotic Effects of Tryptamine Derivatives with the Effects of Mescaline and LSD-25 in Self-Experiments," in *Psychotropic Drugs*, edited by W. Garattini and V. Ghetti. (New York: Elsevier, 1957), 460–67.

6. A. Sai-Halasz, G. Brunecker, and S. Szára, "Dimethyltryptamin: Ein Neues Psychoticum," *Psychiat. Neurol., Basel* 135 (1958): 285–301.

7. A. Sai-Halasz, "The Effect of Antiserotonin on the Experimental Psychosis Induced by Dimethyltryptamine," *Experientia* 18 (1962): 137–38.

8. D. E. Rosenberg, Harris Isbell, and E. J. Miner, "Comparison of Placebo, N-Dimethyltryptamine, and 6-Hydroxy-N-Dimethyltryptamine in Man," *Psychopharmacology* 4 (1963): 39–42.

9. Jonathan Kaplan, Lewis R. Mandel, Richard Stillman, Robert W. Walker, W. J. A. Vandenheuvel, J. Christian Gillin, and Richard Jed Wyatt, "Blood and Urine Levels of N,N-Dimethyltryptamine Following Administration of Psychoactive Dosages to Human Subjects," *Psychopharmacology* 38 (1974): 239–45.

10. Timothy Leary, "Programmed Communication During Experiences with DMT," *Psychedelic Review* 8 (1966): 83–95.

11. This uncertainty about DMT effects helped the drug remain relatively obscure until Terence McKenna began praising it publicly and lavishly in the mid-1980s. More than anyone, McKenna has raised awareness of DMT, through lectures, books, interviews, and recordings, to its present unprecedented level.

12. For an excellent review summarizing the endogenous DMT data, see Steven A. Barker, John A. Monti, and Samuel T. Christian, "N,N-Dimethyltryptamine: An Endogenous Hallucinogen," *International Review of Neurobiology* 22 (1981): 83–110.

13. J. Christian Gillin, Jonathan Kaplan, Richard Stillman, and Richard Jed Wyatt, "The Psychedelic Model of Schizophrenia: The Case of N,N-Dimethyltryptamine," *American Journal of Psychiatry* 133 (1976): 203–8.

14. Despite reservations about the DMT theory of schizophrenia, it is worth noting that in the twenty-five years since scientists abandoned it, there have been no other candidates nearly as well qualified for this role.

15. In this context, it is a fascinating study in how the winds of public and political opinion shape the research community's scientific agenda. There now is a flurry of funding for,

and publications about, the "ketamine model" of schizophrenia. As discussed previously, ketamine is an anesthetic drug, low doses of which produce psychedelic effects. Similar to the "classical" psychedelic drugs, there is overlap between ketamine effects and schizophrenic symptoms. However, there probably are as many differences and similarities between schizophrenia and ketamine as there are between schizophrenia and typical psychedelics.

There are at least two reasons for the current, relatively unimpeded progress in the ketamine field. Many more rating scales now exist that statistically can compare drug-induced to schizophrenic states. These provide more objective, mathematical support for similarities between schizophrenia and ketamine intoxication. This approach may, however, tend to gloss over the real clinical differences between the two conditions. It was these real-life differences that caused earlier investigators to reject the utility of comparing typical psychedelic drug effects with symptoms of schizophrenia.

Another, and probably the more important, difference is that ketamine is a "legal" drug. There are few restrictions limiting its use in human research. Nevertheless, the recent surge in popularity of recreational ketamine use is tightening monitoring and controls over it. In addition, concerns about worsening schizophrenic symptoms with ketamine, and the nature of informed consent for these studies, are raising anxiety about psychedelic ketamine research in ways similar to older psychedelic studies.

16. Making DMT "from scratch" in the laboratory is not complicated. A reasonably skilled chemist can produce it with modest effort in several days. The difficulty in making it is not in the mechanics of doing so, but in obtaining the necessary ingredients, or precursors. Federal drug authorities monitor supplies of these precursors very tightly, and you need a permit to purchase any that might be turned into a known psychedelic drug.

17. Toshihiro Takahashi, Kazuhiro Takahashi, Tatsuo Ido, Kazuhiko Yanai, Ren Iwata, Kiichi Ishiwata, and Shigeo Nozoe, "^{11}C-Labelling of Indolealkylamine Alkaloids and the Comparative Study of Their Tissue Distributions," *International Journal of Applied Radiation and Isotopes* 36 (1985): 965–69; and Kazuhiko Yanai, Tatsuo Ido, Kiichi Ishiwata, Jun Hatazawa, Toshihiro Takahashi, Ren Iwata, and Taiju Matsuzawa, "*In Vivo* Kinetics and Displacement Study of Carbon-11-Labeled Hallucinogen, N,N-[^{11}C]Dimethyltryptamine," *European Journal of Nuclear Medicine* 12 (1986): 141–46.

18. By some unimaginable feat of "pre-literate chemistry," South American natives learned to combine DMT-containing plants with others possessing anti-MAO compounds, or MAO inhibitors. Accompanied by MAO inhibitors, swallowed DMT can withstand enzyme breakdown long enough to enter the bloodstream and exert its psychological effects before MAO recovers sufficiently to dispose of it. This is the secret by which *ayahuasca* succeeds in making DMT orally active. The slower absorption from the stomach and intestines means that DMT effects in *ayahuasca* last 4 to 5 hours, rather than just minutes as with injected DMT.

Chapter 3

1. Willis W. Harman, Robert H. McKim, Robert E. Mogar, James Fadiman, and Myron J. Stolaroff, "Psychedelic Agents in Creative Problem-Solving: A Pilot Study," *Psychological Reports* 19 (1966): 211–27.

2. More than twenty years later, in 1995, I met Dorothy Fadiman at a meeting in Manaus, in the Brazilian Amazon. When she returned home to California, she sent me her 1970s video about light, *Radiance.* The circle finally was complete.

3. The Crown or Thousand-Petaled Lotus *chakra* is not the same as the "third eye." The latter, located in the middle of the forehead just above and between the eyes, anatomically corresponds most closely with the pituitary gland.

4. The relationship of cerebrospinal fluid to consciousness recently got a boost from brain science research. There are very high levels of particular serotonin receptors on the cells lining the ventricles. It is these lining cells that make cerebrospinal fluid. LSD attaches to these receptors with extraordinary vigor. Perhaps psychedelics really do alter our consciousness in such powerful ways by controlling production of this unique brain liquid. Descartes and his followers would certainly get a hearty laugh out of these "modern" discoveries!

5. Rene Descartes, "The Inter-Relation of Soul and Body," in *The Way of Philosophy*, edited by P. Wheelright (New York: Odyssey, 1954), 357.

6. We do not know if the opening in the skull, the fontanel, which is located directly above the *infant's* pineal, allows enough light in to affect the gland.

7. Aaron B. Lerner, James D. Case, Yoshiyata Takahashi, Teh H. Lee, and Wataru Mori, "Isolation of Melatonin, the Pineal Gland Factor That Lightens Melanocytes," *Journal of the American Chemical Society* 30 (1958): 2587.

8. F. Karsch, E. Bittman, D. Foster, R. Goodman, S. Legan, and J. Robinson, "Neuroendocrine Basis of Seasonal Reproduction," *Recent Progress in Hormone Research* 40 (1984): 185–232.

9. The pineal gland becomes full of calcium as we age. The calcified gland is an excellent marker for the mid-line of the brain in skull X-rays and CAT scans. However, little of this calcium collects in the melatonin-producing cells. While melatonin levels do drop as we age, this is independent of the level of pineal calcification.

10. Rick J. Strassman, Clifford R. Qualls, E. Jonathan Lisansky, and Glenn T. Peake, "Elevated Rectal Temperature Produced by All-Night Bright Light Is Reversed by Melatonin Infusion in Men," *Journal of Applied Physiology* 71 (1991): 2178–82.

  Early morning also is when we are most likely to be in dream sleep, and some studies suggested that large doses of melatonin enhanced dreaming. We were unable to examine this in our experiments because subjects needed to stay awake with eyes open for light to suppress melatonin. If melatonin did stimulate dream sleep, we would have expected less vivid dreams in volunteers whose melatonin production was inhibited. Interestingly, drugs that suppress nighttime melatonin formation increase, rather than decrease, dreams.

Chapter 4

1. While DMT may be involved in both spiritual and psychotic experiences, it is important to distinguish between them. There is some overlap between spiritual experiences and psychosis; for example, the thrilling sense of imminence, heightened visual and auditory perceptions, and a change in the passage of time.

  Usually, however, mystical experiences result from a mature and conscious effort toward obtaining them. The practitioner seeks them out, there is an intellectual and moral context supporting and encouraging them, and their expression is socially sanctioned and acceptable.

  On the other hand, symptoms of schizophrenia most often are unexpected, unwelcome, and occur in those with prior behavioral and emotional problems. There is little social support for the experiences, and both the individual and his/her associates wish they would go away.

Just as is the case in our volunteers, set and setting have as much to do with the DMT experience as does the drug itself. How one adapts to the presence of naturally formed DMT in one's life depends upon an even larger context of set and setting: who the person is, his or her experiences and expectations, how he or she interacts with and interprets the effects of DMT, and the social setting in which they occur.

2. Rick J. Strassman, Otto Appenzeller, Alfred J. Lewy, Clifford R. Qualls, and Glenn T. Peake, "Increase in Plasma Melatonin, beta-Endorphin, and Cortisol After a 28.5-Mile Mountain Race: Relationship to Performance and Lack of Effect of Naltrexone," *Journal of Clinical Endocrinology and Metabolism* 69 (1989): 540–45.

The runner's "high" is not just a feeling of euphoria related to endorphin release. There also are sensory changes: shimmering and brightening of the visual field; a sense of body lightness, of almost floating off the ground; a feeling that time dramatically slows. All these effects also are reported by volunteers on a low dose of DMT. Maybe runners and our low-dose DMT volunteers are describing effects of the same biological event: excessive but not fully psychedelic brain levels of DMT. In runners' cases, the massive surge of adrenaline and noradrenaline could stimulate pineal DMT production and cause a naturally occurring low-dose DMT experience. Unfortunately, we were unable to measure DMT at the point, and we could not test this hypothesis.

3. Robin M. Murray, Michael C. H. Oon, Richard Rodnight, James L. T. Birley, and Alan Smith, "Increased Excretion of Dimethyltryptamine and Certain Features of Psychosis. A Possible Association," *Archives of General Psychiatry* 36 (1979): 644–49.

4. L. Bigelow, "Effects of Aqueous Pineal Extract on Chronic Schizophrenia," *Biological Psychiatry* 8 (1974): 5–15.

5. Richard Jed Wyatt, J. Christian Gillin, Jonathan Kaplan, Richard Stillman, Lewis R. Mandel, H. S. Ahn, W. J. A. Vandenheuvel, and R. W. Walker, "N,N-Dimethyltryptamine—A Possible Relationship to Schizophrenia?" *Advances in Biochemical Psychopharmacology* 11 (1974): 299–313.

6. Jace Callaway, "A proposed mechanism for the visions of dream sleep," *Medical Hypotheses* 26 (1988): 119–24.

7. Magnetic fields also may affect consciousness, as in the shifts of awareness one notices in particular geological sites or formations, so-called "power spots." Recent studies describe magnetic fields affecting pineal function, in particular suppressing melatonin formation. These effects may redirect pineal energy and raw materials to make DMT instead.

I propose a relationship between DMT and alien abductions in another chapter. However, this is a good time to note that these experiences sometimes take place near high-intensity power lines, which produce powerful magnetic fields. In addition, alien encounters often occur at particular land locations, also suggesting magnetic field effects.

8. Jane Butterfield English, *Different Doorway: Adventures of a Caesarean Born* (Mt. Shasta, CA: Earth Heart, 1985).

Grof has developed a non-drug "psychedelic" therapy using prolonged hyperventilation. Thirty to 60 minutes of controlled overbreathing results in a highly altered state of consciousness that many compare to a high-dose psychedelic drug experience. Several profound metabolic effects result from this technique: blood chemistry becomes more alkaline, or basic; calcium levels drop; the blood-brain barrier becomes less effective; stress hormone levels rise dramatically. All of these may combine to activate rarely used DMT-synthetic pathways in the pineal. See Stanislav Grof, *The Holotropic Mind* (New York: HarperSanFrancisco, 1993).

Chapter 5

1. Daniel X. Freedman, "On the Use and Abuse of LSD," *Archives of General Psychiatry* 18 (1968): 330–47.

2. We did not collect these urine drug tests as a tool to screen out volunteers. Rather, we were interested in seeing if anyone testing positive had psychedelic experiences different from those of volunteers who were not using recreational drugs. There were only a handful of positive urines in our first study, and these volunteers' data did not differ from those of volunteers with negative urines. In subsequent studies, therefore, we dropped these expensive tests.

3. We asked volunteers to guess which dose they got on each double-blind day. It was easy to tell which was the high dose. But it was intriguing to find out how difficult it was to tell the difference between the intermediates doses, 0.1 and 0.2 mg/kg. Even more surprisingly, many research subjects confused the low dose and saltwater placebo. Our rating scale turned out to be more accurate than the volunteers in ranking, from high to low, the dose received on any given day. That is, the questionnaire reliably showed that 0.2 mg/kg caused a larger psychological response than did 0.1, and 0.05 more than saltwater, even when volunteers' hunches about the dose were wrong.

Chapter 6

1. Rick J. Strassman, "Human Hallucinogenic Drug Research in the United States: A Present-Day Case History and Review of the Process," *Journal of Psychoactive Drugs* 23 (1991): 29–38.

2. The salt form was necessary so the DMT would dissolve in water. It's similar to cocaine—free base doesn't dissolve in water, but various cocaine salts do.

Chapter 8

1. Gillin et al. (1976); and B. Kovacic and Edward F. Domino, "Tolerance and Limited Cross-Tolerance to the Effects of N,N-Dimethyltryptamine (DMT) and Lysergic Acid Diethylamide-25 (LSD) on Food-Rewarded Bar Pressing in the Rat," *Journal of Pharmacology and Experimental Therapeutics* 197 (1976): 495–502.

2. Rick J. Strassman, Clifford R. Qualls, and Laura M. Berg, "Differential Tolerance to Biological and Subjective Effects of Four Closely Spaced Doses of N,N-Dimethyltryptamine in Humans," *Biological Psychiatry* 39 (1996): 784–95.

Chapter 9

1. The results of the dose-response study in which we characterized the effects of different amounts of DMT appeared in published form in 1994 in Dr. Freedman's journal, the *Archives of General Psychiatry*. One paper described the biological data, the other psychological responses and the new rating scale. Freedman took special care to shepherd the articles through, demanding rewrite after rewrite. Sadly, he had been dead a year by the time the papers finally came out. He never had the opportunity to relish seeing a public written record of the fulfillment of his long-held dream: the resumption of human psychedelic research. See Rick J. Strassman and Clifford R. Qualls, "Dose-Response Study of N,N-Dimethyltryptamine in Humans. I: Neuroendocrine, Autonomic, and Cardiovascular Effects," *Archives of General Psychiatry* 51 (1994): 85–97; and Rick J. Strassman, Clifford

R. Qualls, Eberhard H. Uhlenhuth, and Robert Kellner, "Dose-Response Study of N,N-Dimethyltryptamine in Humans. II: Subjective Effects and Preliminary Results of a New Rating Scale," *Archives of General Psychiatry* 51 (1994): 98–108.

Chapter 10

1. We must distinguish this classification from those data we obtained using the Hallucinogen Rating Scale. While I later describe the development and use of the HRS, it is worth mentioning now what the rating scale did measure, and how this differs from the groupings of experiences that are about to follow.

   The mind was the object of the HRS, not the individual volunteer. The HRS provided numerical scores for various aspects of the acute DMT intoxication based upon a theoretical understanding of how the mind works. In this system, a handful of functions, including perception, emotion, body awareness, thinking, and habitual tendencies, blend together seamlessly, resulting in what we routinely experience as our present mental state.

   The classes of effects I propose in this chapter, on the other hand, refer to the person's experience, not just their mind's. The acute effects themselves, of course, constitute that experience, but they do not give it any meaning. It is only within the context of the individual's unique body, spirit, and mind that the sessions take on any real significance.

Chapter 11

1. This idea is a common one in people who use psychedelics for personal growth. It has to do with the purifying and relieving value of catharsis. A powerful, earth-shattering emotional experience might prove more useful than lengthy verbal analysis of the same conflict. In clinical practice, however, both methods of dealing with blocked emotional growth are necessary. Catharsis without any insight may not have much long-term benefit. But insight without emotional contact usually leads to little real progress.

Chapter 12

1. Chaco Canyon is a spectacular ruins site about three hours northwest of Albuquerque. The Anasazi Indians, probable precursors of the contemporary Pueblo tribes, inhabited it for centuries. From where the Anasazi came from, and to where they went upon abandoning this stone city in the mid-thirteenth century, remain two of the world's greatest archeological mysteries. Their astronomical skills were extraordinarily sophisticated, and they supported themselves using irrigation and agricultural techniques that stagger the mind, considering the minimal rainfall with which they had to contend. Chaco Canyon weaves a compelling spell upon any who visit it, and many people make the pilgrimage with an almost mystical fervor.

2. Runes are an ancient Nordic divination tool, similar to the I Ching and the Tarot. Runes date from at least 1000 B.C. and use stones with symbols carved on them, rather than sticks or cards. Modern runes use twenty-five different symbols.

3. "Regular" in Spanish means "regular," "normal," "everyday." The proper pronunciation accents the last syllable.

4. In classical Greek and neo-Platonic philosophy, the Logos is the cosmic reason giving order, purpose, and intelligence to the world.

5. Carlos Castaneda performed anthropology fieldwork in the Mexican desert, spending years with an Indian shaman, Don Juan Matus. Many of the scenes Castaneda describes begin as simple encounters with Don Juan and his friends, in settings similar to that which Sean described. See, for example, Carlos Castaneda, *The Teachings of Don Juan: A Yaqui Way of Knowledge* (Berkeley, CA: University of California, 1998).

Chapter 13

1. Z. Boszormenyi and Stephen I. Szára, "Dimethyltryptamine Experiments with Psychotics," *Journal of Mental Science* 104 (1958): 445–53.

2. Turner and Merlis (1959).

3. Gumby is a character from an American children's television show from the late 1950s and early 1960s. Gumby was composed of a claylike substance molded over metal wire. This made it possible to bend him into all sorts of shapes, something kids loved doing with their own twelve-inch-tall Gumby. Gumby's trusty sidekick was Pokey the horse. The animators bent and moved Gumby's and Pokey's clay bodies, then filmed them using time-lapse photography, thus giving the impression of movement.

Chapter 14

1. John E. Mack, *Abduction* (New York: Ballantine, 1994) and *Passport to the Cosmos* (New York: Crown, 1999).

Chapter 15

1. Raymond A. Moody, *Life After Life* (New York: Bantam Books, 1988); and Kenneth Ring, *Life at Death: A Scientific Investigation of the Near-Death Experience* (New York: Coward, McCann, and Geoghegan, 1980).

2. W. Y. Evans-Wentz, *Tibetan Book of the Dead* (New York: Oxford University Press, 1974).

3. Rinpoche Sogyal, *The Tibetan Book of Living and Dying* (New York: HarperSanFrancisco, 1992). This is a modern rendition of *The Tibetan Book of the Dead.*

4. Dannion Brinkley, *Saved by the Light* (New York: Harper, 1995); and Betty J. Eade, *Embraced by the Light* (New York: Bantam, 1994).

5. Mircea Eliade, *Shamanism: Archaic Techniques of Ecstasy* (Princeton, NJ: Princeton University Press, 1972); and Michael Harner, *The Way of the Shaman* (New York: HarperSanFrancisco, 1990).

Chapter 16

1. Robert Master and Jean Houston, *The Varieties of the Psychedelic Experience* (Rochester, VT: Park Street Press, 2000); William James, *The Varieties of Religious Experience* (New York: Macmillan, 1997); and Robert Forte, ed., *Entheogens and the Future of Religion* (San Francisco: Council on Spiritual Practices, 1997).

Chapter 17

1. It may be a lack of just these considerations that underlies recent reports of adverse reactions in human ketamine research—see Anna Nidecker, "Alleged Abuses Accelerate Reform," *Clinical Psychiatry News* 26 (1998): 1. That is, did the scientists know what they were doing? Had they taken ketamine themselves? How carefully did they control the setting in which their subjects received ketamine? What were their attitudes and responses toward the ketamine-induced state? Of course, it is just these variables that one must think about in reading reports of adverse effects from the first wave of human psychedelic drug research in the 1950s and 1960s.

2. F. Kajtor and Stephen Szára, "Electroencephalographic Changes Induced by Dimethyltryptamine in Normal Adults," *Confinia Neurologica* 19 (1959): 52–61.

3. Sai-Halasz et al. (1958).

4. More recently, Doblin brought to light a highly stressful negative reaction to psilocybin in the famous Good Friday study. The original 1966 article (Walter N. Pahnke and William A. Richards, "Implications of LSD and Experimental Mysticism," *Journal of Religion and Health* 5 (1966): 175–208) described mystical experiences brought on by psilocybin in Harvard Divinity School students. However, we heard nothing about the inebriated fellow whom research team members chased through campus, pinned against a door, and tranquilized with an injection of antipsychotic medication! See Rick Doblin, "The Good Friday Experiment: A Twenty-Five Year Follow-Up and Methodological Critique," *Journal of Transpersonal Psychology* 23 (1991): 1–28.

5. See endnote #1, chapter 11.

Chapter 19

1. The dose of psilocybin that Swiss and German research groups generally use, 0.2 mg/kg, is less than one-half the dose we found would bring on an unmistakable psychedelic response; that is, 0.45 mg/kg. While these groups have published their data as indicating "psychedelic effects of psilocybin," I don't think what they are studying is a typical syndrome. See E. Gouzoulis-Mayfrank, B. Thelen, E. Habermeyer, H. J. Kunert, K.-A. Kovar, H. Lindenblatt, L. Hermle, M. Spitzer, and H. Sass, "Psychopathological, Neuroendocrine and Autonomic Effects of 3,4-Methylenedioxyethylamphetamine (MDE), Psilocybin and d-Methamphetamine in Healthy Volunteers," *Psychopharmacology* 142 (1999): 41–50; and F. X. Vollenweider, K. L. Leenders, C. Scharfetter, P. Maguire, O. Stadelmann, and J. Angst, "Positron Emission Tomography and Fluorodeoxyglucose Studies of Metabolic Hyperfrontality and Psychopathology in the Psilocybin Model of Psychosis," *Neuropsychopharmacology* 16 (1997): 357–72.

   We continued escalating the dose up until 1.1 mg/kg, at which point the two volunteers receiving that quantity felt it was "too much." One became briefly disoriented, and the other experienced a sense of nearly overwhelming "mental pressure." We were going to use 0.9 mg/kg as our high-end dose of psilocybin, more than four times the European "psychedelic dose," before additional circumstances led to my leaving the university.

Chapter 20

1. Rick J. Strassman and Marc Galanter, "The Abhidharma: A Cross-Cultural Application of Meditation," *International Journal Social Psychiatry* 26 (1980): 283–90.

2. This method is quite similar to what Freud called "evenly suspended attention" performed by a trained psychoanalyst. The analyst provides support through mostly silent but present sitting behind and off to the side of the patient's couch. This type of unobtrusive listening and watching mirrors much of what takes place internally during Zen meditation.

3. For example, there are now Spanish, Italian, Russian, Portuguese, German, and Dutch translations of the HRS. Various research groups around the world have used it to measure the effects of ketamine, *ayahuasca*, amphetamines, psilocybin, and MDMA. A German research group has even measured certain features of naturally occurring psychosis with the HRS.

4. As in most monastic religious traditions, Margaret took a new name after joining the priestly order. Since her and others' names are Japanese, and because I know no Japanese and would hate to make up a name that accidentally meant something disgraceful or embarrassing, I've chosen to use English pseudonyms.

5. Rick J. Strassman, "DMT and the Dharma," *Tricycle, The Buddhist Review* 6 (1996): 81–88.

Chapter 21

1. There was little if any contact among the volunteers at the earlier stages of the research. Even when they did meet, either in social settings at my house or in the support group that formed toward the end of the study, volunteers were uniformly shy and uncomfortable discussing their strange being encounters. Neither were Terence McKenna's lectures and writings especially popular when we first started hearing these unusual reports from our research subjects. I often asked volunteers about being familiar with popular accounts of DMT-mediated encounters with elves or insectoid aliens. Few if any were. Thus, I don't think these reports were a type of mass hysteria or a self-fulfilling prophecy. Indeed, if this process was operating, I would have expected an "epidemic" of mystical and near-death experiences instead, because I was expecting and hoping for them.

2. Before television engineers developed the "picture-in-a-picture" option, I could have extended this analogy by saying these levels of reality are mutually exclusive. That is, we could not watch channel 3 and channel 4 at the same time. However, we now can. The picture-in-a-picture concept actually helps with the TV comparison, though, if we recall how many times volunteers opened their eyes to see different levels of reality mix and blend. Oftentimes, too, volunteers would fully engage in the new world to which DMT provided access while still remembering that their bodies were in Room 531 of the University Hospital. They had their feet in several worlds at once, a truly mythic multitasking effort!

3. David Deutsch, *The Fabric of Reality* (New York: Penguin, 1997).

4. David Deutsch, personal communication, January 2000.

5. Ibid, June 1999.

6. Nigel Smith and Neil Spooner, "The Search for Dark Matter," *Physics World* 13 (2000): 4.

7. Why entities or alien intelligences desire to interact with us is, of course, a crucial question. Many of Mack's abduction experiencers describe human-alien hybrid projects intended to repopulate our dying planet. Some of our volunteers also returned with a "breeding" motif, having found themselves in rooms with toys, cribs, and other items from infancy. Additionally, the transfer of information and the "tuning" and "reprogramming" of consciousness follow a similar thread of an advanced race wishing to impart to us some

of what they know. This often relates to the pressing environmental degradation overtaking our planet. Here, too, there are similarities with a few of our volunteers' tales.

Several of our research subjects also refer to the nonmaterial nature of the beings, particularly their lack of emotions of love and relatedness, as crucial to their interest in us. Somehow, by interacting and learning from us, they are able to relearn things forgotten or lost by them long ago. Such descriptions border on "spirit possession" and take on disturbing overtones. On a less sober note, recall the playfulness of some of the figures our volunteers described, bringing to mind fairies, pixies, and elves from our own folkloric past.

8. Karl L. R. Jansen, "The Ketamine Model of the Near-Death Experience: A Central Role for the N-Methyl-D-Aspartate Receptor," *Journal of Near-Death Studies* 16 (1997): 5–26. (I have searched for and been unable to find any data regarding whether DMT is neuroprotective.)

Chapter 22

1. There are examples of religious and scientific models seeming to exist on better terms, such as research occurring within some of the contemporary psychedelic churches, including the Native American peyote- and South American *ayahuasca*-using organizations. However, these are relationships of convenience and not true hybrids of science and religion. Scientific results will not modify the practices and teachings of the churches, nor will the insights and experiences of the religious encounter change the methods of scientific research.

2. Terence McKenna introduced hundreds of people to DMT, and during a visit on his botanical preserve in Hawaii several years ago, we talked about this. He estimated that perhaps 5 percent of people to whom he had given DMT showed nearly no effect. Terence's 5 percent estimate is exactly what we saw in our research: three out of sixty volunteers.

3. F. X. Vollenweider, personal communication, June 1993; and L. Hermle, personal communication, June 1993.

4. Ka-Tzetnik 135633, *Shivitti: A Vision* (Nevada City, CA: Gateways, 1998).

5. Bernard J. Albaugh and Philip O. Anderson, "Peyote in the Treatment of Alcoholism Among American Indians," *American Journal of Psychiatry* 131 (1974): 1247–51; and Charles S. Grob, Dennis J. McKenna, James C. Callaway, Glacus S. Brito, Edison S. Neves, Guilherme Oberlaender, Oswaldo L. Saide, Elizeu Labigalini, Christiane Tacla, Claudio T. Miranda, Rick J. Strassman, and Kyle B. Boone, "Human Psychopharmacology of Hoasca, a Plant Hallucinogen Used in Ritual Context in Brazil," *Journal of Nervous and Mental Disease* 184 (1996): 86–94.

As an example of conflicting models of efficacy, many proponents of ibogaine treatment for addictions suggest a primarily pharmacological basis to its benefits. In fact, members of a National Institute on Drug Abuse ibogaine research panel in which I participated wondered if there were some way to block its psychedelic "side effects" and still maintain its therapeutic ones.